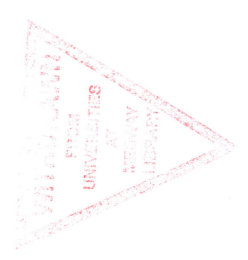

Current Best Practice in Interventional Cardiology

Commissioning Editor: Thomas V. Hartman
Development Editor: Kate Newell
Production Editor: Cathryn Gates
Production Controller: Susan Shepherd

Current Best Practice in Interventional Cardiology

EDITED BY

Bernhard Meier, MD, FACC, FESC

Cardiology
Swiss Cardiovascular Center Bern
University Hospital Bern
Bern
Switzerland

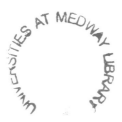

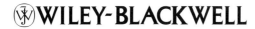

WILEY-BLACKWELL

A John Wiley & Sons, Ltd., Publication

Library of Congress Cataloging-in-Publication Data
Current best practice in interventional cardiology / edited by Bernhard Meier.
p. ; cm.
Includes bibliographical references.
ISBN 978-1-4051-8255-3
1. Heart–Surgery. 2. Heart–Diseases–Treatment. 3. Heart–Interventional radiology.
I. Meier, Bernhard, M.D.
[DNLM: 1. Heart Diseases–surgery. 2. Cardiovascular Diseases–diagnosis. 3. Diagnostic Imaging–methods.
4. Vascular Diseases–surgery. WG 169 C97517 2009]
RD598.C84 2009
617.4'12–dc22

2009014017

ISBN 978-1-4051-8255-3

A catalogue record for this book is available from the British Library.

Set in 9/12pt Meridien by Aptara® Inc., New Delhi, India
Printed and bound in Malaysia by Vivar Printing Sdn Bhd

1 2010

Contents

List of Contributors

Stephan Achenbach, MD, FACC, FESC
Department of Cardiology
University of Erlangen
Erlangen, Germany

Junya Ako, MD
Center for Research in Cardiovascular Interventions
Stanford University Medical Center
Stanford, CA, USA

Yaron Almagor, MD
Interventional Cardiology
Shaare Zedek Medical Center
Jerusalem, Israel

Haran Burri, MD
Cardiology Service
University Hospital of Geneva
Geneva, Switzerland

Paul Chiam, MBBS, MRCP, FACC
Department of Cardiology
National Heart Center
Singapore

Stéphane Cook, MD
Cardiology
Swiss Cardiovascular Center Bern
University Hospital Bern
Bern, Switzerland

Alain Cribier, MD
Department of Cardiology
Hospital Charles Nicolle
University of Rouen
Rouen, France

Pim J. de Feyter, MD
Department of Cardiology
Erasmus University
Rotterdam, The Netherlands

Etienne Delacrétaz, MD, FACC
Cardiology
Swiss Cardiovascular Center Bern
University Hospital Bern
Bern, Switzerland

Helene Eltchaninoff, MD
Department of Cardiology
Hospital Charles Nicolle
University of Rouen
Rouen, France

Peter J. Fitzgerald, MD, PhD
Division of Cardiology
Stanford University Medical Center
Stanford, CA, USA

Otto M. Hess, MD
Cardiology
Swiss Cardiovascular Center
University Hospital
Bern, Switzerland

David Hildick-Smith, MD
Sussex Cardiac Centre
Brighton and Sussex University Hospital NHS Trust
Brighton, UK

Yasuhiro Honda, MD
Division of Cardiology
Stanford University Medical Center
Stanford, CA, USA

Roger Hullin, MD
Départment de Médecine Interne
Centre Hospitalier Universitaire Vaudois
Lausanne, Switzerland

Sriram Iyer, MD, FACC
Department of Cardiac and Vascular Interventional Services
Lenox Hill Heart and Vascular Institute of New York
New York, NY, USA

Pierre-Frédéric Keller, MD
Division of Cardiology
University Hospital of Geneva
Geneva, Switzerland

Simon Koestner, MD
Cardiology
Cardiovascular Department
University Hospital Bern
Bern, Switzerland

David Meerkin, MBBS
Interventional Cardiology
Shaare Zedek Medical Center
Jerusalem, Israel

Bernhard Meier, MD, FACC, FESC
Cardiology
Swiss Cardiovascular Center Bern
University Hospital Bern
Bern, Switzerland

Marco Roffi, MD
Division of Cardiology
University Hospital of Geneva
Geneva, Switzerland

David Rosenmann, MD
Interventional Cardiology
Shaare Zedek Medical Center
Jerusalem, Israel

Gary Roubin, MD, PhD, FACC
Department of Cardiac and Vascular Interventional Services
Lenox Hill Heart and Vascular Institute of New York
New York, NY, USA

Jean-Paul Schmid, MD
Cardiology
Swiss Cardiovascular Center Bern
University Hospital Bern
Bern, Switzerland

Georgios Sianos, MD, PhD, FESC
1st Department of Cardiology
AHEPA University Hospital
Thessaloniki, Greece

Sven Streit, MD
Cardiology
Swiss Cardiovascular Center
University Hospital
Bern, Switzerland

Jean-François Surmely, MD
Cardiology
Clinique de la Source
Lausanne, Switzerland

Jiri Vitek, MD, PhD
Department of Cardiac and Vascular Interventional Services
Lenox Hill Heart and Vascular Institute of New York
New York, NY, USA

Masao Yamasaki, MD
Division of Cardiology
Stanford University Medical Center
Stanford, CA, USA

Preface

A comprehensive textbook on interventional cardiology requires 3 volumes or a DVD. What you hold in your hand is a glimpse at the current best practice of some selected aspects of interventional cardiology.

The book is targeted at a wide spectrum of readers ranging from the accomplished interventional cardiologist, desirous of looking over the fence or filling in some of the few remaining dark spots in his or her knowledge or armamentarium, to the nurse, technician, or physician assistant active in interventional cardiology. A cardiologist referring patients for catheter-based interventions might want to take a look at what is available, and a cardiovascular surgeon might want to find out what is offered to patients before or instead of summoning surgical help. Finally, industry representatives and device developers may use it to keep abreast of the state of the art, remaining shortcomings, and needs that may yet have to be identified.

Part I is the bread-and-butter section: percutaneous interventions for coronary artery disease. Acute coronary syndromes account for more than one-third of patients treated with percutaneous coronary intervention (PCI, introduced under the name PTCA 32 years ago). Stents are an integral part of the procedure, at least intentionally. Globally, 10% to 30% of lesions are still treated without a stent, but this is usually imposed by circumstances rather than the primary plan. Drug-eluting stents are about to supplant the traditional bare metal stents. Their advantage is small but relevant enough to render bare metal stents unattractive, irrespective of the fact that they have done a superb job so far. As for indications, the delineation between bypass surgery and PCI has been concretized by randomized trials. Selected double-vessel disease and triple-vessel disease in-

cluding the left main have been cleared for PCI, albeit only in selected cases. A remaining bastion is chronic total occlusion. The books are still open about how important it is to recanalize it, what the best stepwise approach is, and how much time, radiation, and material should be invested before giving up in favor of medical treatment or bypass surgery. End-stage coronary artery disease carries a stigma almost like end-stage cancer. The respective treatments discussed here are correctly called palliative. So is revascularization, by the way.

In Part II, a variety of noncoronary interventions are discussed, a popular name for them being structural interventions. The most intriguing example is percutaneous replacement of the aortic valve. This is the current phoenix of interventional cardiology and rightfully so. In a very common disease, onerous open heart surgery can be replaced by a catheter intervention, in some cases even under local anesthesia. In contrast to PCI, which started to compete with surgery in the easy case, percutaneous aortic valve replacement is starting with the difficult one. The future looks bright, as percutaneous aortic valve replacement appears to work even in these patients. Closure of atrial shunts preceded PCI by a couple of years. Moreover, it has the potential to become more common than PCI, as every fourth person carries a patent foramen ovale. The medical community is carefully investigating the true value of these procedures, and the respective chapters help with that endeavor. Carotid angioplasty currently involves by default a stent and a protection device. In contrast to PCI the differences between surgery and the percutaneous procedure are small (no thoracotomy, no heart-lung machine). Hence a draw in outcome is not accepted; the percutaneous approach has to be better and safer. We are not there yet, but we hope to be on the right track. Alcohol ablation for hypertrophic cardiomyopathy looks back on more than a decade of clinical use. It has been adopted as a first approach for most patients with this rather rare clinical need.

Part III is dedicated to interventional approaches to left ventricular failure. Biventricular pacing appears to have gained an indelible place for chronic treatment, whereas percutaneous left ventricular assist devices usually serve for short periods of time as bridges to recovery or more definitive treatments. Stem cell therapy is discussed as a glow on the horizon, although it is not quite clear whether the sun is rising on it or has already set on it and we just do not know yet.

Part IV deals with cardiovascular imaging, putting magnetic resonance in the forefront as the recognized technique of the future. Computed tomography and intravascular imaging such as ultrasound and optical coherence tomography are also discussed.

Whether the book is read from cover to cover, used as a hard-copy thesaurus to thumb through when a question comes up, or—why not?—utilized as a picture book to browse through when some spare time is at hand, the authors truly hope that the contact with this book will be interesting, rewarding, and pleasurable.

Bernhard Meier

PART I

Coronary Artery Disease

CHAPTER 1
Acute Coronary Syndromes

Pierre-Frédéric Keller and Marco Roffi
Division of Cardiology, University Hospital of Geneva, Geneva, Switzerland

---

Chapter Overview

- Acute coronary syndromes (ACS) are the acute manifestation of atherosclerotic coronary artery disease. Based on different presentations and management, patients are classified into non–ST-segment elevation ACS (NSTE-ACS) and ST-segment elevation myocardial infarction (STEMI).
- In western countries, NSTE-ACS is more frequent than STEMI.
- Even if the short-term prognosis (30 days) for NSTE-ACS is more favorable than for STEMI, the long-term prognosis is similar or even worse.
- Early invasive strategy is the management of choice in patients with NSTE-ACS, particularly in high-risk subgroups.
- Primary percutaneous coronary intervention (PCI) is the treatment of choice for STEMI. Facilitated PCI is of no additional benefit.
- The reduction of door-to-balloon time in primary PCI is critical for improved outcomes in STEMI patients.
- If fibrinolytic therapy is administered in STEMI, then patients should be routinely transferred for immediate coronary angiography, and if needed, percutaneous revascularization.
- High-risk ACS patients (eg, elderly patients, those in cardiogenic shock) have the greatest benefit from PCI.
- Antithrombotic therapy in ACS is getting more and more complex. The wide spectrum of antiplatelet agents and anticoagulants requires a careful weighing of ischemic and bleeding risks in each individual patient.

ST-Segment Elevation Myocardial Infarction

The term acute coronary syndrome (ACS) has emerged as useful tool to describe the clinical correlate of acute myocardial ischemia. ST-segment elevation (STE) ACS includes patients with typical and prolonged chest pain and persistent STE on the ECG. In this setting, patients will almost invariably develop a myocardial infarction (MI), categorized as ST-segment elevation myocardial infarction (STEMI). The term non–ST-segment (NSTE) ACS refers to patients with signs or symptoms sug-

gestive of myocardial ischemia in the absence of significant and persistent STE on ECG. According to whether the patient has at presentation, or will develop in the hours following admission, laboratory evidence of myocardial necrosis or not, the working diagnosis of NSTE-ACS will be further specified as NSTE-MI or unstable angina.

Recently, MI was redefined in a consensus document [1]. The 99th percentile of the upper reference limit (URL) of troponin was designated as the cut-off for the diagnosis. By arbitrary convention, a percutaneous coronary intervention (PCI)-related MI and coronary artery bypass grafting (CABG)-related MI were defined by an increase in cardiac enzymes more than three and five times the 99th percentile URL, respectively. The application of this definition will undoubtedly increase the number of

---

Current Best Practice in Interventional Cardiology. Edited by B Meier. © 2010 Blackwell Publishing.

events detected in the ACS and the revascularization setting. The impact on public health as well as at the clinical trial level of the new MI definition cannot be fully foreseen.

The extent of cellular compromise in STEMI is proportional to the size of the territory supplied by the affected vessel and to the ischemic length of time. Therefore a quick and sustained restoration of normal blood flow in the infarct-related artery is crucial to salvage myocardium and improve survival.

Primary PCI Versus Thrombolytic Therapy

Primary percutaneous coronary intervention became increasingly popular in the early 1990s. Evidence favoring this strategy in comparison with thrombolytic therapy is substantiated by a meta-analysis of 23 randomized trials demonstrating that

PCI more efficaciously reduced mortality, nonfatal reinfarction, and stroke (Fig. 1.1) [2]. The advantage of primary PCI over thrombolysis was independent of the type of thrombolytic agent used, and was also present for patients who were transferred from one institution to another for the performance of the procedure. Therefore, primary PCI is now considered the reperfusion therapy of choice by all the guidelines [3,4]. With respect to bleeding complications, a recent meta-analysis demonstrated that the incidence of major bleeding complications was lower in patients treated with primary PCI than in those undergoing thrombolytic therapy [2]. In particular intracranial hemorrhage, the most feared bleeding complication, was encountered in up to 1% of patients treated with fibrinolytic therapy and in only 0.05% of primary PCI patients. The algorithm for treatment of patients admitted for a STEMI is presented in Fig. 1.2 [5].

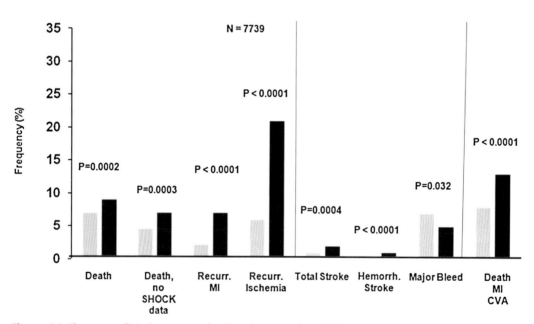

Figure 1.1 Short-term clinical outcomes of patients in 23 randomized trials of primary PCI versus thrombolysis. (Reproduced with permission from [2] Keeley EC, Boura JA, Grines CL. Primary angioplasty versus intravenous thrombolytic therapy for acute myocardial infarction: a quantitative review of 23 randomised trials. *Lancet.* 2003;361:13–20.)

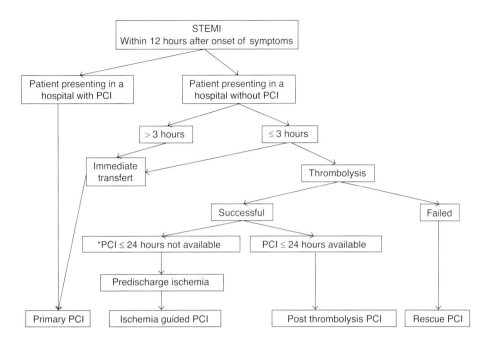

†If thrombolysis is contraindicated or the patient is at high risk, immediate transfer should be considered
*Even after successful thrombolysis, adjunctive PCI should be considered

Figure 1.2 Algorithm for revascularization in STEMI patients with less than 12 hours from symptom onset according to the 2005 ESC guideline for PCI. (Reproduced with permission [5] from Silber S, Albertsson P, Aviles FF, et al. Guidelines for percutaneous coronary interventions. The Task Force for Percutaneous Coronary Interventions of the European Society of Cardiology. *Eur Heart J.* 2005;26:804–847.)

Advantages of Primary PCI

More than 90% of patients treated by primary PCI achieve normal flow (thrombosis in myocardial infarction [TIMI] grade flow 3) at the end of the intervention, while only 65% of patients treated by thrombolytic therapy benefit from this degree of reperfusion (Table 1.1) [6–8]. In addition, thrombolyis is characterized by a rapidly decreased efficacy after 2 hours of symptom onset (Fig. 1.3) [9]. There is a close relationship between the quality of coronary flow obtained after reperfusion therapy and mortality, and the prognosis of patients in whom flow normalization is not achieved is similar to that of patients with persistent vessel occlusion. The classification of TIMI myocardial blush grade allows an estimate of the tissue-level perfusion (Table 1.1). A critical link between lower TIMI myocardial blush grade, expression of a microcirculatory compromise, and mortality has been demonstrated in patients with normal epicardial flow following reperfusion therapy [10]. The improvement of clinical outcomes with primary PCI versus thrombolysis is also the consequence of a lower rate of reocclusion (0–6%). Accordingly, with thrombolytic therapy, reocclusion may occur in over 10% of cases even among patients presenting within the first 2 hours of symptom onset.

Mechanical complications of STEMI, such as acute mitral regurgitation and ventricular septal defect, were reduced by 86% by primary PCI compared with thrombolytic therapy in a meta-analysis of the GUSTO-1 and PAMI trials [11]. Free wall rupture was also significantly reduced by primary PCI [12]. Finally, primary PCI may allow earlier discharge (2–3 days following PCI versus 7 days following fibrinolytic therapy for uncomplicated courses).

Table 1.1 TIMI Classification of Coronary Flow and Perfusion

Flow Grade Classification

TIMI Flow Grade	Definition
0	No antegrade flow beyond the point of occlusion.
1	Faint antegrade coronary flow beyond the occlusion, although filling of the distal coronary bed is incomplete.
2	Delayed or sluggish antegrade flow with complete filling of the distal territory.
3	Normal flow that fills the distal coronary bed completely.

Perfusion Grade Classification

Perfusion Grade	Definition
0	Minimal or no myocardial blush is seen.
1	Dye stains the myocardium; this stain persists on the next injection.
2	Dye enters the myocardium but washes out slowly so that the dye is strongly persistent at the end of the injection.
3	There is normal entrance and exit of the dye in the myocardium so that the dye is mildly persistent at the end of the injection.

Adapted with permission from [7] Gibson CM, Schomig A. Coronary and myocardial angiography: angiographic assessment of both epicardial and myocardial perfusion. *Circulation.* 2004;109:3096–3105; and [8] Schömig A, Mehilli J, Antoniucci D, et al. Mechanical reperfusion in patients with acute myocardial infarction presenting more than 12 hours from symptom onset: a randomized controlled trial. *JAMA.* 2005;293:2865–2872.

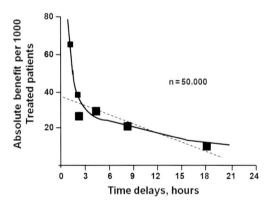

Figure 1.3 Time delays to thrombolysis in STEMI and the absolute reduction in 35-day mortality. (Reproduced with permission from [9] Boersma E, Maas AC, Deckers JW, Simoons ML. Early thrombolytic treatment in acute myocardial infarction: reappraisal of the golden hour. *Lancet.* 1996;348:771–775.)

Decreasing the Time to Reperfusion in Primary PCI

The survival benefit of reperfusion associated with thrombolytic therapy shrinks with increasing delay in the administration of the agent. For stable patients undergoing primary PCI, no association between symptom-onset-to-balloon time and mortality was observed in the U.S. NRMI registry [13]. In contrast, a significant increase in mortality was detected for patients with a door-to-balloon-time greater than 2 hours [14]. Therefore, the findings of primary PCI trials may be only applicable to hospitals with established primary PCI programs, experienced teams of operators, and a sufficient volume of interventions. Indeed, an analysis of the NRMI-2 registry demonstrated that hospitals with less than 12 primary PCIs per year have a higher rate of mortality than those with more than 33 primary PCIs per year [13]. Useful tools to decrease the door-to-balloon time are described in Table 1.2 [15].

Challenging Groups of Patients

Concomitant High-Grade Non-Culprit Lesions

The timing of revascularization of severe non-culprit lesion treatment in patients with multivessel

Table 1.2 Strategies to Reduce the Door-to-Balloon Time in Primary PCI

- Emergency medicine physicians activate the catheterization laboratory (mean reduction in door-to-balloon time, 8.2 minutes)
- Having a single call to a central page operator activate the laboratory (13.8 minutes)
- Having the emergency department activate the catheterization laboratory while the patient is en route to the hospital (15.4 minutes)
- Expecting staff to arrive in the catheterization laboratory within 20 minutes after being paged (vs. >30 minutes) (19.3 minutes)
- Having an attending cardiologist always on site (14.6 minutes),
- Having staff in the emergency department and the catheterization laboratory use real-time data feedback (8.6 minutes).

From [15] Bradley EH, Herrin J, Wang Y, et al. Strategies for reducing the door-to-balloon time in acute myocardial infarction. *N Engl J Med.* 2006;355:2308–2320.

disease undergoing primary PCI has long been debated. Multivessel PCI in stable STEMI patients was found to be an independent predictor of major adverse cardiac events (MACE) at 1 year [16]. However, a recent study suggested that systematic revascularization of multivessel disease at the time of primary PCI in contrast to ischemia-driven revascularization may be of advantage because incomplete revascularization was found to be a strong and independent risk predictor for death and MACE [17]. Another study supported the notion that complete revascularization improved clinical outcomes in STEMI patients with multivessel disease [18]. Accordingly, the study showed a significant lower rate of recurrent ischemic events and acute heart failure during the indexed hospitalization. Nevertheless, current American College of Cardiology/American Heart Association (ACC/AHA) guidelines recommend that PCI of the non-infarct artery should be avoided in the acute setting in patients without hemodynamic instability [19].

Cardiogenic Shock

The incidence of cardiogenic shock in acute MI patients is in decline, accounting for approximately 6% of all cases [20]. As the result of the increasing use of primary PCI, the shock-related mortality has decreased. Accordingly, a U.S. analysis showed mortality rates in shock of 60% in 1995 and 48% in 2004, while the corresponding primary PCI rates were 27% to 54% [21]. In the SHOCK trial, early revascularization was associated with a significant survival advantage [22]. In the study, approximately two-thirds of patients in the invasive arm were revascularized by PCI and one-third by CABG surgery. Thrombolysis was administered in 63% of patients allocated to the medical stabilization arm. Early revascularization is strongly recommended for shock patients younger than 75 years. In older patients, revascularization may be considered in selected patients [23].

In the last two decades, hemodynamic support devices have been developed to limit end-organ failure in the setting of cardiogenic shock. The intraaortic balloon pump (IABP) is the most commonly used mechanical support device. Percutaneous left atrial-to-femoral arterial bypass assistance, and more recently the Impella Recover microaxial left ventricular and/or right ventricular assist device, have been developed to increase cardiac output. However, no randomized clinical data exist to support the benefit of this device. Percutaneous cardiopulmonary bypass support using extracorporeal membrane oxygenation (ECMO) can be used in cardiogenic shock for a longer period of time than the other devices just described. However, while ECMO has excellent oxygenation properties, it provides only limited cardiac output support.

Elderly Patients

Elderly patients present more frequently with non–ST-segment elevation myocardial infarction (NSTEMI) than with STEMI. As many as 80% of all deaths related to MI occur in persons older than 75 years of age. With respect to STEMI, up to two-thirds may occur in patients older than 65 years of age. Although, fibrinolytic therapy has been shown to be as effective in the elderly as in younger patients for achieving TIMI-3 flow, the percentage of patients eligible for this therapy decreases with advancing age due to comorbid conditions. The Senior PAMI trial randomized 483 patients ≥ 70 years old who were eligible for thrombolysis to primary PCI versus thrombolytic therapy [24]. A substantial benefit of PCI was seen in patients aged 70 to 80 with a 37% reduction in death, and a 55% reduction in the composite end point of death, MI, or stroke. Among patients older than 80 years of age, the prognosis was poor in both the PCI and thrombolytic arms. Based on these findings and on the increased delay of reperfusion observed in this population, primary PCI is the preferred revascularization approach.

Late Presentation

Few studies have evaluated whether mechanical reperfusion is beneficial in patients presenting >12 hours from symptom onset. The OAT trial demonstrated in patients randomized to conservative medical therapy or late PCI that stable patients do not clinically benefit from late invasive strategy after MI [25]. This was confirmed with the DECOPI trial [26]. However, in the latter trial at 6 months, left ventricular ejection fraction was 5% higher in the invasive compared with the medical group ($p = 0.013$), suggesting that mechanical revascularization may improve ventricular remodeling and function. The BRAVE-2 investigators randomized 365 patients with STEMI (between 12 and 48 hours from symptom onset) to PCI with abciximab versus conservative care [28]. Infarct size measured by sestamibi was smaller in the invasive group, with a favorable trend with respect to composite clinical end points. These data suggest that the benefit of primary PCI may extend beyond the traditional 12-hour window.

Rescue and Urgent PCI Following Thrombolytic Therapy

Because of the high rate of primary failure of fibrinolysis, in the absence of reperfusion rescue PCI must be considered 60 to 90 minutes after thrombolytic therapy [27]. Suggestive of primary failure are persistent, severe, or worsening chest pain, dyspnea, diaphoresis, persistent or worsening ST segment elevation, and hemodynamic or rhythmic instability. According to the ACC/AHA guidelines, reduction of > 50% of the initial ST segment elevation on ECG at 60 to 90 minutes after thrombolytic therapy is suggestive of reperfusion, and > 70% reduction is considered as complete resolution [4]. Among 1398 STEMI patients presenting within 6 hours of symptom onset, the 35-day mortality rate for complete, partial (30–70%), or no resolution of ST segment elevation at 3 hours was 2.5%, 4.3%, and 17.5%, respectively ($p < 0.0001$) [28]. This relationship was observed in both anterior and inferior wall infarction. In the study, the degree of ST segment resolution was the most powerful clinical predictor of 35-day mortality. In the InTIME-II trial, the prognostic impact of ST segment resolution at 60 versus 90 minutes was compared among 1797 patients [29]. Patients with ST segment resolution at 60 minutes had a lower mortality rate at 30 days and 1 year compared to those with resolution at 90 minutes. These findings suggest that ST segment should be routinely reassessed at 60 minutes and, in the absence of reperfusion, patients should undergo rescue PCI.

Facilitated PCI

Facilitated PCI refers to the administration of an urgent pharmacologic therapy (ie, thrombolysis, GP IIb/IIIa inhibitor, or a combination) followed by systematic early PCI. Although the international European Society of Cardiology (ESC) and ACC/AHA guidelines recommended a door-to-balloon time for primary PCI of less than 90 minutes, a survey of 4278 patients transferred for primary PCI from the U.S. NRMI registry found that only 4% and 15% of them were treated within 90 and 120 minutes, respectively [30]. In the CAPITAL AMI trial, 170 high-risk STEMI patients were randomized to full-dose tenecteplase or full-dose

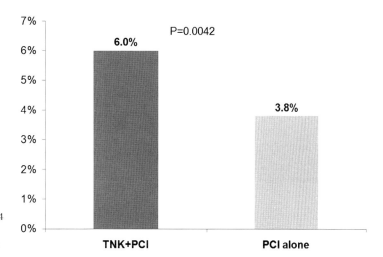

Figure 1.4 Thirty-day mortality following primary or facilitated PCI by using tenecteplase [TNK] among the 1663 patients involved in the ASSENT-4 trial. (Data extracted with permission from the ASSENT-4 investigators [32].)

tenecteplase followed by immediate transfer for PCI [31]. The composite primary end point of death, recurrent MI, recurrent unstable ischemia, or stroke at 6 months was significantly decreased by facilitated PCI (11.6% vs. 24.4 %, $p = 0.04$). The reduction was driven by a decrease in recurrent ischemia.

The ASSENT-4 trial randomized 4000 patients with STEMI of less than 6 hours from symptom onset to full dose tenecteplase or placebo prior to primary PCI. The composite primary end point was death, heart failure, or shock within 90 days. The study was stopped prematurely because of a significant increase in mortality in the tenecteplase group (6% vs. 3%, $p = 0.0105$) (Fig. 1.4) [32]. A meta-analysis of facilitated PCI trials showed that GP IIb/IIIa inhibitor-facilitated PCI had no advantages in term of post-procedure TIMI 3 grade flow and clinical end points [33]. Similarly, no benefit in terms of ischemic event reduction but a greater bleeding risk was observed in facilitated PCI with abciximab and half-dose reteplase compared with primary PCI. Therefore, facilitated PCI should be avoided.

Adjunctive PCI After Successful Thrombolysis

In the CARESS-in-AMI trial, among 600 high-risk STEMI patients treated with reteplase, randomization to immediate transfer for urgent PCI was associated with a significant decrease in the compos-

ite end point of death, reinfarction, or refractory ischemia at 30 days compared to a conservative approach [34]. In the TRANSFER-AMI trial, high-risk STEMI patients were randomized to tenecteplase or tenecteplase and transfer for PCI within 6 hours of fibrinolysis [35]. The 30-day composite primary end point of death, recurrent MI, congestive heart failure, severe recurrent ischemia, or shock occurred in 16.6% of patients in the control group and in 10.6% of patients in the invasive group ($p = 0.0013$). No difference was noted in bleeding complications. The optimal timing of routine angiography and possible PCI after fibrinolytic therapy for STEMI has not been determined. Evidence from the GRACIA-2 trial suggests that PCI within 3 to 12 hours after fibrinolysis is both safe and effective [36]. Therefore following fibrinolytic therapy, patients should be routinely transferred for immediate coronary angiography.

Transfer for Primary PCI

The DANAMI-2 trial compared primary PCI and fibrinolysis, specifically addressing the impact of patients transferred to primary PCI centers [37]. The primary composite end point of death, reinfarction, or disabling stroke was significantly decreased by primary PCI compared with fibrinolysis in the overall study cohort (13.7% vs. 8%, $p < 0.001$) as well as among patients treated in centers without catheterization facilities. The greatest benefit of primary PCI was found in patients with a delay of more than 4 hours from symptom onset to reperfusion. The mean duration of inter-hospital transportation by ambulance was short (32 minutes). These benefits of primary PCI over thrombolytic therapy persisted at 3 years [38]. Overall, primary PCI is to be considered superior to thrombolytic therapy if it can be performed within 110 minutes of admission to the first hospital.

Delayed PCI

It has been suggested that delayed reperfusion compared to medical therapy prevents unfavorable ventricular remodeling. However, the TOAT study (N = 66) suggested that late recanalization of occluded infarct-related arteries (1 month post STEMI) in symptom-free patients had an adverse effect on remodeling despite showing a trend to improved exercise tolerance and quality of life [39]. The recent OAT study (N = 2166) demonstrated that late PCI (3 to 28 days post STEMI) in stable patients did not reduce the occurrence of death, reinfarction, or heart failure compared to medical management, with a trend toward an excess of reinfarction in the intervention group at 4-year follow-up [25]. The BRAVE-2 trial including 365 asymptomatic patients found a significant smaller infarct size by scintigraphy among individuals randomized to PCI between 12 and 48 hours following a STEMI compared to those treated optimal medical therapy alone (infarct size 8% vs. 13%, $p < 0.001$) [28]. In conclusion, delayed PCI following a STEMI should be considered in patients at high risk such as those with heart failure, left ventricular dysfunction, or moderate to severe ischemia.

Techniques of Reperfusion and Adjunctive Pharmacologic Treatments

Bare-Metal and Drug-Eluting Stents

The CADILLAC trial compared balloon angioplasty and stenting in the setting of STEMI [40]. No difference in mortality or reinfarction rates was noted, but a significant decrease in ischemic target vessel revascularization (TVR) at 6 months favored stenting. The TYPHOON study randomized 712 patients to sirolimus-eluting stents or bare-metal

stents (BMS) [41]. The composite primary end point defined as target vessel–related death, recurrent MI, or TVR was significantly lower in the drug-eluting stent (DES) group than in the BMS group at 1 year (7.3% vs. 14.3%, $p = 0.004$). There was no significant difference between the two groups in the rate of death, reinfarction, or stent thrombosis. At 2 years, the benefit persisted. A similar benefit was observed in the MULTISTRATEGY trial comparing sirolimus-eluting stents and bare-metal stents among 672 STEMI patients. Therefore, drug-eluting stents appear to be beneficial also in the STEMI setting [42].

Embolic Protection Devices and Thrombus Aspiration

Distal embolization, a frequent phenomenon in the setting of primary PCI, is associated with reduced epicardial and/or tissue-level perfusion and late mortality. Neverthelesss, a strategy based on distal emboli protection did not reduce events in the STEMI setting in two randomized trials (EMERALD [43] and PROMISE [44]). The use of thrombectomy with the AngioJet device was not beneficial in the AiMI trial but the strategy will be assessed again in the JETSTENT trial in patients with large thrombotic burden [45]. The TAPAS study randomized 1701 STEMI patients prior to angiography to thrombectomy with an aspiration catheter or conventional primary PCI [46]. The study demonstrated a significant increase in rate of complete resolution of ST-segment elevation with the use of aspiration catheters. While the use of distal protection devices is not recommended, aspiration catheter-based thrombectomy should be routinely performed in the presence of a sizable thrombus.

Antithrombotic Therapy

A detailed description of antithrombotic agents will follow in the NSTEMI section of the chapter. With respect to STEMI, an initial loading dose of 162 to 325 mg of uncoated acetylsalicylic acid should be given immediately and continued indefinitely at a dose of 75 to 162 mg/day [3]. The recommendations for clopidogrel were extrapolated from the PCI and the NSTEMI setting because no randomized trial has been performed in the primary

PCI setting. Patients should be loaded with 300 to 600 mg of clopidogrel prior to PCI, and the treatment should be continued for up to 1 year at 75 mg/day. Prasugrel is discussed below.

Glycoprotein IIb/IIIa Inhibitors

The use of glycoprotein (GP) IIb/IIIa receptor inhibitors is well established and supported by a meta-analysis demonstrating a MACE reduction at 30 days and 6 months [47]. In addition, multiple registries have shown a mortality reduction associated with the use of this class of agents [48,49]. Although the most-studied compound in STEMI has been abciximab, a high-bolus dose of tirofiban may be equally effective [42]. Recently however, the BRAVE-3 study questioned the value of GP IIb/IIIa inhibitors in STEMI patients pretreated with clopidogrel [50]. Among 800 patients there was no difference in left ventricular infarct size assessed by nuclear imaging. The HORIZONS AMI trial studied 3602 patients with STEMI randomized to either bivalirudin with provisional use of a GP IIb/IIIa inhibitor, or to unfractionated heparin (UFH) plus a GP IIb/IIIa inhibitor prior to primary PCI [51]. There was a significant reduction in the primary end point of net adverse clinical events in the group receiving bivalirudin at 30 days, and even a reduction in 30-day mortality. Bivalirudin appears to be a valid alternative to UFH plus GP IIb/IIIa inhibitors in selected patients.

Summary of Guidelines

Primary PCI, if performed in a timely fashion, is the reperfusion therapy of choice in patients with STEMI. However, since not all hospitals have the ability to perform primary PCI, the choice of reperfusion strategy should take into account the delay between primary PCI in another institution and immediate thrombolysis. PCI should be considered as the preferred strategy if it can be achieved within 90 minutes from the first medical contact. The 2007 ACC/AHA/SCAI PCI guidelines concluded that facilitated PCI is harmful. However, facilitated PCI using regimens other than full-dose fibrinolytic therapy might be considered in patients with a low bleeding risk and if PCI is not available within 90 minutes. The optimal timing of routine angiography and possible PCI after fibrinolytic therapy for STEMI has not been determined, though a procedure at 3 to 12 hours appears to be both safe and effective. Mechanical thrombectomy using an aspiration catheter at the time of primary PCI is recommended.

Non–ST-Elevation Acute Coronary Syndromes

Epidemiology and Risk Stratification

In western countries, the ratio between NSTE-ACS and STEMI has switched over time, and currently NSTE-ACS is more frequent than STEMI. Registries and surveys have estimated that the annual incidence of hospital admissions for NSTE-ACS is in the range of 3 per 1000 inhabitants. With respect to gender, approximately 40% of ACS patients in the United States are women. Overall, the in-hospital mortality is generally higher for STEMI than for NSTE-ACS (approximately 7% and 5%, respectively). However, while in STEMI most events occur before or shortly after presentation, in NSTE-ACS adverse events continue over days and weeks. As a consequence, the mortality rates at 6 months of both conditions become comparable (approximately 12% and 13%, respectively). At 4 years, a two-fold higher rate in the NSTE-ACS population compared to STEMI has been reported. The difference in mid- and long-term evolution may be due to different patient profiles. NSTE-ACS patients are generally older, have more comorbidities such as diabetes and renal failure, and may have a more advanced stage of CAD and vascular disease.

A variety of parameters have been shown to have independent predictive power for long-term ischemic events in patients with ACS. Clinical parameters include age, heart rate, blood pressure, Killip class, diabetes, history of prior MI, history of CAD, ECG changes such as ST-depression, laboratory parameters such as troponin, measurements of renal function, BNP or NT-proBNP, and high-sensitivity CRP. Some of them have been grouped to form multiple risk stratification scores. However, only a limited number of scores are simple enough to be useful in everyday practice. The GRACE risk score, recommended by the ESC 2007 ACS guidelines as the preferred risk stratification tool, is based upon a large unselected international population of patients presenting with NSTE-ACS and STEMI and has been validated in several registries for prediction of in-hospital deaths and postdischarge deaths at 6 months [52,53]. However, score calculation is complex and hardly doable at the bedside. As alternative is the TIMI risk score, which includes 7 variables: age > 65 years; > 3 risk factors for coronary artery disease; prior coronary stenosis > 50%; ST-segment deviation on ECG at presentation; > 2 anginal events in the 24 hours prior to admission; use of acetylsalicylic acid in the 7 days prior to admission; and elevated serum cardiac biomarkers [54].

Anti-Ischemic Medications

Independently of the revascularization strategy chosen, pharmacologic options in ACS include antianginal medication, anticoagulants, and antiplatelet agents. The role of antianginal medications in the acute setting of NSTE-ACS is limited. No randomized data support the use of nitrates for prognostic reasons. Two randomized trials have compared beta-blockers to placebo in unstable angina, showing a modest 13% reduction in the risk of progression to STEMI. The value of beta-blockade in the acute phase of ACS was further shaken by the recent COMMIT study, a mega-trial showing no benefit of an early and aggressive beta-blocker treatment in STEMI patients [55]. Only small randomized studies have tested calcium channel blockers in NSTE-ACS, and a meta-analysis failed to document a reduction in the progression to STEMI or mortality. Nicorandil and ivabradine have not been tested in ACS.

Anticoagulants

A pooled analysis of six trials testing UFH or low-molecular-weight heparin (LMWH) versus placebo or untreated controls in the setting of NSTE-ACS demonstrated a significant 33% risk reduction at 7 days for death or MI. [56] A meta-analysis of the six trials comparing UFH and enoxaparin including almost 22,000 patients found no difference in mortality but a modest, though statistically significant based on the large sample size, 9% relative risk re-

duction in the combined end point of death or MI at 30 days in favor of enoxaparin [57]. No significant differences in blood transfusions or in major bleeding were observed.

Fondaparinux is the only selective factor Xa inhibitor approved for ACS. In the OASIS-5 trial, among 20,078 patients with NSTE-ACS, fondaparinux or enoxaparin conveyed similar reduction in ischemic events at 9 days [58]. However, fondaparinux therapy was associated with halving in major bleeding episodes. As a result, the composite outcome of death, MI, refractory ischemia, or major bleeding was significantly reduced with fondaparinux (7.3% vs. 9.0%). In addition, the mortality was lower in the fondaparinux group both at 30 days (2.9% vs. 3.5%, HR 0.83, $p = 0.02$) and at 6 months (5.8% vs. 6.5%, HR 0.89, $p = 0.05$). In the study most of the patients were treated conservatively. However, also among the 6238 patients who underwent PCI, fondaparinux halved major bleeding compared to enoxaparin (2.4% vs. 5.1%, HR 0.46, $p < 0.00001$) [59]. In the presence of similar rates of ischemic events among the two arms, this resulted in a superior net clinical benefit for fondaparinux (death, MI, stroke, major bleeding: 8.2% vs. 10.4%, HR 0.78, $p = 0.004$). A source of great concern was the observation that catheter thrombus formation was more common in patients receiving fondaparinux (0.9%) than enoxaparin (0.4%), despite an additional intravenous dose of fondaparinux at the time of cardiac catheterization.

The direct thrombin inhibitor bivalirudin was assessed in 13,819 patients with moderate- to high-risk NSTE-ACS undergoing early angiography within the ACUITY trial, a randomized, open-label study [60]. Three primary 30-day end points included composite ischemia (death from any cause, MI, or unplanned revascularization for ischemia), major bleeding, and net clinical outcome (composite of ischemic events and major bleeding). Patients were randomized to one of three treatment groups: UFH or LMWH with GP IIb/IIIa inhibitors; bivalirudin with GP IIb/IIIa inhibitor; or bivalirudin alone. In a subsequent randomization process, GP IIb/IIIa inhibitors were administered either upstream or at the time of PCI. There was no significant difference between standard UFH/LMWH plus GP IIb/IIIa inhibitors and the combination of bivalirudin and GP IIb/IIIa inhibitors for the composite ischemia end point at 30 days (7.3% vs. 7.7%, respectively), or for major bleeding (5.7% vs. 5.3%). Bivalirudin alone was shown to be non-inferior to the standard UFH/LMWH combined with GP IIb/IIIa inhibitors as to the composite ischemia end point (7.8% vs. 7.3%, respectively) in the presence of a significantly lower rate of major bleeding (3.0% vs. 5.7%, RR 0.53, $p < 0.001$). As a consequence, the rate of 30-day net clinical outcome was significantly lower (10.1% vs. 11.7%, RR 0.86, $p = 0.015$) with bivalirudin alone versus UFH/LMWH plus GP IIb/IIIa inhibitors.

In both the 2007 ESC and the 2007 ACC/AHA guidelines on ACS, the use of an anticoagulant drug (UFH, enoxaparin, bivalirudin, or fondaparinux) is a class IA recommendation. In the context of early invasive or conservative strategy, fondaparinux was given a prominent place (class I recommendation) by both societies, notably in patients at risk of bleeding. Fondaparinux was preferred over enoxaparin (class IA vs. IIa-B) in the ESC guidelines, regardless of initial strategy (excluding urgent revascularization for life-threatening conditions). In the ACC/AHA guidelines, fondaparinux was considered the drug of choice in conservative strategy. In fondaparinux patients undergoing invasive procedures, it was recommended to add unfractionated heparin. For patients taken immediately to the catheterization laboratory, the ESC 2007 guidelines recommend either UFH or bivalirudin as first choice [53]. In patients treated with a therapeutic dose of enoxaparin, PCI can be safely performed within 6 to 8 hours following the last subcutaneous dose. If a longer delay is present, then an additional intravenous bolus of enoxaparin is recommended.

Antiplatelet Agents

Acetylsalicylic Acid and Clopidogrel

Acetylsalicylic acid reduces the risk of MI, ischemic stroke, and cardiovascular death in patients with NSTE-ACS and is recommended in all patients as acute and long-term treatment. Clopidogrel has an established role in NSTE-ACS based on results of the CURE trial, which randomized 12,562 patients

with NSTE-ACS to receive clopidogrel or placebo in addition to acetylsalicylic acid [61]. Clopidogrel was administered in a loading dose of 300 mg, followed by 75 mg/day for 3 to 12 months. The composite of cardiovascular death, nonfatal MI, or stroke occurred significantly less often in the clopidogrel group (9.3% vs. 11.4%, RR 0.80, $p < 0.001$). Major bleeding occurred in 3.7% of patients in the clopidogrel group and 2.7% of patients in the placebo group (RR 1.38, $p = 0.001$). Among the 2658 patients in the CURE trial who underwent PCI, the incidence of cardiovascular death or MI was reduced by one-third in the clopidogrel group [62].

The appropriate loading dose of clopidogrel before PCI has been the subject of debate. In the ARMYDA-2 study, 255 patients undergoing planned PCI were randomized to loading doses of 300 or 600 mg of clopidogrel. Patients allocated to the higher dose had a $> 50\%$ risk reduction in the 30-day incidence of MI, a difference due entirely to a reduction in periprocedural MI, with no excess of bleeding [63]. A pharmacologic study failed to prove that a 900-mg loading dose offers an additional advantage over the 600-mg dose in terms of platelet aggregation inhibition [64].

GP IIb/IIIa Receptor Inhibitors

In the pre-clopidogrel era, the administration of GP IIb/IIIa inhibitors has been associated with a 30-day mortality reduction compared with placebo in a meta-analysis involving 20,186 patients undergoing PCI (OR 0.73, $p = 0.024$) [65]. In the setting of NSTE-ACS, the degree of benefit derived from these agents has been related to the revascularization strategy used. For patients treated mainly conservatively, the benefit of GP IIb/IIIa inhibitors has been modest. Accordingly, a meta-analysis detected a 9%, albeit statistically significant, relative risk reduction in death or nonfatal MI at 30 days compared with placebo [66]. However, in the subgroup of patients undergoing PCI while on study drug in this analysis, a significant 26% reduction in death or MI was detected. A far greater benefit was observed in the subgroup of diabetic patients, with a significant mortality reduction at 30 days associated with active treatment [67]. With respect to interventional studies in the setting of ACS, the most

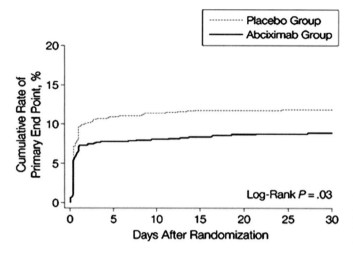

Figure 1.5 Kaplan-Meier analysis of cumulative incidence of death, myocardial infarction, or urgent target vessel revascularization in the ISAR-REACT 2 trial. (Reproduced with permission from [70] Kastrati A, Mehilli J, Neumann FJ, et al. Abciximab in patients with acute coronary syndromes undergoing percutaneous coronary intervention after clopidogrel pretreatment: the ISAR-REACT 2 randomized trial. *JAMA.* 2006;295:1531–1538.)

studied agent has been abciximab. Among 7290 patients enrolled in three trials, allocation to abciximab was associated with a significant reduction in cardiac events at 30 days as well as a significant late mortality benefit (HR 0.71, $p = 0.003$) [68].

The benefit of GP IIb/IIIa receptor inhibitors in the clopidogrel era has been recently questioned [69]. However, the ISAR-REACT-2 study demonstrated among 2022 high-risk NSTE-ACS patients that abciximab was beneficial in patients pretreated with clopidogrel 600 mg [70]. Accordingly, the 30-day composite end point of death, MI, or urgent TVR occurred significantly less frequently in abciximab-treated patients versus placebo (8.9% vs. 11.9%, RR 0.75, $p = 0.03$) (Fig. 1.5). The effect was more pronounced in troponin-positive patients (13.1% vs. 18.3%, RR 0.71, $p = 0.02$). The benefit of abciximab in addition to acetylsalicylic acid and clopidogrel was sustained at 1 year, with a combined incidence of death, MI, or TVR of 23.3% in the abciximab group and 28.0% in the placebo group (RR 0.80, $p = 0.012$). The combined incidence of death or MI was 11.6% and 15.3%, respectively (RR 0.74, $p = 0.015$) [71].

The value of upstream versus in-laboratory GP IIb/IIIa inhibitor therapy still needs to be fully elucidated. In the ACUITY trial, upstream use of GP IIb/IIIa inhibitors resulted in a lower rate of ischemic events but a higher rate of bleeding such

that the net clinical benefit was similar for the two strategies [72]. However, the major limitation of this analysis is that the time of administration prior to PCI in the upstream group was short (median 5 hours). The EARLY ACS trial demonstrated that high dose regiment fo GP IIb/IIIa receptor inhibitors eptifibatide 12 hours or more before angiography was not superior to the provisional use of eptifibatide after angiography (insert Ref: [Giugliano RP, White JA, Bode C, et al.; EARLY ACS Investigators. *N Engl J Med.* 2009 May 21:360(21):2176–2190]).

Prasugrel

In the TRITON-TIMI 38 trial, 13,608 moderate- to high-risk patients with NSTE-ACS or STEMI undergoing PCI were randomized to receive prasugrel or clopidogrel for 6 to 15 months [73]. The composite end point of death from cardiovascular causes, nonfatal MI, or nonfatal stroke occurred in 12.1% of patients randomized to clopidogrel and 9.9% of patients randomized to prasugrel (HR 0.81, $p < 0.001$). There were also significant reductions in the rates of MI, urgent TVR, and stent thrombosis among patients randomized to prasugrel. The rate of major bleeding was higher in the prasugrel group (2.4% vs. 1.8%, HR 1.32, $p = 0.03$). The somewhat overdosed prasugrel and underdosed clopidogrel may account for most of the difference.

Recommendations

The ESC 2007 guidelines have made following recommendations [53]. Acetylsalicylic acid is recommended as acute and long-term treatment for all patients with NSTE-ACS, independently of the chosen revascularization strategy. Clopidogrel is recommended for acute treatment at a dose of 300 mg, followed by 12 months of treatment at 75 mg/day. Treatment with eptifibatide or tirofiban in addition to oral antiplatelet therapy is recommended for initial early treatment in patients at intermediate to high risk; in high-risk patients undergoing PCI not pretreated with a GP IIb/IIIa inhibitor, abciximab is recommended immediately following angiography. Bivalirudin may be considered an alternative to GP IIb/IIIa inhibitors plus UFH/LMWH.

Invasive Versus Conservative Strategy

The more recent meta-analysis of randomized trials comparing early invasive versus conservative strategy including six studies and 7962 patients demonstrated a significant 16% reduction at 1 year in death or MI associated with the early invasive treatment (Fig. 1.6) [53]. This analysis also included the ICTUS trial, a study that challenged the paradigm of superior outcome with routine invasive strategy. In this trial, 1200 patients were randomized to an early invasive strategy versus a more conservative (selective) approach [74]. In the routine invasive arm, revascularization was performed within 48 hours of randomization in 56% of patients and during initial hospitalization in 76% of cases. While there was no difference in the incidence of the

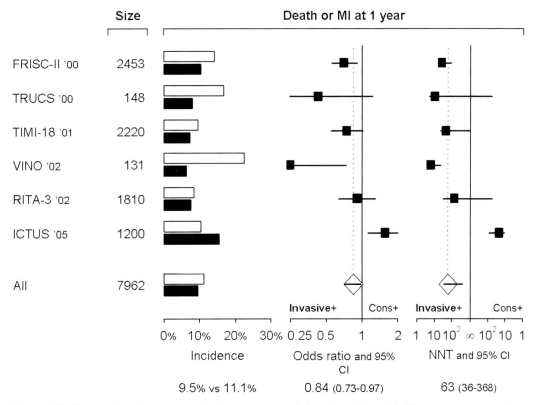

Figure 1.6 Meta-analysis of randomized trials comparing early invasive strategy (*dark bars*) versus conservative strategy (*open bars*). (Reproduced with permission from [53] Bassand JP, Hamm CW, Ardissino D, et al. Guidelines for the diagnosis and treatment of non-ST-segment elevation acute coronary syndromes. *Eur Heart J.* 2007;28:1598–1660.)

primary composite end point of death, MI, or re-hospitalization for angina within 1 year (22.7% in the early invasive vs. 21.2% in the selective invasive arm), routine angiography was associated with a significant early hazard. Accordingly, MI was significantly more frequent in the early invasive group (15.0% vs. 10.0%, RR 1.5, $p = 0.005$) and in two-thirds of cases was a periprocedural event. The discrepancy between this and previous trials could be attributed in part to the small difference in revascularization rates between the two study groups and the high overall rate of revascularization before discharge (76% in the routine invasive and 40% in the selective group). In addition, the criterion for diagnosis of MI (any CK-MB elevation above ULN as opposed to more than three times ULN) differs between studies. Furthermore, the selection of patients may have been biased, as some studies included all consecutive patients admitted while others did not enter severely unstable patients.

Additional data supporting the long-term benefit of an early invasive strategy come from the RITA-3 trial. At 5 years, 16.6% of patients in the invasive arm and 20.0% of patients in the conservative arm died or had nonfatal MI (OR 0.78, $p = 0.044$), with a similar benefit for cardiovascular death or MI (OR 0.74, $p = 0.030$) [75]. The mortality reduction associated with an invasive treatment barely missed statistical significance (2% vs. 15%, OR 0.76, $p = 0.054$). In the highest-risk group, a highly significant 56% reduction in death or nonfatal MI was observed. The 5-year follow-up of the FRISC-II study confirmed a benefit of an early invasive strategy in terms of death or MI 19.9% in the invasive arm and 24.5% in the conservative arm (RR 0.81; $p = 0.009$) [76]. While mortality did not differ among the groups, the rate of MI was 12.9% in the invasive arm and 17.7% in the conservative group (RR 0.73; $p = 0.002$). In all randomized trials, a large proportion of patients in the conservative arm eventually underwent revascularization (crossover). This phenomenon represents a failure of conservative therapy and dilutes the benefit of revascularization. Even in the FRISC-2 study, a study with hard requirements for the conservative arm to get investigated with coronary angiography and if needed revascularization, 43% of patients in the conservative arm had to be revascularized in the first year.

Timing of Angiography

The ESC ACS 2007 guidelines stratify the degree of urgency of an early invasive strategy depending on the risk of the patient into urgent, early, or elective (Fig. 1.7) [53]. In low-risk patients, either an elective angiography or a noninvasive assessment of inducible ischemia may be performed. While the time window in the American and previous European guidelines to perform early invasive strategy was 48 hours, it has been extended to 72 hours in the current ESC guidelines. However, controversy remains as to the optimal timing between hospital admission, initiation of medical therapy, and invasive evaluation. Support for immediate angiography came from the small ISAR-COOL study [77]. In 410 consecutive high-risk patients with either ST-segment depression (65%) or elevated troponin (67%) enrolled in the trial, deferral of intervention did not improve outcome. On the contrary, patients randomized to immediate PCI (on average 2.4 hours after admission) had a lower incidence of death or MI at 30 days than patients randomized to deferred PCI (86 hours after admission and medical therapy) (5.9% vs. 11.6%, RR 1.96, $p = 0.04$). No early hazard was observed among patients undergoing PCI in ISAR-COOL as well as in TACTICS-TIMI-18, in which the mean delay for PCI was 22 hours and all patients had upstream treatment with GP IIb/IIIa inhibitors [78]. The timing issue was investigated retrospectively in the SYNERGY trial (N = 9978) [79]. In the study 92% of patients underwent coronary angiography, 63% within 48 hours. Unadjusted and adjusted rates of death/MI increased with increasing time to angiography. The adjusted odds ratio for death/MI in patients receiving angiography in ≤ 6 hours was 0.56 (95% CI 0.41 to 0.74), whereas after 30 hours, there was no significant benefit compared with further delayed angiography.

Bleeding Complications and Outcomes

It is estimated that 2% to 8% of patients with NSTE-ACS suffer a major bleeding episode during

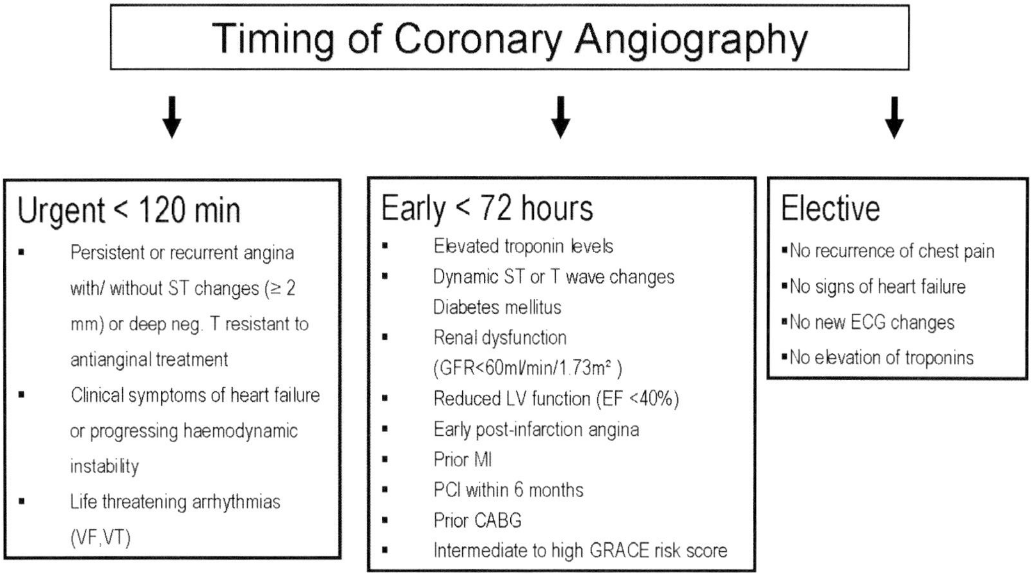

Timing of Coronary Angiography

Urgent < 120 min

- Persistent or recurrent angina with/ without ST changes (≥ 2 mm) or deep neg. T resistant to antianginal treatment
- Clinical symptoms of heart failure or progressing haemodynamic instability
- Life threatening arrhythmias (VF,VT)

Early < 72 hours

- Elevated troponin levels
- Dynamic ST or T wave changes Diabetes mellitus
- Renal dysfunction (GFR<60ml/min/1.73m^2)
- Reduced LV function (EF <40%)
- Early post-infarction angina
- Prior MI
- PCI within 6 months
- Prior CABG
- Intermediate to high GRACE risk score

Elective

- No recurrence of chest pain
- No signs of heart failure
- No new ECG changes
- No elevation of troponins

Figure 1.7 Timing of coronary angiography according to the 2007 Guidelines of the European Society of Cardiology. (VF, ventricular fibrillation; VT, ventricular tachycardia; GFR, glomerular filtration rate; LV, left ventricular; EF, ejection fraction; MI, myocardial infarction; CABG, coronary artery bypass surgery.) (Modified with permission from [53] Bassand JP, Hamm CW, Ardissino D, et al. Guidelines for the diagnosis and treatment of non-ST-segment elevation acute coronary syndromes. *Eur Heart J.* 2007;28:1598–1660.)

hospitalization. The main predisposing factors are the type and dose of antithrombotic and antiplatelet therapies and whether or not the patient underwent an invasive procedure. With respect to clinical variables, advanced age, female gender, renal insufficiency, and history of bleeding have all been shown to independently predict a bleeding event. In recent years, the link between bleeding and poor outcomes in ACS patients has become evident. Pooled data from four multicenter randomized clinical trials of patients with ACS documented a stepwise increase in the risk of death at 30 days and 6 months, according to the severity of bleeding. At 1 month, the hazard ratios for death were 1.6, 2.7, and 10.6 for mild, moderate, and severe bleeding, and at 6 months, the hazard ratios were 1.4, 2.1, and 7.5, respectively [80]. In the OASIS-5 trial, the risk of ischemic events was strongly influenced by major bleeding. The rate of 30-day death was 12.9% versus 2.8%, the risk of MI 13.9% versus 3.6%, and the risk of stroke 3.6% versus 0.8% for patients who suffered major bleeding versus no bleeding, respectively [58]. Nonpharmacologic

strategies to reduce access site bleeding complications include the use of closure devices and the radial approach.

Secondary Prevention

Measures and therapies that may reduce the risk of recurrence of events after ACS include lifestyle changes such as smoking cessation; regular physical exercise; and a healthy diet based on low salt intake, reduced intake of saturated fats, and regular intake of fruit and vegetables. Additional measures include weight reduction and optimal blood pressure, diabetes mellitus, and lipid control. The ESC guidelines recommend that beta-blocker therapy should be initiated in all ACS patients and maintained indefinitely in the case of reduced LV function, with or without symptoms of heart failure, unless formal contraindications exist [81]. In other patients, beta-blockers may be useful, but evidence of their long-term benefit is not established. ACE inhibitors have, in addition to the beneficial properties for patients with heart failure or left ventricular dysfunction, anti-atherogenic properties, quantified in meta-analyses in a 14% risk reduction for death at 4 years. The applicability of these findings, although documented in the context of stable coronary artery disease, has been extended to all ACS. A meta-analysis including 13 trials and 17,963 patients revealed that early initiation of statin therapy reduced major cardiovascular events at 2 years (HR 0.81, $p < 0.001$) [82]. The advantage of early initiation of aggressive (atorvastatin 80 mg) vs. moderate (pravastatin 40 mg) lipid-lowering therapy in ACS was assessed in the PROVE-IT trial [83]. At 2 years, the primary composite end point (death, MI, unstable angina requiring rehospitalization, revascularization, or stroke) was significantly reduced by 16% in the atorvastatin arm compared with the pravastatin arm. Current recommendations support early initiation of statin therapy for all ACS patients.

References

1. Thygesen K, Alpert JS, White HD. Universal definition of myocardial infarction. *Eur Heart J.* 2007;28:2525–2538.
2. Keeley EC, Boura JA, Grines CL. Primary angioplasty versus intravenous thrombolytic therapy for acute myocardial infarction: a quantitative review of 23 randomised trials. *Lancet.* 2003;361:13–20.
3. Van de Werf F, Ardissino D, Betriu A, *et al.* Management of acute myocardial infarction in patients presenting with ST-segment elevation. The Task Force on the Management of Acute Myocardial Infarction of the European Society of Cardiology. *Eur Heart J.* 2003;24:28–66.
4. Antman EM, Hand M, Armstrong PW, *et al.* 2007 Focused update of the ACC/AHA 2004 guidelines for the management of patients with ST-elevation myocardial infarction: a report of the American College of Cardiology/American Heart Association Task Force on Practice Guidelines. Developed in collaboration with the Canadian Cardiovascular Society; endorsed by the American Academy of Family Physicians 2007 Writing Group to review new evidence and update the ACC/AHA 2004 guidelines for the management of patients with ST-elevation myocardial infarction, writing on behalf of the 2004 Writing Committee. *Circulation.* 2008;117:296–329.
5. Silber S, Albertsson P, Aviles FF, *et al.* Guidelines for percutaneous coronary interventions. The Task Force for Percutaneous Coronary Interventions of the European Society of Cardiology. *Eur Heart J.* 2005;26:804–847.
6. Grines CL, Browne KF, Marco J, *et al.* A comparison of immediate angioplasty with thrombolytic therapy for acute myocardial infarction. The Primary Angioplasty in Myocardial Infarction Study Group. *N Engl J Med.* 1993;328:673–679.
7. Gibson CM, Schomig A. Coronary and myocardial angiography: angiographic assessment of both epicardial and myocardial perfusion. *Circulation.* 2004;109:3096–3105.
8. Schömig A, Mehilli J, Antoniucci D, *et al.* Mechanical reperfusion in patients with acute myocardial infarction presenting more than 12 hours from symptom onset: a randomized controlled trial. *JAMA.* 2005;293:2865–2872.
9. Boersma E, Maas AC, Deckers JW, Simoons ML. Early thrombolytic treatment in acute myocardial infarction: reappraisal of the golden hour. *Lancet.* 1996;348:771–775.
10. Costantini CO, Stone GW, Mehran R, *et al.* Frequency, correlates, and clinical implications of myocardial perfusion after primary angioplasty and stenting, with and without glycoprotein IIb/IIIa inhibition, in acute myocardial infarction. *J Am Coll Cardiol.* 2004;44:305–312.
11. Kinn JW, O'Neill WW, Benzuly KH, Jones DE, Grines CL. Primary angioplasty reduces risk of myocardial rupture compared to thrombolysis for acute myocardial infarction. *Cathet Cardiovasc Diagn.* 1997;42:151–157.
12. Moreno R, Lopez-Sendon J, Garcia E, *et al.* Primary angioplasty reduces the risk of left ventricular free wall rupture compared with thrombolysis in patients with acute myocardial infarction. *J Am Coll Cardiol.* 2002;39:598–603.
13. Canto JG, Every NR, Magid DJ, *et al.* The volume of primary angioplasty procedures and survival after acute myocardial infarction. National Registry of Myocardial Infarction 2 Investigators. *N Engl J Med.* 2000;342:1573–1580.
14. Cannon CP, Gibson CM, Lambrew CT, *et al.* Relationship of symptom-onset-to-balloon time and door-to-balloon time with mortality in patients undergoing angioplasty for acute myocardial infarction. *JAMA.* 2000;283:2941–2947.
15. Bradley EH, Herrin J, Wang Y, *et al.* Strategies for reducing the door-to-balloon time in acute myocardial infarction. *N Engl J Med.* 2006;355:2308–2320.
16. Corpus RA, House JA, Marso SP, *et al.* Multivessel percutaneous coronary intervention in patients with

multivessel disease and acute myocardial infarction. *Am Heart J.* 2004;148:493–500.

17. Kalarus Z, Lenarczyk R, Kowalczyk J, *et al.* Importance of complete revascularization in patients with acute myocardial infarction treated with percutaneous coronary intervention. *Am Heart J.* 2007;153:304–312.

18. Qarawani D, Nahir M, Abboud M, Hazanov Y, Hasin Y. Culprit only versus complete coronary revascularization during primary PCI. *Int J Cardiol.* 2008;123:288–292.

19. Smith SC Jr., Feldman TE, Hirshfeld JW Jr., et al. ACC/AHA/SCAI 2005 guideline update for percutaneous coronary intervention—summary article: a report of the American College of Cardiology/American Heart Association Task Force on Practice Guidelines (ACC/AHA/SCAI Writing Committee to update the 2001 guidelines for percutaneous coronary intervention). *Circulation.* 2006;113:156–175.

20. Goldberg RJ, Gore JM, Thompson CA, Gurwitz JH. Recent magnitude of and temporal trends (1994–1997) in the incidence and hospital death rates of cardiogenic shock complicating acute myocardial infarction: the second national registry of myocardial infarction. *Am Heart J.* 2001;141:65–72.

21. Babaev A, Frederick PD, Pasta DJ, Every N, Sichrovsky T, Hochman JS. Trends in management and outcomes of patients with acute myocardial infarction complicated by cardiogenic shock. *JAMA.* 2005;294:448-454.

22. Hochman JS, Sleeper LA, White HD, *et al.* One-year survival following early revascularization for cardiogenic shock. *JAMA.* 2001;285:190–192.

23. Antman EM, Anbe DT, Armstrong PW, *et al.* ACC/AHA guidelines for the management of patients with ST-elevation myocardial infarction—executive summary. A report of the American College of Cardiology/American Heart Association Task Force on Practice Guidelines (Writing Committee to revise the 1999 guidelines for the management of patients with acute myocardial infarction). *J Am Coll Cardiol.* 2004;44:671–719.

24. Grines C. A prospective randomized trial of primary angioplasty and thrombolytic therapy in elderly patients with acute myocardial infarction (SENIOR-PAMI). Presented at Transcatheter Cardiovascular Therapeutics 2005, Washington, DC, October 2005.

25. Hochman JS, Lamas GA, Buller CE, *et al.* Coronary intervention for persistent occlusion after myocardial infarction. *N Engl J Med.* 2006;355:2395–2407.

26. Steg PG, Thuaire C, Himbert D, *et al.* DECOPI (DEsobstruction COronaire en Post-Infarctus): a randomized multi-centre trial of occluded artery angioplasty after acute myocardial infarction. *Eur Heart J.* 2004;25:2187–2194.

27. The GUSTO Angiographic Investigators. The effects of tissue plasminogen activator, streptokinase, or both on coronary-artery patency, ventricular function, and survival after acute myocardial infarction. *N Engl J Med.* 1993;329:1615–1622.

28. Schröder R, Wegscheider K, Schröder K, Dissmann R, Meyer-Sabellek W. Extent of early ST segment elevation resolution: a strong predictor of outcome in patients with acute myocardial infarction and a sensitive measure to compare thrombolytic regimens. A substudy of the International Joint Efficacy Comparison of Thrombolytics (INJECT) trial. *J Am Coll Cardiol.* 1995;26:1657–1664.

29. de Lemos JA, Antman EM, Giugliano RP, *et al.* Comparison of a 60- versus 90-minute determination of ST-segment resolution after thrombolytic therapy for acute myocardial infarction. InTIME-II Investigators. Intravenous nPA for teatment of infarcting myocardium early-II. *Am J Cardiol.* 2000;86:1235–1237.

30. Nallamothu BK, Bates ER, Herrin J, Wang Y, Bradley EH, Krumholz HM. Times to treatment in transfer patients undergoing primary percutaneous coronary intervention in the United States: National Registry of Myocardial Infarction (NRMI)-3/4 analysis. *Circulation.* 2005;111:761–767.

31. Le May MR, Wells GA, Labinaz M, *et al.* Combined angioplasty and pharmacological intervention versus thrombolysis alone in acute myocardial infarction (CAPITAL AMI study). *J Am Coll Cardiol.* 2005;46:417–424.

32. Assessment of the Safety and Efficacy of a New Treatment Strategy with Percutaneous Coronary Intervention (ASSET-4PCI) investigators. Primary versus tenecteplase-facilitated percutaneous coronary intervention in patients with ST-segment elevation acute myocardial infarction (ASSENT-4 PCI): randomised trial. *Lancet.* 2006;367:569–578.

33. Keeley EC, Boura JA, Grines CL. Comparison of primary and facilitated percutaneous coronary interventions for ST-elevation myocardial infarction: quantitative review of randomised trials. *Lancet.* 2006;367:579–588.

34. Di Mario C, Dudek D, Piscione F, *et al.* Immediate angioplasty versus standard therapy with rescue angioplasty after thrombolysis in the Combined Abciximab REteplase Stent Study in Acute Myocardial Infarction

(CARESS-in-AMI): an open, prospective, randomised, multicentre trial. *Lancet.* 2008;371:559–568.

35. Cantor WJ, Fitchett D, Borgundvaag B, *et al.* Routine early angioplasty after fibrinolysis for acute myocardial infarction. *N Engl J Med.* 2009;360:2705–2718.

36. Fernandez-Aviles F, Alonso JJ, Pena G, *et al.* Primary angioplasty vs. early routine post-fibrinolysis angioplasty for acute myocardial infarction with ST-segment elevation: the GRACIA-2 non-inferiority, randomized, controlled trial. *Eur Heart J.* 2007;28:949–960.

37. Andersen HR, Nielsen TT, Rasmussen K, *et al.* A comparison of coronary angioplasty with fibrinolytic therapy in acute myocardial infarction. *N Engl J Med.* 2003;349:733–742.

38. Busk M, Maeng M, Rasmussen K, *et al.* The Danish multicentre randomized study of fibrinolytic therapy vs. primary angioplasty in acute myocardial infarction (the DANAMI-2 trial): outcome after 3 years follow-up. *Eur Heart J.* 2008;29:1259–1266.

39. Yousef ZR, Redwood SR, Bucknall CA, Sulke AN, Marber MS. Late intervention after anterior myocardial infarction: effects on left ventricular size, function, quality of life, and exercise tolerance: results of the Open Artery Trial (TOAT Study). *J Am Coll Cardiol.* 2002;40:869–876.

40. Stone GW, Grines CL, Cox DA, *et al.* Comparison of angioplasty with stenting, with or without abciximab, in acute myocardial infarction. *N Engl J Med.* 2002;346:957–966.

41. Spaulding C, Henry P, Teiger E, *et al.* Sirolimus-eluting versus uncoated stents in acute myocardial infarction. *N Engl J Med.* 2006;355:1093–1104.

42. Valgimigli M, Campo G, Percoco G, *et al.* Comparison of angioplasty with infusion of tirofiban or abciximab and with implantation of sirolimus-eluting or uncoated stents for acute myocardial infarction: the MULTISTRATEGY randomized trial. *JAMA.* 2008;299:1788–1799.

43. Stone GW, Webb J, Cox DA, *et al.* Distal microcirculatory protection during percutaneous coronary intervention in acute ST-segment elevation myocardial infarction: a randomized controlled trial. *JAMA.* 2005;293:1063–1072.

44. Gick M, Jander N, Bestehorn HP, *et al.* Randomized evaluation of the effects of filter-based distal protection on myocardial perfusion and infarct size after primary percutaneous catheter intervention in myocardial infarction with and without ST-segment elevation. *Circulation.* 2005;112:1462–1469.

45. Ali A, Cox D, Dib N, *et al.* Rheolytic thrombectomy with percutaneous coronary intervention for infarct size reduction in acute myocardial infarction: 30-day results from a multicenter randomized study. *J Am Coll Cardiol.* 2006;48:244–252.

46. Svilaas T, Vlaar PJ, Van Der Horst IC, *et al.* Thrombus aspiration during primary percutaneous coronary intervention. *N Engl J Med.* 2008;358:557–567.

47. Kandzari DE, Hasselblad V, Tcheng JE, *et al.* Improved clinical outcomes with abciximab therapy in acute myocardial infarction: a systematic overview of randomized clinical trials. *Am Heart J.* 2004;147: 457–462.

48. Tornvall P, Nilsson T, Lagerqvist B. Effects on mortality of abciximab in ST-elevation myocardial infarction treated with percutaneous coronary intervention including stent implantation. *J Intern Med.* 2006;260:363–368.

49. Srinivas VS, Skeif B, Negassa A, Bang JY, Shaqra H, Monrad ES. Effectiveness of glycoprotein IIb/IIIa inhibitor use during primary coronary angioplasty: results of propensity analysis using the New York State Percutaneous Coronary Intervention Reporting System. *Am J Cardiol.* 2007;99:482–485.

50. Mehilli J. Abciximab in patients with AMI undergoing primary PCI after clopidogrel pre-treatment. BRAVE-3 trial. Presented at the American College of Cardiology, Scientific Sessions, Chicago, 2008.

51. Stone GW, Witzenbichler B, Guagliumi G, *et al.* Bivalirudin during primary PCI in acute myocardial infarction. *N Engl J Med.* 2008;358:2218–2230.

52. Eagle KA, Lim MJ, Dabbous OH, *et al.* A validated prediction model for all forms of acute coronary syndrome: estimating the risk of 6-month post-discharge death in an international registry. *JAMA.* 2004;291:2727–2733.

53. Bassand JP, Hamm CW, Ardissino D, *et al.* Guidelines for the diagnosis and treatment of non-ST-segment elevation acute coronary syndromes. *Eur Heart J.* 2007;28:1598–1660.

54. Antman EM, Cohen M, Bernink PJ, *et al.* The TIMI risk score for unstable angina/non-ST elevation MI: A method for prognostication and therapeutic decision making. *JAMA.* 2000;284:835–842.

55. Chen ZM, Pan HC, Chen YP, *et al.* Early intravenous then oral metoprolol in 45,852 patients with acute myocardial infarction: randomised placebo-controlled trial. *Lancet.* 2005;366:1622–1632.

56. Eikelboom JW, Anand SS, Malmberg K, Weitz JI, Ginsberg JS, Yusuf S. Unfractionated heparin and low-molecular-weight heparin in acute coronary

syndrome without ST elevation: a meta-analysis. *Lancet.* 2000;355:1936–1942.

57. Petersen JL, Mahaffey KW, Hasselblad V, *et al.* Efficacy and bleeding complications among patients randomized to enoxaparin or unfractionated heparin for antithrombin therapy in non-ST-segment elevation acute coronary syndromes: a systematic overview. *JAMA.* 2004;292:89–96.

58. Yusuf S, Mehta SR, Chrolavicius S, *et al.* Comparison of fondaparinux and enoxaparin in acute coronary syndromes. *N Engl J Med.* 2006;354:1464–1476.

59. Mehta SR, Granger CB, Eikelboom JW, *et al.* Efficacy and safety of fondaparinux versus enoxaparin in patients with acute coronary syndromes undergoing percutaneous coronary intervention: results from the OASIS-5 trial. *J Am Coll Cardiol.* 2007;50:1742–1751.

60. Stone GW, White HD, Ohman EM, *et al.* Bivalirudin in patients with acute coronary syndromes undergoing percutaneous coronary intervention: a subgroup analysis from the Acute Catheterization and Urgent Intervention Triage strategy (ACUITY) trial. *Lancet.* 2007;369:907–919.

61. Yusuf S, Zhao F, Mehta SR, *et al.* Effects of clopidogrel in addition to aspirin in patients with acute coronary syndromes without ST-segment elevation. *N Engl J Med.* 2001;345:494–502.

62. Mehta SR, Yusuf S, Peters RJ, *et al.* Effects of pretreatment with clopidogrel and aspirin followed by long-term therapy in patients undergoing percutaneous coronary intervention: the PCI-CURE study. *Lancet.* 2001;358:527–533.

63. Patti G, Colonna G, Pasceri V, Pepe LL, Montinaro A, Di Sciascio G. Randomized trial of high loading dose of clopidogrel for reduction of periprocedural myocardial infarction in patients undergoing coronary intervention: results from the ARMYDA-2 (Antiplatelet therapy for Reduction of MYocardial Damage during Angioplasty) study. *Circulation.* 2005;111: 2099–2106.

64. von Beckerath N, Taubert D, Pogatsa-Murray G, Schomig E, Kastrati A, Schomig A. Absorption, metabolization, and antiplatelet effects of 300-, 600-, and 900-mg loading doses of clopidogrel: results of the ISAR-CHOICE (Intracoronary Stenting and Antithrombotic Regimen: Choose Between 3 High Oral Doses for Immediate Clopidogrel Effect) Trial. *Circulation.* 2005;112:2946–2950.

65. Kong DF, Hasselblad V, Harrington RA, *et al.* Meta-analysis of survival with platelet glycoprotein IIb/IIIa antagonists for percutaneous coronary interventions. *Am J Cardiol.* 2003;92:651–655.

66. Roffi M, Chew DP, Mukherjee D, *et al.* Platelet glycoprotein IIb/IIIa inhibition in acute coronary syndromes. Gradient of benefit related to the revascularization strategy. *Eur Heart J.* 2002;23: 1441–1448.

67. Roffi M, Chew DP, Mukherjee D, *et al.* Platelet glycoprotein IIb/IIIa inhibitors reduce mortality in diabetic patients with non-ST-segment-elevation acute coronary syndromes. *Circulation.* 2001;104:2767–2771.

68. Anderson KM, Califf RM, Stone GW, *et al.* Long-term mortality benefit with abciximab in patients undergoing percutaneous coronary intervention. *J Am Coll Cardiol.* 2001;37:2059–2065.

69. Roffi M, Mukherjee D. Platelet glycoprotein IIb/IIIa receptor inhibitors-end of an era? *Eur Heart J.* 2008;29:429-431.

70. Kastrati A, Mehilli J, Neumann FJ, *et al.* Abciximab in patients with acute coronary syndromes undergoing percutaneous coronary intervention after clopidogrel pretreatment: the ISAR-REACT 2 randomized trial. *JAMA.* 2006;295:1531–1538.

71. Ndrepepa G, Kastrati A, Mehilli J, *et al.* One-year clinical outcomes with abciximab vs. placebo in patients with non-ST-segment elevation acute coronary syndromes undergoing percutaneous coronary intervention after pre-treatment with clopidogrel: results of the ISAR-REACT 2 randomized trial. *Eur Heart J.* 2008;29:455–461.

72. Stone GW, Bertrand ME, Moses JW, *et al.* Routine upstream initiation vs deferred selective use of glycoprotein IIb/IIIa inhibitors in acute coronary syndromes: the ACUITY Timing trial. *JAMA.* 2007;297: 591–602.

73. Wiviott SD, Braunwald E, McCabe CH, *et al.* Prasugrel versus clopidogrel in patients with acute coronary syndromes. *N Engl J Med.* 2007;357:2001–2015.

74. de Winter RJ, Windhausen F, Cornel JH, *et al.* Early invasive versus selectively invasive management for acute coronary syndromes. *N Engl J Med.* 2005;353:1095–1104.

75. Fox KA, Poole-Wilson P, Clayton TC, *et al.* 5-year outcome of an interventional strategy in non-ST-elevation acute coronary syndrome: the British Heart Foundation RITA 3 randomised trial. *Lancet.* 2005;366:914–920.

76. Lagerqvist B, Husted S, Kontny F, Stahle E, Swahn E, Wallentin L. 5-year outcomes in the FRISC-II randomised trial of an invasive versus a non-invasive strategy in non-ST-elevation acute coronary syndrome: a follow-up study. *Lancet.* 2006;368:998–1004.

77. Neumann FJ, Kastrati A, Pogatsa-Murray G, *et al.* Evaluation of prolonged antithrombotic pretreatment ("cooling-off" strategy) before intervention in patients with unstable coronary syndromes: a randomized controlled trial. *JAMA.* 2003;290: 1593–1599.

78. Cannon CP, Weintraub WS, Demopoulos LA, *et al.* Comparison of early invasive and conservative strategies in patients with unstable coronary syndromes treated with the glycoprotein IIb/IIIa inhibitor tirofiban. *N Engl J Med.* 2001;344:1879–1887.

79. Tricoci P, Lokhnygina Y, Berdan LG, *et al.* Time to coronary angiography and outcomes among patients with high-risk non ST-segment elevation acute coronary syndromes: results from the SYNERGY trial. *Circulation.* 2007;116:2669–2677.

80. Rao SV, O'Grady K, Pieper KS, *et al.* Impact of bleeding severity on clinical outcomes among patients with acute coronary syndromes. *Am J Cardiol.* 2005;96:1200–1206.

81. Smith SC Jr., Allen J, Blair SN, *et al.* AHA/ACC guidelines for secondary prevention for patients with coronary and other atherosclerotic vascular disease: 2006 update: endorsed by the National Heart, Lung, and Blood Institute. *Circulation.* 2006;113: 2363–2372.

82. Hulten E, Jackson JL, Douglas K, George S, Villines TC. The effect of early, intensive statin therapy on acute coronary syndrome: a meta-analysis of randomized controlled trials. *Arch Intern Med.* 2006;166:1814–1821.

83. Cannon CP, Braunwald E, McCabe CH, *et al.* Intensive versus moderate lipid lowering with statins after acute coronary syndromes. *N Engl J Med.* 2004;350:1495–1504.

CHAPTER 2
Modern Coronary Stenting

Stéphane Cook

Cardiology, Swiss Cardiovascular Center Bern, University Hospital Bern, Bern, Switzerland

---

Chapter Overview

- Drug-eluting stents (DES) effectively addressed the problem of restenosis inherent to bare-metal stents by reducing target-lesion revascularization from 20% to 30% to less than 10%.
- DES were used in > 80% of percutaneous coronary interventions in the United States at the end of 2006.
- DES are associated with increased incidence of very late stent thrombosis (>1 year after implantation) in comparison to BMS.
- Very late stent thrombosis raised concern about the global safety profile of DES, which climaxed in the "ESC firestorm" in 2006 and was followed by indentation in the DES sales curves (50–60% of stent market).
- Subsequent research confirmed the good safety profile of DES up to 5 years in elective patients, as well as in other patients.
- Registries and underpowered randomized controlled trials suggest that PCI with DES is a valuable alternative to coronary artery grafting surgery in patient with left main coronary artery disease.
- Mechanical interventions on vulnerable, active plaques have been promulgated in order to seal the lesion before rupture happened. To date, however, DES implantation in nonobstructive lesions remains an unproved strategy.
- Passive modern stents appeared in the shadow of DES and could challenge DES in selected patients.

Coronary artery stents have emerged as the preferred tool for percutaneous coronary interventions (PCI) during the past decade. Their ubiquitous acceptance results from the ease and speed of applicability, the improved safety by elimination of abrupt closure and the need for urgent coronary artery bypass grafting, and the angiographically pleasing result.

Restenosis has been the principal limitation of PCI since its inception. The recent advent of drug-eluting stents (DES) with antiproliferative drugs generally immobilized via biocompatible polymers on the stent surface to reduce smooth muscle proliferation and the response to vascular injury has successfully addressed the problem of restenosis inherent to bare metal stents. The interventional cardiologist had embraced DES with a growing enthusiasm since 2002, and dreamed about conquering even more of the remaining surgical strongholds.

During the last couple of years, a general recognition of a logical, unavoidable, and anticipated [1] yet snubbed bane of DES emerged: very late stent thrombosis. This recognition led to an inappropriately fabricated panic about DES safety and stimulated powerful research leading to significant improvement not only in patient care (better selection, better follow-up) but also in research tools (Academic Research Consortium consensus) [2].

This chapter will review the key reports relevant to DES published during the past years, present its use in special subsets of lesions (plaque sealing)

Current Best Practice in Interventional Cardiology. Edited by
B Meier. © 2010 Blackwell Publishing.

and patients (left main), and discuss new options in passive modern stenting using conventional stents.

First-Generation Drug-Eluting Stents

Drug-Eluting Stents and the Risk of Very Late Stent Thrombosis

Stent thrombosis is a rare but dreaded complication of a drug-eluting stent (DES) or bare metal stent (BMS), that is, a thrombotic formation in the implant leading to a partial or complete obstruction of the cross-sectional vascular area [3]. While stent thrombosis was observed in 5% to 7% of patients treated with BMS in the early 90s, modifications in the indications and improvement in stent techniques, as well as the launch of dual antithrombotic regimens, led to an important reduction of the rate of stent thrombosis to 0.5% to 2% with modern BMS.

Outcome after stent thrombosis is similar for BMS and DES. It is estimated that stent thrombosis is associated with large myocardial infarction or death in about 90% of the detected cases [4].

Since various studies used divergent definitions of stent thrombosis, an Academic Research Consortium (ARC) recently worked out a uniform definition [2]. Stent thromboses are classified as definite (proven by angiography or autopsy), probable (sudden cardiac death up to 30 days, as well as myocardial infarction in the territory of the implanted stent without angiographic confirmation of stent thrombosis, independently of the duration), and possible (cardiac sudden death after 30 days). The ARC pointed out that the combination of adjudicated definite and probable stent thrombosis is the most appropriate to quantify the risk of stent thrombosis. Another instrument of classification is classification of stent thrombosis according to the temporal appearance after implantation of the stent. Thus, stent thromboses that appear in the first month after implantation are classified as early, those occurring between 1 month and

1 year as late, and those occurring after 1 year as very late.

Early and Late Stent Thrombosis: No Overall Difference Between DES and BMS

In a meta-analysis of 6 studies including 2963 patients, the incidence of *early* (0–1 month after implantation) stent thrombosis amounted 0.5% for SES and 0.6% for BMS (RR= 0.76, 95% CI 0.30–1.88, $p = 0.55$) [5]. Similar results appeared in a meta-analysis of five studies including 3513 patients comparing PES (0.5%) to BMS (0.6%) (RR = 0.74 risk, 95% CI 0.31–1.80, $p = 0.51$) [6].

Although the phenomenon of *late* (1–12 months after implantation) stent thrombosis was around with BMS, it was largely neglected. Four observation studies including a total of 9465 patients demonstrated an incidence of late stent thrombosis of 1%. The Bern Registry [7,8] demonstrated a similar incidence of stent thrombosis up to 6 months (Fig. 2.1). A meta-analysis did not show any difference in the incidence of late stent thrombosis (up to 1 year) between DES (0.2%, 2602 patients) and BMS (0.3%, 2428 patients; odds ratio = 0.99; confidence interval of 95% 0.35–2.84, $p = 1.00$).

Very Late Stent Thrombosis: Higher Incidence in DES than BMS

In opposition to early and late stent thrombosis, very late stent thrombosis (>1 year) seems to occur more frequently after DES than BMS.

The first respective data appeared in the long-term follow-up of 826 patients included in the BASKET-LATE study: an increased incidence of very late stent thrombosis was indicated to explain the results in which the mortality and myocardial infarction rate 1 year after discontinuation of clopidogrel were higher in the group assigned to DES than in the group treated with BMS [9]. The frequency and the temporal distribution of definite stent thromboses after implantation of DES were examined in the Bern-Rotterdam registry, which included 8146 consecutive patients [10]. While the incidence of early stent thrombosis (1.1%) was comparable with former studies with BMS, the long-term follow-up showed a continued risk of

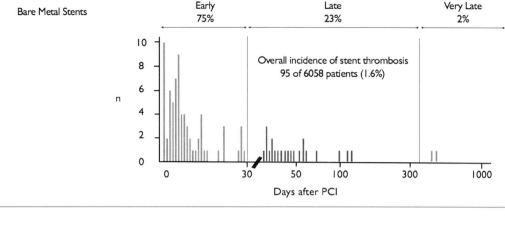

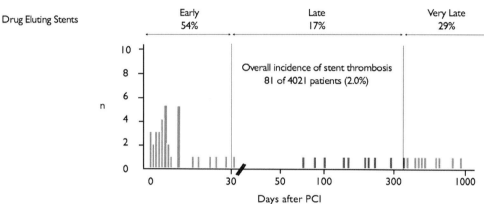

Figure 2.1 Incidence of stent thrombosis (n = number of stent thromboses per day) following bare metal stent and drug-eluting stent implantation. Early stent thrombosis ≤ 1 month; late stent thrombosis > 1 month but ≤ 1 year; very late stent thrombosis if > 1 year. (Redrawn with permission from Wenaweser P, Rey C, Eberli FR, et al. Stent thrombosis following bare-metal stent implantation: success of emergency percutaneous coronary intervention and predictors of adverse outcome. *Eur Heart J.* 2005;26:1180–1187; and unpublished data on incidence of stent thrombosis at Swiss Cardiovascular Center, Bern, Switzerland.)

late stent thrombosis of approximately 0.6% per year up to 4 years after implantation of a DES. Therefore and unlike with BMS, the risk of ST did not seem to wane with time after implantation of at least the first generation of DES (Fig. 2.2).

It should be stressed that these studies recorded only definite primary stent thromboses (without intercurrent revascularization), while secondary stent thromboses—appearing following intercurrent revascularization procedures for restenosis—were partly censured, which consequently favored BMS. Taking secondary stent thrombosis into account and in the light of the new definitions of the ARC, no longer a significant difference in the total (primary + secondary) incidence of stent thrombosis could be demonstrated long term (up to 4 years) between BMS and DES [11].

In 2006, two independent meta-analyses claimed that first-generation DES increase mortality. Nordmann suggested that sirolimus- (but not paclitaxel-) eluting stents were associated with a small but significant increase in noncardiac mortality at 2 and 3 years of follow-up. Camenzind

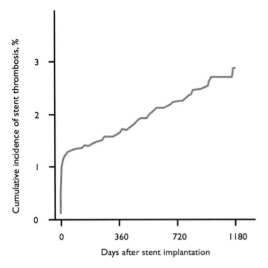

Figure 2.2 Kaplan-Meier survival curve showing the cumulative incidence of stent thrombosis in patients with sirolimus-eluting or paclitaxel-eluting stents during long-term follow-up. The slope of the linear portion of the cumulative incidence curve between 30 days and 3 years was 0.6 %/year. (Redrawn from reference Wenaweser P, Daemen J, Zwahlen M, et al. Incidence and correlates of drug-eluting stent thrombosis in routine clinical practice: 4-year results from a large 2-institutional cohort study. *J Am Coll Cardiol.* 2008;52:1134–1140, with permission.)

found that the mortality rate of patients treated with DES was higher than that of those treated with BMS. The (small) increase in the rate of death and myocardial infarction was observed in patients followed 18 months to 3 years after stent implantation [unpublished data]. These led to an unwarranted panic about DES thrombosis, coined the "ESC 2006 firestorm." This stimulated a very powerful research on DES safety by looking at clinical outcome after DES implantation in various study models.

Net Clinical Safety Profile of First-Generation Drug-Eluting Stents

On one hand, DES prevent neointimal formation, restenosis, and target lesion revascularization. On the other hand, DES slightly increase the risk of very late primary stent thrombosis. Therefore, the total safety profile of DES must be judged on indubitable clinical outcomes, such as the rate of

death and myocardial infarction. The body of evidence currently consists of several "real-world" registries with adjustments for patient characteristics, registries with propensity score matched pairs, and finally results of meta-analyses from randomized controlled trials.

Data from "Real-World" and "Propensity Score Matched Pairs" Registries

A Swedish observation's study (SCAAR registry) [12] compared the clinical follow-up of 6033 patients treated with DES to 13,738 patients treated with BMS. After 3 years, no significant difference was found for the primary end point (death and myocardial infarction) between DES and BMS. However, temporal differences appeared in a landmark analysis with a trend to fewer events in DES patients within the first 6 months after stent implantation (HR = 0.94, 95% CI 0.83–1.06), followed by a higher risk in the next time interval (HR = 1.20, 95% CI 1.05–1.57). The mortality at 3 years was similar in both stent groups (RR = 1.18, 95% CI 1.04–1.35). However, there were highly significant differences between the baseline patient characteristics of both groups, such as the incidence of type 2 diabetes mellitus, prior revascularization, number of implanted stents, as well as stent length and diameter. The most recent analysis of the SCAAR registry, including the year 2005 and up to 35,266 patients (BMS 21,480 patients, DES 13,786 patients) showed no significant difference in mortality (RR 1.03, 95% CI 0.94–1.14) or the combined outcome death or myocardial infarction (RR 1.01, 95% CI 0.94–1.09) between DES and BMS [13]. Other real-world registries, including a total of 49,052 patients, showed either a comparable mortality between the two groups, as in the study of the National Heart, Lung, and Blood Institute [14] (DES 1460 patients, BMS 1763 patients); or an even lower mortality rate in patients treated with DES, as in the DESCover registry (DES 397 patients, BMS 6509 patients), the REAL registry [15] (DES 3064 patients, BMS 7565 patients), the Wake Forest University [16] (DES 1164 patients, BMS 1285 patients), the Western Denmark (DES 3548 patients, BMS 8847 patients), the STENT registry (DES 1377 patients, BMS 5631 patients), or the study of Thoraxcenter (SES 976 patients, PES 2776 patients, BMS 2287 patients). These last registries have results very similar to the two registries with propensity score matched pairs, adding 17,484 patients to them. Ontario [17] demonstrated a reduction in the absolute mortality from 2.3% at 3-year follow-up, and Massachusetts [18] showed a absolute reduction of 2.5% in 2-year mortality, both in favor of DES patients.

Data from Meta-Analyses

The rates of mortality and myocardial infarctions resulting from randomized controlled trials and meta-analyses comparing DES with BMS are more valuable in the evaluation of the DES safety profile. Stone, Kastrati, and their associates investigated the mortality rate and the rate of myocardial infarction in one meta-analysis of all individual data from four double-blind trials in which 1748 patients were randomly assigned to receive either SES or BMS, and five double-blind trials in which 3513 patients were randomly assigned to receive either PES or BMS. There were no significant differences in the cumulative rates of death or myocardial infarction at 4 years [19,20].

Currently, the best evaluation of the safety profile of DES is provided by a network meta-analysis of all randomized controlled trials of first-generation DES published hitherto (38 studies, 18,023 patients) [21]. In this study, no difference in mortality was present between the stent types in the long-term follow-up, up to 4 years (SES versus BMS: HR = 1.00, 95% CI 0.82–1.25; PES versus BMS: HR = 1.03, 95% CI 0.84–1.22; SES versus PES: HR = 0.96, 95% CI 0.83–1.24). The rate of myocardial infarction was slightly smaller in the SES group than in the BMS group (HR = 0.81, 95% CI 0.66–0.97) or the PES group (HR = 0.83, 95% CI 0.71–1.00). In this work, a subanalysis was performed according to the diabetic status and also confirmed the results for diabetics: no significant difference in mortality (SES versus BMS: HR = 1.24, 95% CI 0.74–1.87; PES versus BMS: HR = 1.16, 95% CI 0.78–1.84; SES versus PES: HR = 1.06, 95% CI 0.76–1.59), and no difference for the combined rate of death and myocardial infarction (SES versus BMS: HR = 1.03, 95% CI 0.79–1.35;

PES versus BMS: HR = 1.08, 95% CI 0.79–1.43; SES versus PES: HR = 0.96, 95% CI 0.69–1.31).

In summary, these three individual meta-analyses do not show any difference in mortality between DES and BMS up to 4 years for PES and 5 years for SES. The only difference consisted of a smaller rate of myocardial infarction in patients treated with SES rather than BMS or PES.

Late Stent Thrombosis in DES Area: New Pathophysiologic Insights

Whereas the cause of very late ST remains largely unknown and is possibly multifactorial, hypersensitivity reaction has been a concern. It was first evoked by the pathologist Renu Virmani, who conducted autopsies on stent patients and found hypersensitivity reaction at the vicinity of DES, leading to necrosis, aneurysmatic dilatation of the vessel border, and stent thrombosis.

Joner and associates [22] presented the histopathologic comparison of 32 DES with 36 bare metal stents in 23 and 25 patients, respectively, who died more than 1 month after stent implantation. Late stent thrombosis was defined as an acute thrombus within a stent > 30 days old. Of 23 patients with DES > 30 days old, 14 had evidence of LST. SES and PES showed greater delayed healing characterized by persistent fibrin deposition (fibrin score 2.3 ± 1.1 versus 0.9 ± 0.8, $p < 0.0001$), and poorer endothelialization ($55.8 \pm 26.5\%$) compared with BMS (89.8 ± 20.9, $p < 0.0001$). Moreover, DES with LST showed more delayed healing compared with patent DES. In 5 of 14 patients suffering LST, antiplatelet therapy had been withdrawn. Additional procedural and pathologic risk factors for LST were (1) local hypersensitivity reaction, (2) ostial and/or bifurcation stenting, (3) malapposition/incomplete apposition, (4) restenosis, and (5) strut penetration into a necrotic core.

The main study limitation is also its strength: the group observed is highly selected and consisted only of the rare patients who have had a fatal event. Its main limitation is that these findings cannot be generalized to the complete DES population. However, the strength of this study is that it focused on patients suffering from sudden

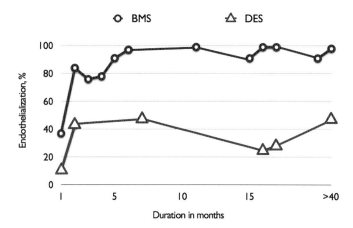

Figure 2.3 Line chart comparing the percentage of endothelialization in drug-eluting stents (DES) versus bare-metal stents (BMS) as a function of time. Note that DES (lower curve) consistently show less endothelialization compared with BMS (upper curve) regardless of time point. Even beyond 40 months, DES are not fully endothelialized, whereas BMS are completely covered by 6 to 7 months. (Redrawn from Joner M, Finn AV, Farb A, et al. Pathology of drug-eluting stents in humans: delayed healing and late thrombotic risk. *J Am Coll Cardiol*. 2006;48:193–202, with permission.)

cardiac death and late stent thrombosis. This highly selected population consisted of 23 patients with DES: from these, 19 had a cardiac death (13 due to late stent thrombosis), 1 suffered a late stent thrombosis but died from cerebrovascular hemorrhage (indirectly linked to LST), and the last 3 died from noncardiac death. This study demonstrates that compared to BMS, DES result in delayed arterial healing and incomplete endothelialization. Whereas BMS are fully endothelialized and display a low chronic inflammation at the vicinity of stent struts by 6 months, DES endothelialization seems to plateau at 40% (Fig. 2.3), and DES are associated with greater inflammatory reaction, including fibrin deposition giant cell, lymphocytes, eosinophils, and macrophages, lasting for more than 40 months.

Interestingly, DES patients who suffered stent thrombosis also had higher fibrin scores and lower endothelialization scores than DES patients who did not have stent thrombosis. It seems, therefore, that in this special population, an inflammatory gradient could be drawn not only between BMS and DES but also between patients who died from late stent thrombosis and patients with patent stents, which suggests that the more inflammation, the higher is the risk of stent thrombosis in DES patients.

The question arises how to pick out DES patients with an exaggerated inflammatory reaction who are thus at risk of late stent thrombosis.

In order to identify structural differences of the stented segment between patients with and with-

out very late ST (>1 year) [23], we used intravascular ultrasound studies (IVUS) [23]. The findings in 13 patients with very late ST at a mean of 630 ±166 days after DES implantation who underwent IVUS were compared with IVUS routinely obtained 8 months after DES implantation in 144 control patients, who did not experience ST for > 2 years. Compared with DES controls, patients with very late ST had longer lesions (23.9 ± 16.0 versus 13.3 ± 7.9 mm, $p < 0.001$) and stents (34.6 ± 22.4 mm versus 18.6 ± 9.5 mm, $p < 0.001$), more stents per lesion (1.6 ± 0.9 versus 1.1 ± 0.4, $p < 0.001$), and stent overlap (39% versus 8%, $p < 0.001$). Vessel cross-sectional area was similar for the reference segment (EEM-CSA: 18.9 ± 6.9 mm^2 versus 20.4 ± 7.2 mm^2, $p = 0.46$) but significantly larger for the in-stent segment (28.6 ± 11.9 mm^2 versus 20.1 ± 6.7 mm^2, $p = 0.005$) in very late ST patients compared with DES controls. Incomplete stent apposition (ISA) was present in 10 (77%) patients with very late ST, but in only 21 (12%) DES controls ($p < 0.001$). Multivariate logistic regression analysis identified ISA and stent overlap as independent variables associated with very late ST [23].

Previous IVUS studies with BMS and DES failed to identify late incomplete stent apposition (ISA) as a predictor for clinical adverse events. However, the predictive accuracy of these studies may have been limited by the small number of patients with late ISA (13–90 patients), the limited follow-up period of only 12 months (earliest moment for very

0

late stent thrombosis) in patients after DES implantation, and the inherently unlikely occurrence of very late stent thrombosis in such patients.

The present study focused on the rare patients presenting with very late stent thrombosis and systematically performed IVUS prior to emergency PCI. ISA was highly prevalent (77%) in patients with very late stent thrombosis as compared to only 12% in the DES control group. This suggests a causal role of ISA in the pathogenesis of this adverse event. In addition, the extent of ISA, both in terms of length and depth, was more pronounced in very late stent thrombosis patients compared to controls. This finding suggests that small areas of ISA may be clinically silent, whereas large areas of ISA may increase the risk of stent thrombosis.

The results of this study apply only to patients with very late stent thrombosis following DES implantation, but together with the previous study

from Joner and associates [22] ask for more adequate management of patients displaying ultrasonic coronary aneurysm and/or large stent malapposition (Fig. 2.4) [23].

First Generation of Drug-Eluting Stents in Acute Coronary Syndromes

There have been a number of specific concerns about using DES (thrombogenic material) in acute myocardial infarction (pro-thrombotic state), particularly after studies and case reports relating DES thrombosis occurring in patients having suffered from acute coronary syndrome. For instance, McFadden and colleagues [24] reported that the majority of late stent thrombosis occurred when a DES was placed in patients with acute coronary syndrome. Moreover, the preliminary results of the PREMIER registry displayed a 3-fold higher mortality rate in the group treated with DES (SES) compared to the group treated with BMS. Based

Incomplete stent apposition due to positive vessel remodelling

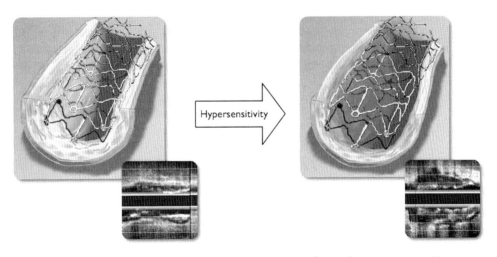

Successful implantation of stent.

Incomplete stent apposition by aneurysmal dilation of the stented arterial segments

Figure 2.4 Schematic representation of mechanisms leading to incomplete stent apposition by positive arterial remodeling. An exaggerated peri-stent inflammatory response (hypersensitivity) with increase of external elastic membrane out of proportion to the increase in peri-stent plaque and media, leads to incomplete stent

apposition of an initially well-apposed stent. (Reproduced with permission from Cook S, Wenaweser P, Togni M, et al. Incomplete stent apposition and very late stent thrombosis following drug eluting stent implantation. *Circulation.* 2007;115:2426–2434.)

on these data, a cautionary approach has been pro-mulgated to refrain from systematic use of DES in the setting of STEMI until the publication of the two first large randomized controlled trials (TY-PHOON and PASSION), which are summarized next.

The TYPHOON trial [25] was a single-blind, mul-ticenter, prospectively randomized trial to com-pare SES with BMS in primary PCI for acute my-ocardial infarction with ST-segment elevation. The trial included 712 patients at 48 medical centers. The primary end point was target-vessel failure at 1 year after the procedure, defined as target-vessel–related death, recurrent myocardial infarc-tion, or target-vessel revascularization. A follow-up angiographic substudy was performed at 8 months among 174 patients from selected centers. In this study, the rate of the primary end point was signif-icantly lower in the SES group than in the BMS group (7.3% versus 14.3%, $p = 0.004$). This re-duction was driven by a decrease in the rate of target-vessel revascularization (5.6% and 13.4%, respectively; $p < 0.001$). There was no significant difference between the two groups in the rate of death (2.3% and 2.2%, respectively; $p = 1.00$), re-infarction (1.1% and 1.4%, respectively; $p = 1.00$), or stent thrombosis (3.4% and 3.6%, respectively; $p = 1.00$).

The PASSION trial [26] randomly assigned 619 patients presenting with an acute myocardial in-farction with ST-segment elevation to receive ei-ther a PES or BMS. The primary end point was a composite of death from cardiac causes, recurrent myocardial infarction, or target-lesion revascular-ization at 1 year and did not reach the significance level. There was, however, a trend toward a lower rate of serious adverse events in the PES group than in the BMS group (8.8% versus 12.8%; adjusted relative risk, 0.63; 95% CI, 0.37 to 1.07; $p = 0.09$). A nonsignificant trend was also detected in favor of the PES group, as compared with the BMS group, in the rate of death from cardiac causes or recur-rent myocardial infarction (5.5% versus 7.2%, $p = 0.40$) and in the rate of target-lesion revasculariza-tion (5.3% versus 7.8%, $p = 0.23$). The incidence of stent thrombosis during 1 year of follow-up was the same in both groups (1.0%).

TYPHOON and PASSION trials ultimately at-test to the safety and efficacy of both SES and PES as compared to BMS in the setting of ST-elevation myocardial infarction. Although the stud-ies were designed and conducted differently, the re-sults were remarkably similar (Table 2.1).

Because of differences in study design and def-initions of end points, side-by-side comparisons were not possible. Both stents proved not to be inferior to BMS but only SES proved some su-periority. The TYPHOON trial showed a statisti-cally significant reduction in target vessel failure and revascularization, but SES failed to achieve re-duction in cardiac death and nonfatal myocardial infarction.

Table 2.1 Randomized Trials of DES Versus BMS in ST-Elevation Acute Myocardial Infarction

		TYPHOON			PASSION		
		Active Arm (n = 355)	Control Arm (n = 357)	p-value	Active Arm (n = 355)	Control Arm (n = 357)	p-value
Study design	No. of Centers Involved	48			2		
	Adjudication	Independent			Authors		
Results	TVF (Death, MI, TVR) (%)	7.3	14.3	0.04	8.8	12.8	0.09
	TVR (%)	5.6	13.4	< 0.001	5.3	7.8	0.23
	Cardiac Death (%)	2.0	1.4	0.58	3.9	6.2	0.20
	Myocardial Infarction (%)	1.1	1.4	1.0	1.7	2.0	0.74
	Angiographically Proven Stent Thrombosis (%)	2.0	3.4	0.35	1.0	1.0	1.0

These Figures support data from the STRAT-EGY trial [27] published in 2005, which verified that single high-dose bolus tirofiban plus DES (sirolimus-eluting stent) was safer than abciximab plus bare-metal stenting with regard to binary restenosis and TVR; again, there was no change in mortality.

So what do we know to date? Based on these three last studies, one can consider that for up to 1 year, DES implantation in patients suffering acute myocardial infarction is safe for both first-generation DES, and that in addition SES has proved to be clinically more effective than BMS and equally cost-effective in this setting. However, considering that most of the concerns were about whether patients suffering from acute coronary syndromes treated with DES would be at higher risk for late stent thrombosis than patients treated with BMS, one must regret the short duration of follow-up (12 months) and the deficient statistical power of both studies to address this issue. Long-term follow-up data from very large trials and registries are therefore mandated before coming to definite conclusions. Longer follow-up of TYPHOON and PASSION studies would be appreciated but have not been announced to date; alternatives, such as the STENT thrombosis study, the e-SELECT registry, and the HORIZONS AMI trial, will undoubtedly address the problem. The STENT (Strategic Transcatheter Evaluation of New Therapies) thombosis study, which would be the continuation of the registry, aims to follow approximately 10,000 new patients undergoing DES implantation over 2 years, in order to address the incidence and try to find contributing factors leading to stent thrombosis after DES (sirolimus-eluting stent and paclitaxel-eluting stent) implantation. The e-SELECT registry and the INSIGHT randomized trial aim to follow 30,000 patients assigned to standard versus long-duration clopidogrel treatment. The HORIZONS AMI trial is a randomized trial in 3400 patients with acute ST-elevation myocardial infarction, aiming to compare unfractionated heparin or bivalirudin with a GpIIb/IIIa inhibitor, and primary angioplasty with paclitaxel-eluting stent versus bare metal stent implantation.

New Generation of Drug-Eluting Stents

After Medtronic's Endeavor stent, which elutes zotarolimus and has been commercially available since April 2005, the Promus and Xience V stents (identical products, sold respectively by Boston Scientific and Abbott) using everolimus hit the market in October 2006. Biomatrix and Nobori stents (identical products sold by Biosensors and Terumo), eluting biolimus A9, received Conformité Européenne (CE) approval in January 2008.

Moreover, two additional stents eluting paclitaxel have been introduced: Axxion from Biosensors and CoStar from Conor MedSystems (since bought by Cordis and abandoned). Furthermore, a new generation of DES (Cypher Select and Taxus Liberté) was launched in both Europe and the United States and provides better deliverability and crossing rate than the first generation did.

Table 2.2 summarizes the DES currently available in the European and U.S. market.

Biolimus
The identical Biomatrix and Nobori coronary stents use a biodegradable polymer. They were designed with an asymmetric, abluminal coating, which releases biolimus A9 into the vessel wall while the polylactic acid polymer is being resorbed.

In the STEALTH trial [28], 120 patients with 122 de novo coronary lesions (2.75–4.0 mm vessels, $\leq$ 24 mm lesion length) were prospectively randomized in a 2:1 ratio to receive the biolimus stent (n = 80, 82 lesions) or the control uncoated stent (n = 40). Baseline lesion and angiographic characteristics were similar between groups. At 6-month follow-up, late lumen loss was significantly decreased with the biolimus stent in the stent (0.26 $\pm$ 0.43 versus 0.74 $\pm$ 0.45 mm, $p < 0.001$) and in the segment (0.14 $\pm$ 0.45 versus 0.40 $\pm$ 0.41 mm, $p = 0.004$). In-stent restenosis was 3.9% in the biolimus stent group versus 7.7% in the control group ($p = 0.40$).

These findings were echoed by the Nobori 1 trial presented at Transcatheter Cardiovascular Therapeutics in November 2006. The Nobori 1 phase I trial was a 2:1 noninferiority randomized

Table 2.2 Drug-Eluting Stents

Drug	Name	Manufacturer	Stent Material	Polymer	Status
Biolimus-A9	BioMatrix	Biosensors	Stainless steel	Bioabsorbable	CE mark
	Nobori	Terumo	Stainless steel	Bioabsorbable	CE mark
Everolimus	Champion	Guidant	Stainless steel	Bioabsorbable	—
	Xience V	Guidant	Cobalt chromium	Durable	CE mark
Sirolimus	Sirolimus-eluting stent Select	Cordis	Stainless steel	Durable	CE mark
	Sirolimus-eluting stent Neo	Cordis	Cobalt chromium	Durable	
Tacrolimus	Janus	Sorin	Stainless steel	None	CE mark
Zotarolimus	Endeavor	Medtronic	Cobalt chromium	Durable	CE mark
	ZoMaxx	Abbott	Tantalum/stainless steel	Durable	—
Paclitaxel	Axxion	Biosensors	Stainless steel	None	CE mark
	CoStar	Biotronik/Conor	Cobalt chromium	Bioabsorbable	CE mark
	Infinnium	SMT	Stainless steel	Bioabsorbable	CE mark
	Paclitaxel-eluting stent Liberté	Boston Scientific	Stainless steel	Durable	CE mark

multicentric trial involving 120 patients comparing biolimus A9 to paclitaxel-eluting stents. The trial focused on late loss and found that both the in-stent late loss at nine months (primary endpoint) and the total major adverse cardiac events (MACE) rate were statistically significantly lower in the Nobori group compared with the paclitaxel-eluting stent group.

However, the potent accomplishment in preventing neointimal formation and the presence of late-acquired coronary aneurysm in one patient of the STEALTH study should warrant caution regarding a possible increased risk of hypersensitivity, arterial remodeling, and its corollary, stent thrombosis. Larger-scale studies, such as the LEADERS randomized (1:1 comparing with Cypher Select), single blind, multicenter "real-world" clinical trial are mandatory, and so far showed noninferiority of the Biosensor Stent up to 1 year with slight clinical advantages [29].

Zotarolimus

Apart from the ENDEAVOR Sprint coronary stent, which elutes zotarolimus from a nonresorbable phosphorylcholine (PC) polymer within 28 days, Medtronic developed and launched in 2007 a new system based on a new polymer (BioLink), which elutes the drug more slowly.

In the ENDEAVOR II trial [30], 1197 patients with single coronary artery stenosis were enrolled in a prospective, randomized, double-blind study and randomly assigned to receive the Endeavor zotarolimus-eluting phosphorylcholine polymer-coated stent (ZES, n = 598) or a similar BMS (n = 599). The primary end point was target vessel failure (TVF) at 9 months, defined as a composite of target vessel revascularization (TVR), Q- and non-Q-wave myocardial infarction, or cardiac death. TVF was reduced from 15.1% with BMS to 7.9% with ZES ($p < 0.0001$), and the rate of major adverse cardiac events was reduced from 14.4% with BMS to 7.3% with ZES ($p < 0.0001$). Target lesion revascularization was 4.6% with ZES compared with 11.8% with BMS ($p < 0.0001$). The rate of stent thrombosis was 0.5% for ZES and 1.2% for BMS. An angiographic follow-up was performed in 531 patients. The in-stent late loss was reduced from 1.03 ± 0.58 to 0.61 ± 0.46 ($p < 0.001$), and the rate of in-segment binary restenosis was reduced from 35.0% to 13.2% with ZES ($p < 0.0001$). Differences in clinical outcome were maintained at 12 and 24 months ($p < 0.0001$).

In the ENDEAVOR III trial [31], 436 patients with single coronary artery disease were enrolled in a prospective, multicenter, single-blind, randomized trial. The primary end point of in-segment late loss did not meet the noninferiority criteria of a 0.20-mm difference with a late loss of 0.34 mm in ZES and 0.13 mm in SES ($p < 0.001$ for superiority). The same holds true for the in-stent late loss, which was also larger in the ZES group (0.60 mm) than in the SES group (0.15 mm, $p < 0.001$), as well as the binary restenosis both in-stent (9.2% versus 2.1%, $p = 0.02$) and in-segment (11.7% versus 4.3%, $p = 0.04$). At 9-month follow-up, the composite of target vessel failure did not differ by treatment group (12.0% versus 11.5%, $p = 1.0$), nor did death (0.6% versus 0%) or target lesion revascularization (6.3% versus 3.5%, $p = 0.34$). The 2-year clinical data were recently reported. The rate of major adverse cardiac events—a composite safety measure of death, repeat procedures, and myocardial infarction (MI)—was reported to be 9.3% for ZES and 11.6% for SES ($p = 0.47$). There was no statistically significant difference in the need for repeat procedures, target lesion revascularization (ZES 7.0% versus SES 4.5%; $p = 0.50$), or all-cause mortality (ZES 1.6% versus SES 4.5%; $p = 0.14$).

The history of the Endeavor Sprint (zotarolimus-eluting stent) is appealing. It basically demonstrates that even if the angiographic end points of late loss and binary restenosis were substantially higher for zotarolimus-eluting stents than those usually seen in sirolimus-eluting and paclitaxel-eluting stents, there was apparently no clinical disadvantage: the target vessel failure—defined as a composite of target vessel revascularization, recurrent Q-wave or non–Q-wave MI, or cardiac death—was comparable to similar end points found in sirolimus-eluting and paclitaxel-eluting stent trials. This implies a cleavage between angiographic measures and clinical follow-up (probably within certain limits).

Based on these results, the authors of Endeavor II proposed that accepting a "mild degree of restenosis might offer a reasonable compromise between safety and efficacy." However, we should consider that the major impact of DES has been among high-risk subgroups, such as patients suffering from multivessel disease and/or diabetes mellitus, and that restenosis, especially if occlusive, is closely correlated with long-term mortality in such patients. One hundred and six diabetics were included in the Endeavor II study and the differences between

the groups regarding binary restenosis and target lesion revascularization rates were no more statistically significant in patients under insulin therapy (9-month TLR rate by IDDM: 11.5% versus 13.6%, ZES versus BMS).

Direct comparison between DES is mandatory, and apart from ENDEAVOR IV, which aims to compare ZES to PES, Medtronic announced that it will begin a large (8000 patients) multicentric, randomized, controlled trial, named the PROTECT study, which aims to compare the safety profile (stent thrombosis, death, and nonfatal myocardial infarction) of zotarolimus-eluting stents with sirolimus-eluting stents.

In conclusion, by permitting higher late loss and possibly better endothelialization than the competitors, Endeavor Sprint probably lessens the rate of stent thrombosis in a low-risk population, which is in itself a salutary virtue. However, and like a double-edged sword, we should exercise caution in high-risk patients, in whom binary restenosis is typically associated with TLR and death. To overcome this problem, Medtronic launched the ZES Resolute, and the first data demonstrate smaller late loss than expected (0.12 mm at 4-month follow-up in 30 patients included in the RESOLUTE trial).

Drug-Eluting Stents in the Treatment of Intermediate Lesions

The lack of linear relation between stenosis severity and the probability of developing an acute coronary syndrome (ACS) is well recognized. Indeed, the majority of plaques leading to ACS are angiographically not significant. This is due to the fact that thrombosis is more dependent on the presence of a thin-cap fibroatheroma than on the tightness of stenosis. Infarction may even be caused by a segment without visible stenosis as the plaque may bulge abluminally due to medial atrophy or overall (positive) remodeling of the vessel wall. This implies that the potential for plaque erosion, fissure, or rupture is the salient point, and that the hemodynamic significance of the stenosis is prognostically of secondary importance.

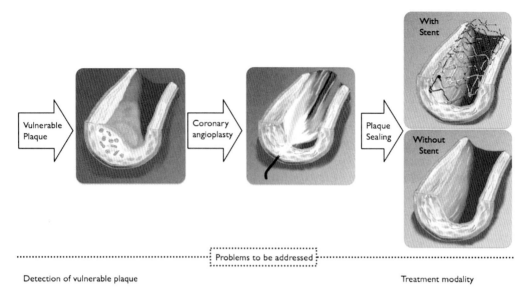

Figure 2.5 The concept of plaque sealing aims at detecting and treating unstable (vulnerable) atherosclerotic plaques before plaque rupture. However, this raises two concerns: (1) how to detect and document vulnerability and (2) the modality of treatment.

Therefore, in order to prevent ACS and boast a prognostic impact, coronary intervention should be aimed not only at stenoses of hemodynamical significance, but also at treating (sealing) vulnerable, active lesions (Fig. 2.5).

The first challenge will be to distinguish the stable from the vulnerable plaque. Several techniques are available to help the interventionist in differentiating these two states; structural changes can be detected by angiography, intravascular ultrasound with or without virtual histology, optical coherence tomography, angioscopy, ultrafast computerized tomography, or magnetic resonance imaging. Functional changes can be detected by elastography, palpography, or thermography. However, none of these techniques are currently reliable, and most of them are used for research purposes only. Furthermore, they provide snapshots with limited validity over time, and gathering of information using intracoronary devices may itself render plaques vulnerable.

The second challenge will be the way to treat such lesions. Whereas medical therapy remains the mainstay of treatment, mechanical plaque sealing has been promulgated by a few. While plain balloon angioplasty (Fig. 2.5) has been traditionally used for plaque sealing, introduction of DES into clinical practice is appealing. They virtually eliminate the risk of transforming a nonsignificant lesion into a significant lesion by restenosis after balloon angioplasty. On the other hand, they introduce the ominous risk of late thrombosis, which may well match that of leaving the lesion untreated.

In a subanalysis from pooled data from four different randomized trials (SIRIUS, TAXUS-IV, and the FUTURE-I and -II trials), Moses and colleagues [32] found that treatment of intermediate lesions (QCA $< 50\%$, mean 44%) with DES (sirolimus-eluting stent, paclitaxel-eluting stent, or zotarolimus-eluting stent) was associated with lower rates of revascularization (target-lesion revascularization 1.2% versus 20.3%, $p < 0.0001$; target-vessel revascularization 3.2% versus 19.4%, $p < 0.004$), myocardial infarction (3.2% versus 20.0%, $p = $ ns), and cumulative composite adverse cardiac events (4.1% versus 23.5%, $p = 0.001$) than with bare metal stents.

To stent or not to stent intermediate lesions? No study clearly was so far designed to answer this question. Based on three studies that deferred similar lesions (QCA < 50%), one could estimate the 12- to 36-month MACE rate at 4% to 9%, which is similar to the one found in this paper (4.1% at 12 months). Therefore, the only conclusion to be drawn is that DES implantation in intermediate lesions is probably not harmful up to 1 year.

Mechanical interventions on intermediate, non–flow-limiting plaques remain an unproved strategy, and larger, randomized trials with longer follow-up duration are mandatory.

Comparison of Modern PCI with Bypass Surgery

Although percutaneous coronary intervention (PCI) has long surpassed coronary artery bypass grafting (CABG) as the most common revascularization strategy in patients with coronary artery disease, current recommendations still favor CABG in the treatment of multivessel disease and unprotected left main coronary artery disease. Restenosis and the need for repeat revascularization remain the major limitations of PCI for such patients. By significantly reducing restenosis and the need for repeat revascularization in patients treated with DES, emerging data have, however, suggested that CABG may not have the advantage over PCI in the era of drug-eluting stents: In the second arm from the Arterial Revascularization Therapy Study (ARTS II) published in 2005, in which 607 patients with multivessel disease were treated with sirolimus-eluting stent, Serruys and coworkers [33] found better 12-month clinical outcomes in these patients when compared to historical controls of the ARTS I trial. Finally, a growing body of evidence resulting from registries suggests that the implantation of DES for unprotected left main coronary artery lesions is a feasible and safe approach. The recently published SYNTAX trial, however, sets things straight insofar as the advanced triple-vessel disease should remain a surgical domain while selected cases can be treated with DES [34].

Real-World Registries

Data comparing the efficacy of DES with CABG in the management of the unprotected left main coro-

nary artery are still in the early stages, with mostly 1-year follow-up available to date. These data have been presented at national conferences, and only three retrospective, nonrandomized, single-center experiences and one small randomized-controlled study have been published so far.

Chieffo and colleagues [35] investigated 249 patients with LMCA stenosis treated with either PCI and DES implantation (n = 107) or coronary artery bypass grafting (n = 142), in a single center, between March 2002 and July 2004. A propensity analysis was performed to adjust for baseline differences between the two cohorts. At 1 year, there was no statistical difference in the occurrence of death in PCI versus CABG both for the unadjusted (OR 0.291; 95% CI 0.054–1.085; $p = 0.0710$) and adjusted analyses (OR 0.331; 95% CI 0.055–1.404; $p = 0.1673$). PCI was correlated to a lower occurrence of the composite end points of death and myocardial infarction (unadjusted OR 0.235; 95% CI 0.048–0.580; $p = 0.0002$; adjusted OR 0.260; 95% CI 0.078–0.597; $p = 0.0005$) and death, myocardial infarction, and cerebrovascular events (unadjusted OR 0.300; 95% CI 0.102–0.617; $p = 0.0004$; adjusted OR 0.385; 95% CI 0.180–0.819; $p = 0.01$). No difference was detected in the occurrence of major adverse cardiac and cerebrovascular events in the unadjusted (OR 0.675; 95% CI 0.371–1.189; $p = 0.1891$) and adjusted analyses (OR 0.568; 95% CI 0.229–1.344; $p = 0.23$).

In the study, Chieffo and associates found that on the one hand DES treatment was associated with a lower rate of the composite end points of death and myocardial infarction, as well as death, myocardial infarction, and cerebrovascular events (MACCE), when compared with surgery during both hospitalization and at 1-year follow-up. On the other hand, surgery was associated with a lower rate of target vessel revascularization (TVR) during follow-up.

In the second registry, Lee and associates [36] compared 50 patients with DES implantation to 123 patients who underwent CABG for left main coronary artery disease and found very similar results: Even when the PCI group was composed of patients with higher risk (more female, higher Parsonnet score), both 1-year survival rates and

MACCE rates were not different, with a tendency towards better outcomes in the PCI-group.

Finally, the registry from Sanmartin and associates [37] paralleled the results of the first two registries: 96 patients treated by PCI versus 245 by CABG. In this particular study, both types of procedures were exemplary: almost 100% of LIMA graft in the surgical group and 90% PCI performed with only one DES. The cumulative MACE rate were low in both groups up to 1 year (PCI 10.4% versus CABG 11.4%; $p = 0.50$) with slightly higher mortality rate in the CABG group (PCI 5.2% versus CABG 8.4%; $p = 0.37$) and more revascularization in the PCI group (TVR-PCI 5.2% versus CABG 0.8%; $p = 0.02$).

DES for Unprotected Left Main Coronary Disease

These data are consistent with several registries investigating efficacy and safety of DES in unprotected left main coronary stenosis. The pooled data from eight current registry studies are depicted in Figure 2.6 and show that one should expect one-year TVR and mortality rates from 8% and 4%, respectively, which are very close to the Figures after CABG.

More importantly, two studies underlined that the outcome after PCI with DES for unprotected left main disease (ULM-PCI) was similar or even better than predicted by EuroScore.

Vecchio and associates [38] showed in 114 patients treated by ULM-PCI that the long-term follow-up (up to 17 months) was good (100% sur-

vival) for the patients having a EuroScore lower than 11 points (30-day mortality $< 24\%$). Dubois made the same observation in a cohort of 143 patients, and demonstrated moreover that ULM-PCI was better than the predicted EuroScore for patients having a predicted mortality $< 50\%$. Among patients whose operational risk was higher than 50%, the EuroScore was directly predictive for the observed mortality.

Therefore, good surgical candidates, such as the ones included in the study from Erglis and associates [39], have a very low MACE rate (6-month death rate 2%, TLR 2%, cumulative MACE 13%).

Finally, few data are available on long-term follow-up after DES ULM-PCI. Briefly, the registry from the John Radcliffe Hospital [40] investigated the 3-year follow-up of 100 patients. The patients were divided into three groups, based on the local indication for ULM-PCI: group 1 was deemed operable or inoperable, group 2 contained patients with ongoing STEMI or cardiogenic shock, and group 3 consisted of patients with acute coronary syndrome, favorable anatomy, and patient agreement. In this particular group, they found very encouraging results with 100% survival at 3 years.

DES ULM-PCI Versus CABG: Randomized Controlled Study

The only modern-day, randomized controlled study to compare unprotected left main stenting with CABG for left main disease was published in 2008 [41]. In this study (Le Mans) 52 patients were randomized to PCI and 53 patients were assigned

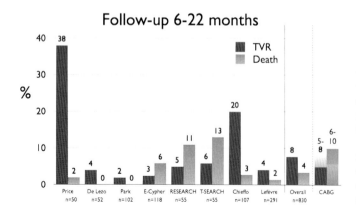

Figure 2.6 Target vessel revascularization (TVR) and mortality (*Death*) rates at end of follow-up (6–22 months) in eight registries investigating the efficacy and safety of drug-eluting stents (DES) in unprotected left main coronary stenosis. The pooled data from the eight current registry studies (*Overall*) show 1-year TVR and mortality rates from 8% and 4%, respectively, which come close to the incidences initially expected after coronary artery bypass grafting (CABG).

to CABG. Interestingly, DES were implanted only in vessels with diameter < 3.8 mm (35% of patients in the PCI group), whereas 79% of patients in the CABG group received LIMA graft. The primary end point was a composite of LVEF, functional capacity, and angina status. After 12 months, there was no difference within the groups with regards to angina status and exercise testing. However, the patients in the PCI groups had a statistically significant increase in systolic LV function. The secondary end points included major adverse cardiac events (MACE), survival, and any major adverse events (MAEs), defined as any MACE, procedure-related infection, bleeding, or renal or respiratory insufficiency. Patients within the PCI group had fewer early complications with significantly fewer MACE at 30 days, but the same survival rate at 12 months.

Summary

In conclusion, early evidence from registries demonstrated exciting results from DES implantation for left main coronary disease with low rate of binary restenosis and favorable short-term clinical outcome up to 1 year. Recent studies found no difference in outcome between percutaneous interventions and CABG for left main coronary disease. Based on these data, routine DES implantation should currently be the preferred strategy when percutaneous coronary intervention is undertaken for left main coronary artery disease. However, the benefit of drug-eluting stent implantation in the long term (>1 year) and the incidence of major adverse cardiovascular events in this setting remain largely unknown. Some very late stent thrombosis and very late target lesion restenosis have been reported and raised concerns about the safety of percutaneous procedures for left main coronary artery disease. Randomized controlled trials with long follow-up observation duration are mandatory. The results from the COMBAT trial should be available in 2011.

Modern Passive Stents (BMS) and Bioactive Stents

Passive modern stents appeared (in the shadow of DES) with advanced design allowing improved per-formance compared to former generations: smaller strut thickness, and different scaffolding and configuration, improve the flexibility and stent crossing profile, together with improved radial support and improved side branch accessibility. There are also gains in safety with secure delivery-balloon technology and new vessel surface coverage.

New surface coatings have been developed to further improve the crossing profile and lessen the restenosis rate. Moreover, it is known that the stent surface plays a key role in the inflammatory response after stent implantation, and that by modulating the surface material, both the neointimal hyperplasia and the risk of thrombotic event could be decreased. Various biologically inert surface materials have been investigated so far, such as carbon, platinum, phosphorylcholine, or gold, without clinically proven effect in human trials. Of the new materials, titanium is especially interesting, while it is extremely biocompatible and could be combining to nitric oxide, which has well-known antiproliferative effects.

Mosseri and associates [42] presented the results from a registry investigating the 6-month outcomes of patients treated with titanium nitric-oxide coated stainless steel stents. A total of 333 Titan stents were implanted in 296 patients. At 180 days, 6.3% of patients had a total of 7.6% MACE including 5.4% TLR, 0.7% MI, 0.7% stent thrombosis, and 0.7% death. One should, however, stress that this registry included only a moderate number of patients, had a short follow-up period, and the adjudication of adverse events was performed by the authors. Nevertheless, the clinical outcome shows potential and could compete with drug-eluting stents. Accordingly, unpublished data from the Israel Cypher stent registry showed comparable TLR (3.9%) and MACE (5.7%) rates after identical follow-up duration in a similar population treated with sirolimus-eluting stents.

In light of these promising results, the time is coming for randomized study allowing direct comparison between modern bioactive bare metal stents and DES.

The elegant concept of seeding stents with antibodies targeted at CD 40 endothelial cell ligands is under clinical testing but will likely be a stillbirth.

References

1. Togni M, Windecker S, Meier B. Treatment of restenosis. *Curr Interv Cardiol Rep*. 2001;3:306–310.

2. Cutlip DE, Windecker S, Mehran R, *et al.* Clinical endpoints in coronary stent trials: a case for standardized definitions. *Circulation*. 2007;115:2344–2351.

3. Windecker S, Meier B. Late coronary stent thrombosis. *Circulation*. 2007;116:1952–1965.

4. Stone GW, Ellis SG, Colombo A, *et al.* Offsetting impact of thrombosis and restenosis on the occurrence of death and myocardial infarction after paclitaxel-eluting and bare metal stent implantation. *Circulation*. 2007;115:2842–2847.

5. Bavry AA, Kumbhani DJ, Helton TJ, Bhatt DL. Risk of thrombosis with the use of sirolimus-eluting stents for percutaneous coronary intervention (from registry and clinical trial data). *Am J Cardiol*. 2005;95:1469–1472.

6. Bavry AA, Kumbhani DJ, Helton TJ, Bhatt DL. What is the risk of stent thrombosis associated with the use of paclitaxel-eluting stents for percutaneous coronary intervention? A meta-analysis. *J Am Coll Cardiol*. 2005;45:941–946.

7. Wenaweser P, Morger C, Cook S, *et al.* Late and very late stent thrombosis in patients with drug-eluting stents. *J Am Coll Cardiol*. 2006(suppl):2902–2974.

8. Wenaweser P, Daemen J, Zwahlen M, *et al.* Incidence and correlates of drug-eluting stent thrombosis in routine clinical practice: 4-year results from a large 2-institutional cohort study. *J Am Coll Cardiol*. 2008;52:1134–1140.

9. Pfisterer M, Brunner-La Rocca HP, Buser PT, *et al.* Late clinical events after clopidogrel discontinuation may limit the benefit of drug-eluting stents: an observational study of drug-eluting versus bare-metal stents. *J Am Coll Cardiol*. 2006;48:2584–2591.

10. Daemen J, Wenaweser P, Tsuchida K, *et al.* Early and late coronary stent thrombosis of sirolimus-eluting and paclitaxel-eluting stents in routine clinical practice: data from a large two-institutional cohort study. *Lancet*. 2007;369:667–678.

11. Mauri L, Hsieh WH, Massaro JM, *et al.* Stent thrombosis in randomized clinical trials of drug-eluting stents. *N Engl J Med*. 2007;356:1020–1029.

12. Lagerqvist B, James SK, Stenestrand U, *et al.* Long-term outcomes with drug-eluting stents versus bare-metal stents in Sweden. *N Engl J Med*. 2007;356:1009–1019.

13. James S, Carlsson J, Lindbäck J, *et al.* Swedish Coronary Angiography and Angioplasty Registry (SCAAR) Group. Long-term outcomes with drug-eluting stents vs. bare-metal stents in Sweden: one additional year of follow-up. Presented at European Society of Cardiology Congress, September 2007, Vienna.

14. Abbott JD, Voss MR, Nakamura M, *et al.* Unrestricted use of drug-eluting stents compared with bare-metal stents in routine clinical practice: findings from the National Heart, Lung, and Blood Institute Dynamic Registry. *J Am Coll Cardiol*. 2007;50:2029–2036.

15. Marzocchi A, Saia F, Piovaccari G, *et al.* Long-term safety and efficacy of drug-eluting stents: two-year results of the REAL (REgistro AngiopLastiche dell'Emilia Romagna) multicenter registry. *Circulation*. 2007;115:3181–3188.

16. Applegate RJ, Sacrinty MT, Kutcher MA, *et al.* Comparison of drug-eluting versus bare metal stents on later frequency of acute myocardial infarction and death. *Am J Cardiol*. 2007;99:333–338.

17. Tu JV, Bowen J, Chiu M, *et al.* Effectiveness and safety of drug-eluting stents in Ontario. *N Engl J Med*. 2007;357:1393–402.

18. Mauri L. Long-term clinical outcomes following drug-eluting and bare metal stenting in Massachusetts. AHA special session, Orlando, November 4th, 2007.

19. Stone GW, Moses JW, Ellis SG, *et al.* Safety and efficacy of sirolimus- and paclitaxel-eluting coronary stents. *N Engl J Med*. 2007;356:998–1008.

20. Kastrati A, Mehilli J, Pache J, *et al.* Analysis of 14 trials comparing sirolimus-eluting stents with bare-metal stents. *N Engl J Med*. 2007;356:1030–1039.

21. Stettler C, Wandel S, Allemann S, *et al.* Outcomes associated with drug-eluting and bare-metal stents: a collaborative network meta-analysis. *Lancet*. 2007;370:937–948.

22. Joner M, Finn AV, Farb A, *et al.* Pathology of drug-eluting stents in humans: delayed healing and late thrombotic risk. *J Am Coll Cardiol*. 2006;48:193–202.

23. Cook S, Wenaweser P, Togni M, *et al.* Incomplete Stent apposition and very late stent thrombosis following drug eluting stent implantation. *Circulation*. 2007;115:2426–2434.

24. McFadden EP, Stabile E, Regar E, *et al.* Late thrombosis in drug-eluting coronary stents after discontinuation of antiplatelet therapy. *Lancet*. 2004;364:1519–1521.

25. Spaulding C, Henry P, Teiger E, *et al.* Sirolimus-eluting versus uncoated stents in acute myocardial infarction. *N Engl J Med*. 2006;355:1093–1104.

26. Laarman GJ, Suttorp MJ, Dirksen MT, *et al.* Paclitaxel-eluting versus uncoated stents in primary

percutaneous coronary intervention. *N Engl J Med*. 2006;355:1105–1113.

27. Valgimigli M, Percoco G, Malagutti P, *et al.* Tirofiban and sirolimus-eluting stent versus abciximab and bare-metal stent for acute myocardial infarction: a randomized trial. *JAMA*. 2005;293:2109–2117.

28. Costa RA, Lansky AJ, Abizaid A, *et al.* Angiographic results of the first human experience with the bi-olimus A9 drug-eluting stent for de novo coronary lesions. *Am J Cardiol*. 2006;98:443–446.

29. Windecker S, Serruys PW, Wandel S, *et al.* Biolimus-eluting stent with biodegradable polymer versus sirolimus-eluting stent with durable polymer for coronary revascularisation (LEADERS): a randomised non-inferiority trial. *Lancet*. 2008;372:1163–1173.

30. Fajadet J, Wijns W, Laarman GJ, *et al.* Random-ized, double-blind, multicenter study of the endeavor zotarolimus-eluting phosphorylcholine-encapsulated stent for treatment of native coronary artery lesions: clinical and angiographic results of the ENDEAVOR II trial. *Circulation*. 2006;114:798–806.

31. Kandzari DE, Leon MB, Popma JJ, *et al.* Com-parison of zotarolimus-eluting and sirolimus-eluting stents in patients with native coronary artery dis-ease: a randomized controlled trial. *J Am Coll Cardiol*. 2006;48:2440–2447.

32. Moses JW, Stone GW, Nikolsky E, *et al.* Drug-eluting stents in the treatment of intermediate lesions: pooled analysis from four randomized trials. *J Am Coll Cardiol*. 2006;47:2164–2171.

33. Serruys PW, Colombo A, Morice MC, *et al.* Arterial revascularisation therapies study part II - sirolimus-eluting stents for the treatment of patients with mul-tivessel de novocoronary artery lesions. *EuroInterven-tion*. 2005;1:147–156.

34. Serruys PW, Mohr FW, on behalf of the SYNTAX in-vestigators. The synergy between percutaneous coro-nary intervention with TAXUS and cardiac surgery: the SYNTAX study. *N Engl J Med*. 2009;359: in press.

35. Chieffo A, Morici N, Maisano F, *et al.* Percuta-neous treatment with drug-eluting stent implan-tation versus bypass surgery for unprotected left main stenosis: a single-center experience. *Circulation*. 2006;113:2542–2547.

36. Lee MS, Kapoor N, Jamal F, *et al.* Comparison of coro-nary artery bypass surgery with percutaneous coro-nary intervention with drug-eluting stents for unpro-tected left main coronary artery disease. *J Am Coll Car-diol*. 2006;47:864–870.

37. Sanmartín M, Baz JA, Claro R, *et al.* Compari-son of drug-eluting stents versus surgery for unpro-tected left main coronary artery disease. *Am J Cardiol*. 2007;100:970–973.

38. Vecchio S, Chechi T, Vittori G, *et al.* Outlook of drug-eluting stent implantation for unprotected left main disease: insights on long-term clinical predictors. *J In-vas Cardiol*. 2007;19:381–387.

39. Erglis A, Narbute I, Kumsars I, *et al.* A random-ized comparison of paclitaxel-eluting stents versus bare-metal stents for treatment of unprotected left main coronary artery stenosis. *J Am Coll Cardiol*. 2007;50:491–497.

40. Schrale RG, van Gaal W, Channon KM, *et al.* Long-term outcomes of percutaneous coronary interven-tion for unprotected left main coronary artery disease. *Int J Cardiol*. 2008;130:185–189.

41. Buszman PE, Kiesz SR, Bochenek A, *et al.* Acute and late outcomes of unprotected left main stenting in comparison with surgical revascularization. *J Am Coll Cardiol*. 2008;51:538–545.

42. Mosseri M, Miller H, Tamari I, *et al.* The titanium-NO stent: results of a multicentre registry. *EuroInterven-tion*. 2006;6:192–196.

43. Wenaweser P, Rey C, Eberli FR, *et al.* Stent throm-bosis following bare-metal stent implantation: suc-cess of emergency percutaneous coronary interven-tion and predictors of adverse outcome. *Eur Heart J*. 2005;26:1180–1187.

CHAPTER 3
Chronic Total Occlusion

David Rosenmann, David Meerkin and Yaron Almagor

Interventional Cardiology, Shaare Zedek Medical Center, Jerusalem, Israel

---

Chapter Overview

- Chronic total occlusion (CTO) remains a very challenging issue, with a prevalence of about 10% to 15% of cases treated in a routine interventional practice.
- Despite the debate in the literature, it appears that PCI to CTO results in improved morbidity and mortality.
- Technical and procedural success rates have been reported to be about 70% to 75%.
- The periprocedural complication rate is similar to that in non-CTO cases.
- Over recent years, multiple advances have been made in both technique and specialized devices to improve acute and long-term outcomes.

Percutaneous recanalization of chronically occluded coronary vessels remains a field laden with challenges, techniques, novel technologies, and most of all dilemmas. In spite of the breathtaking progress that continues to occur in the field of interventional cardiology, one of the unconquered territories remains the treatment of chronic total occlusions. The field has, however, not been neglected. Significant progress has been made with understanding of the pathophysiology of the condition, and as such a wealth of novel devices and techniques have been developed attempting to improve procedural success while reducing complications. The broad range of options reminds us, however, that there is a lack of a single solution with outstanding success.

The aim of this chapter is to review the current status of this clinical and angiographic challenge, with particular emphasis on approaches to maximize procedural success rates and most importantly optimize clinical outcomes.

Current Best Practice in Interventional Cardiology. Edited by B Meier. © 2010 Blackwell Publishing.

Definition

CTO of a coronary artery refers to the complete obstruction of a coronary artery. Antegrade flow may be completely interrupted, "a true total occlusion," or the occlusion may be "functional" with minimal contrast passage as represented by TIMI grade I flow [1].

Different authors have used variable criteria for the temporal definition of this condition, varying from 2 weeks to 3 or more months [2–4]. For obvious reasons, the age of the CTO is often indeterminate. In some patients, however, with careful history-taking, a clinical syndrome such as sudden change in angina pattern can be used to estimate the duration of the CTO.

Prevalence

In experienced catheterization laboratories, approximately 10% to 15% of patients undergoing angioplasty procedures are treated for a chronic total occlusion. In the National Cardiovascular Registry of the American College of Cardiology, PCI for CTO was attempted in 12% of 100,292 patients at 130 U.S. hospitals undergoing PCI from January 1998 through September 2000 [5]. A slightly higher incidence (15.6%) was reported in the NHLBI Dynamic Registry report in 1997 to 1998 [6].

The finding of a CTO following reperfusion therapy for acute myocardial infarction has also been reported. In patients treated with thrombolytic therapy, approximately 30% will have an angiographically proven total occlusion 3 to 6 months after the acute event [7]. For patients treated with primary PCI, however, only 5.2% had an occlusion at 6 to 7 months if a stent was deployed. This compared favorably with the 12.2% of occlusions noted when angioplasty alone was performed [8].

Pathologic Features

Understanding the pathologic processes taking place at the vessel occlusion site can provide important insights potentially allowing for a tailoring of approach depending upon specific lesion features such as type, length, and age. Srivasta and associates described the histologic correlates of CTO and the influence of occlusion duration on neovascular channel patterns and plaque composition. Cholesterol and foam cell-laden intimal plaque was more frequent in younger lesions, while fibrocalcific intimal plaque was more frequent in older CTO lesions [9]. In most cases, a chronic occlusion arises from arterial thrombotic occlusion with subsequent organization of the thrombus [10]. The eventual atherosclerotic plaque of CTOs consists of intracellular and extracellular lipids, smooth muscle cells, extracellular matrix, and calcium [11]. Interestingly angiographic total occlusions frequently correspond to less than complete occlusion by histologic criteria. Moreover, there is often very little relationship between the severity of the histopathologic lumen stenosis and either plaque composition or lesion age [1].

Another important feature of CTO is the extensive neovascularization that occurs in older lesions with more severe capillary density and angiogenesis. In CTOs older than 1 year, the number and size of capillaries in the intima have increased to a

similar or greater extent than those present in the adventita, where the formation of new capillaries is greatest [1]. It appears that as the lesion matures, the new capillary formation that occurs predominantly in the adventitia in lesions less than 1 year old becomes more pronounced in the intima, particularly in lesions greater than 1 year of age.

Clinical Presentation

One of the clinical challenges that chronic total occlusions present is the difficulty correlating their angiographic presence with a clinical syndrome. Although different patterns of angina have been reported in patients with CTOs, there are no exclusive patterns of angina that can be attributed to such findings. Nevertheless, many patients describe angina occurring at the onset of physical activities that improves during "warming up," possibly due to recruitment of collaterals. Other patients might complain of less specific symptoms such as shortness of breath or diminishing exercise tolerance. The spectrum of clinical syndromes is extremely broad, varying from severe limiting angina to a silent incidental angiographic finding. The decision to intervene will be very dependent upon the clinician's understanding regarding the correlation of the angiographic finding with the clinical scenario.

Rationale and Indications for Recanalization

Several benefits of CTO revascularization have been proposed to justify PCI in these patients. Relief of angina pectoris is certainly the most accepted. Other theoretical benefits of CTO revascularization have been proposed, including survival improvement, improved left ventricular function, reduced risk of ventricular arrhythmias, and improved tolerance during contralateral vessel occlusion.

Four retrospective studies have been published comparing survival in patients after successful PCI in CTO. All four studies demonstrated favorable results in the population that underwent successful

PCI. In a consecutive series of 2007 patients with CTO who underwent PCI between 1980 and 1999, Suero and colleagues reported technical success rates of 74.4% with procedural success in 69.9%. The group with successful procedures showed improvement over time without an increase in MACE. The in-hospital MACE for patients with successful PCI was 3.2%, compared with the patients with failed PCI, who showed a MACE of 5.4% ($p = 0.023$). There was no significant difference in cumulative 10-year survival of 71.2% of the study cohort group compared with a matched non-CTO cohort that had a survival of 71.4%. The most significant finding in this study was the improved better long-term survival of 10 years in the cohort of patients with successful PCI, 73.5% versus 65.0% in the group with failed PCI. By multivariate analysis, successful PCI to CTO was an independent predictor of survival (hazard ratio 0.7; $p < 0.0003$) [12].

A similar time-independent benefit of successful PCI was reported in the British Columbia Cardiac Registry. Among 1458 patients who underwent PCI for CTO, successful recanalization was associated with a 56% reduction of mortality over the 7 year follow-up period [13].

In a prospective multicenter observational study—Total Occlusion Angioplasty Study (TOAST-GISE)—that included 20 Italian hospitals, Olivari and colleagues reported a technical and a procedural success rate of 77.2% and 73.3%, respectively. At 12 months, patients with a successful procedure had a lower incidence of cardiac death or myocardial infarction (1.1% vs. 7.2%, $p = 0.005$), a reduced need for surgical revascularization (2.5% vs. 15.7%, $p < 0.00001$), and were more frequently free of angina (88.7% vs. 75%, $p = 0.008$) when compared with patients who had an unsuccessful procedure [14].

Finally, in the Percutaneous Coronary Intervention for Chronic Total Occlusions, a retrospective study that included 543 patients with a mean follow-up of 1.7 years, successful PCI was achieved in 69.4% of the cohort, and was associated with a significant reduction of mortality rate. Death for CTO success patients was 2.5% compared to 7.3% in CTO failure patients. The crude hazard ratio for

death with CTO failure was 3.92 (95% confidence interval, 1.56–10.07; $p = 0.004$) [15].

Left Ventricular Function after PCI

Several studies have shown significant improvements in left ventricular function in patients following successful CTO recanalization. Sirnes and associates showed improvement in left ventricular function in a population of 95 patients with CTO and angina or proven ischemia. Ejection fraction was measured on left ventriculogram performed during cardiac catheterization. The duration of CTO was relatively short (median duration, 4.3 months). Left ventricular ejection fraction increased from 0.62 ± 0.13 at baseline to 0.67 ± 0.11 at follow-up ($p < 0.001$) [16].

Recently MRI has been reported to predict left ventricular function, identifying ischemic and viable myocardium. In a study by Baks and colleagues, 47 patients underwent MRI at 16 ± 16 days before PCI for CTO with DES and 27 patients repeated MRI after the procedure. The mean vessel occlusion duration was 7 ± 5 months [17].

Mean end-systolic volume index decreased significantly, from 34 ± 13 mL/m^2 to 31 ± 13 mL/m^2 ($p = 0.02$), and mean end-diastolic volume index decreased significantly, from 84 ± 15 mL/m^2 to 79 ± 15 mL/m^2 ($p < 0.002$). Overall ejection fraction did not change significantly. The extent of the segments in the left ventricle that were dysfunctional but viable before PCI was related to improvement in end-systolic volume index (R = 0.46; $p = 0.01$) and ejection fraction (R = 0.49, $p = 0.01$) but not to the end-diastolic volume index (R = 0.10; $p = 0.53$). Segmental wall thickening improved significantly in segments with transmural extent of infarction of less than 25% and did not improve with transmural extent of infarction of more than 75%.

In contrast to CTO patients, the OAT study recently published should be mentioned [18]. This study included 2166 patients who had experienced a myocardial infarction due to occlusion of a coronary vessel. All included patients were stable and were randomized to receive optimal medical therapy alone or in conjunction with late reperfusion, with PCI performed 3 to 28 days after the acute episode.

After an average of 3 years follow-up, there was no difference between the PCI group and the medical group in the primary end point that included a composite of death, reinfarction, or heart failure. These results support the routine use of aggressive secondary prevention without revascularization. Although the results of this study may be not relevant to true CTO populations because these patients did not have a chronic lesion, the message of doing revascularization of an occluded vessel only if there is evidence of ischemia in that specific territory should be taken.

Patient Selection

CTOs represent about 10% to 15% of the total number of angioplasty procedures of catheter laboratory activity; this percentage depends obviously on the selection of cases. At selected referral centers it constitutes about 20% of all angioplasty procedures [19], whereas in most centers about 10% of PCIs are performed for CTO [20,21].

The decision to intervene on a CTO is based upon the same formula interventionalists use to tackle any lesion: how great are the chances of success that will lead to what degree of clinical benefit, with respect to the chances of failure and at what clinical risk. As such, the decision to attempt PCI in these patients depends on a variety of clinical and angiographic criteria. Personal operator experience plays a major role in the decision to tackle these lesions. PCI for a CTO is indicated when the following three conditions are all present: (1) The lesion is judged to be responsible for the patient's symptoms, (2) the territory of the occluded artery has viability, and (3) there is a moderate to high likelihood of success of the procedure (> 60%) with reasonably low risk of complication (myocardial infarction < 5% and death < 1%) [1].

In patients with CTO and multivessel disease, the decision to refer the patient for coronary bypass or to attempt PCI depends on similar criteria but the tendency to send for CABG is certainly higher, particularly in the presence of left main disease,

proximal occlusion of the left anterior descending coronary artery, triple-vessel disease, insulin-dependent diabetes, and multiple obstructions with low chance of success cases [1].

Complications

Complications of PCI in patients with CTO are not rare despite the fact that the procedure has been mistakenly considered by some physicians to be of lower risk than procedures in patients without an occluded vessel [1]. Periprocedural myocardial infarction has been reported to be about 1% to 2%, urgent CABG 1% to 2%, and death 1% (Table 3.1) [12,14].

One of the most common complications is dissection of the occluded vessel seen after probing of a subintimal channel. Hydrophilic wires used frequently in these cases have a propensity for subintimal rupture and vessel wall perforation, which may occasionally result in cardiac tamponade and other complications.

Other reported complications include guidewire fracture with or without entrapment and perforation [22].

In rare cases due to aggressive wiring and guide catheter techniques, treatment of CTOs can be complicated with dissection of left main or ostial right coronary arteries with proximal vessel occlusion, aortic root dissection, and perforation of the sinus of Valsalva [23].

The complex nature of these interventions, involving the application of multiple devices, wires, balloons, and alternative techniques, results in long radiation exposure times, large volumes of contrast material, and relatively expensive procedures [24].

The large volume of contrast injected in many CTO cases may result in a compromise of renal function. Several authors have reported increases in serum creatinine levels following PCI for complex and long procedures. Baumgart and associates reported on 25 consecutive patients (age 56 ± 10 years) with normal renal and cardiac function receiving > 500 mL of the nonionic dimeric contrast medium iodixanol during complex coronary interventions. Mean serum creatinine rose from

	CTO (n = 2007)	Non-CTO (n = 2007)	p Value
Death	27(1.3)	17 (0.8)	0.13
Q-wave MI	10 (0.5)	12 (0.6)	0.67
Non-Q-wave MI	38 (1.9)	48 (2.4)	0.27
Urgent CABG	15 (0.7)	22 (1.1)	0.25
Urgent Re-PCI	30 (1.5)	40 (2.0)	0.23
Any dissection	357 (17.8)	267 (13.3)	<0.001
CVA	1 (0.01)	3 (0.1)	0.63
Vascular	34 (1.7)	50 (2.5)	0.08
MACE	76 (3.8)	75 (3.7)	0.9

Table 3.1 In-Hospital Complications for CTO and Non-CTO Cohorts

Data listed as number of patients (percent of group).
CABG = coronary artery bypass grafting; CIO = chronic total coronary artery occlusion; CVA = cerebrovascular accident; MACE = major adverse coronary event: MI = myocardial infarction; Re-PCI = repeat percutaneous coronary intervention.

0.9 ± 0.2 mg/dL to 1.1 ± 0.2 mg/dL ($p < 0.05$) 2 days after coronary intervention [25].

Bell and coworkers reported on the increased radiation doses delivered during percutaneous treatment of CTOs. They compared radiation exposure associatied with the procedure in 90 consecutive patients undergoing PCI for CTO to 100 consecutive patients who underwent PCI for subtotal stenosis. Angioplasty was successful in 60% of the CTO group and in 94% of the other patients. They found that although there was no significant difference in cineangiographic time, a marked prolongation of fluoroscopic time was reported (Table 3.2) [24].

This prolonged fluoroscopic exposure, often performed in a single view, can result in high radiation doses to localized areas of skin, causing severe damage. Kawakami and coworkers reported on 3 patients who had undergone lengthy interventions for difficult and complex lesions. Following the pro-

Table 3.2 Prolongation of Fluoroscopic Time in CTO. Reproduced with permission from Bell MR, Berger PB, Menke KK, Holmes DR, Jr. Balloon angioplasty of chronic total coronary artery occlusions: what does it cost in radiation exposure, time, and materials? Cathet Cardiovasc Diagn 1992;25:10–15.

	CTO	non CTO	p
Fluoroscopy	34+/−17min	23+/−15min	0.0004
Cineangiography	1.5+/1.0min	1.6+/−0.6min	NS

cedures, they were found to have skin eruptions characterized by an atrophic rectangular plaque on the left upper back, presenting as mottled hyper- and hypopigmentation with reticulate telangiectasia. Histologically, the eruption demonstrated epidermal atrophy, hyalinized and irregularly stained collagen, and telangiectasia of superficial vessels in the dermis [26].

Outcome and Trends

In spite of technological advances and broadening operator experience, several studies have recently been published demonstrating that the treatment of CTOs remains challenging with suboptimal success rates [1]. The Mayo Clinic published a retrospective comparative analysis of patient outcomes for CTOs treated with PCI during eras of different treatment strategies (Table 3.3) [27]. This study evaluated the outcomes of 1262 patients who underwent PCI for a CTO over a 25-year period, dividing the study population into four groups according to the time of their intervention: PCI only, early stent era, BMS era, and DES era. They found acute procedural success rates of 51%, 72%, 73%, and 70%, respectively. In-hospital mortality improved comparing the four periods (2%, 1%, 0.4%, and 0%; $p = 0.009$) Emergency coronary artery bypass grafting also was significantly reduced (15%, 3%, 12%, and 0.7%; $p < 0,001$) In-hospital major adverse cardiac

Table 3.3 In-Hospital Outcomes

Variable	1979–1989, n = 169 (%)	1990–1996, n = 459 (%)	1997 to March 2003, n = 482 (%)	April 2003 to July 2005, n = 152 (%)	p Value
Death	4 (2.4)	6 (1.3)	2 (0.4)	0 (0)	0.009
Any myocardial infarction	17 (10)	41 (9)	39 (8)	7 (5)	0.081
Q-wave myocardial infarction	4 (2.4)	9 (2.0)	12 (2.5)	5 (3.3)	0.48
CABS	26 (15)	16 (3)	8 (1.7)	1 (0.7)	<0.001
MACE	13 (8)	21 (6)	16 (3.3)	6 (3.9)	0.052

The p values are test for trend across time groups.
CABG = coronary artery bypass grafting: MACE = major adverse cardiac event.

events—defined as in-hospital death, Q-wave myocardial infarction, urgent or emergent CABG during the index hospitalization, and cerebrovascular accident—also showed borderline reduction (8%, 5%, 3%, and 4%; $p = 0.052$). Interestingly, at multivariate analysis technical failure was not an independent predictor of mortality (HR 1.16, with 95% confidence interval 0.9–1.5; $p = 0.25$).

It appears that the introduction of DES significantly reduced the need for target vessel revascularization. The authors comment about a slightly greater survival at 6 years after PCI taking all four eras together due to a potential benefit of restoring coronary patency and myocardial perfusion on ventricular function. Alternatively, patients with a failed procedure may reflect more severe disease including fibrosis and calcification of vessels. From this registry it appears that the introduction of stents contributed significantly to the impressive advances we have seen in interventional cardiology. However, the introduction of other new devices has had a less pronounced impact on procedural success rates.

Recent Developments: Retrograde Approach

In spite of continued improvements in PCI equipment and techniques for CTO, including increasing operator experience, there remains an acute failure rate of approximately 30% to 40%. This has motivated interventional cardiologists to broaden their approach. As the principal cause for failure is the inability to adequately cross the lesion with a wire, most efforts have been invested in crossing the occlusion. Based on the presumption that the most resistant portion of the occlusion to cross is the proximal cap, several reports have been recently published describing a technique where the occlusion is approached and crossed from the distal vessel to its proximal portion (Figs. 3.1 to 3.3) [28–30]. Access to the distal vessel is usually attained via contralateral collateral vessels; however, a bypass graft can also be used. Once wire position has been established, a wire is passed in the antegrade fashion alongside the initial wire, allowing for standard angioplasty techniques to be used. Additional mechanisms have also been postulated to explain the success of this approach. These include the possibility that following failed attempts to cross the lesion antegrade may induce intimal dissection and subsequent vessel distortion. Alternatively, the entry point into the anterograde channel may be incorrect, without the ability to establish entrance back into the vessel lumen [29]. Indications for the use of this technique include failed antegrade approach or an inability to determine the site of the ostium of the occluded vessel. We have also used an extension of this technique in an instance where a protruding stent prevented catheter cannulation to a right coronary artery. Calling this the one-wire retrograde technique, following wire passage from the LAD through a septal to the RCA, the lesion was crossed and the wire passed into the aorta. Here it was snared and externalized through a right guiding catheter. This wire was then used for angioplasty and stenting of the vessel through the right guide. Following completion of the procedure,

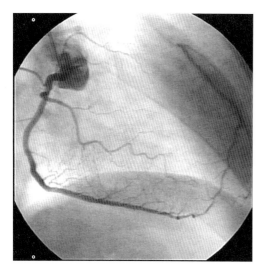

Figure 3.1 Angiography showing filling of RCA and retrograde filling of LAD through collaterals.

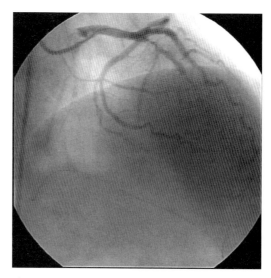

Figure 3.2 Anterograde filling of occluded LAD. Wire crossing from RCA through collaterals into LAD and entering into ascending aorta.

the wire was removed back through the septals and LAD.

The most comprehensive report from Saito and associates summarizes the authors' experience in 45 patients from January 2006 to January 2007. The procedures were performed at different medical institutions, following the failure of the antegrade approach. The septal branch was the route used in 93% of cases.

The retrograde wire was successfully passed distal to the lesion in 37 patients (82%), with final PCI success achieved in 31 patients (69%). No major complications were observed. Six patients had dissection of the target artery or minor perforation and/or dissection of a septal artery due to the guidewire tip [29].

The retrograde approach seems to offer an alternative option with reasonably high success rates following failure of the more standard approaches.

Long-Term Prognosis: Restenosis Rate and Late Patency

Is DES indicated after successful CTO recanalization? The role of DES in patients undergoing PCI for CTO has not yet been fully elucidated; however, several small studies without control groups have

been published in this subgroup of lesions. These have demonstrated that when compared to historical controls with BMS, DES-treated patients have less restenosis and less MACE.

Migliorini and associates studied 92 of a total of 104 patients with CTO who underwent successful

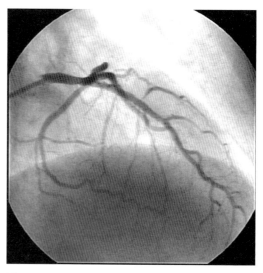

Figure 3.3 Final result showing patent LAD after stent deployment.

PCI with either sirolimus-eluting or placlitaxel-eluting stents [31]. A case-matched control group of 26 patients were selected from a prospectively acquired PCI database.

There was no difference in baseline clinical or angiographic characteristics. The majority of CTOs were located in the right coronary artery. The mean lesion length was 39 ± 22 mm in the DES group and 40 ± 19 mm in the BMS group ($p = 0.212$).

There was no significant difference in the DES group regarding stent distribution; 47 patients (57 CTO lesions) received placlitaxel-eluting stents and 45 patients (47 CTO lesions) received serolimus-eluting stents. There were no periprocedural MACE. There was a lower incidence of target vessel revascularization in the DES group (7.6 % vs. 23%, $p = 0.027$), and therefore lower incidence of MACE (9.8% vs. 23 %, $p = 0.072$) in the same group. There was an 80% angiographic follow-up in the DES group and 81% in the BMS group, with a significantly reduced restenosis rate of 19% in the DES group compared to 45% in the BMS group. No difference was noted between the different DES stents.

The only two predictors of angiographic restenosis in the DES group were stent length and a reference vessel diameter of less than 2.5 mm. The authors concluded that use of DES stent CTO as compared with BMS is associated with an improved outcome as determined by less restenosis and target vessel revascularization.

The SICTO (Sirolimus-Eluting Stent in Chronic Total Occlusion) study [32] was a multicenter, prospective, nonrandomized study performed to assess feasibility and restenosis and reocclusion rates of coronary stenting with a sirolimus-eluting stent in patients with CTO. All patients were planned to undergo repeat angiography at 6 months as well as IVUS examination prior to and following stent deployment as well as at 6-month follow-up.

Primary end point was angiographic in-stent late loss at 6-month follow-up determined by quantitative coronary angiography. Five medical centers in Europe and Israel participated in the study. Secondary end points were major adverse cardiac advents, in-stent and in-lesion minimum lumen diameter, angiographic binary restenosis after 6 months, in-stent volume of restenosis determined by IVUS follow-up at 6 months, and target vessel revascularization at 6 months postprocedure.

All patients were treated with sirolimus-eluting stents and only stent lengths of 8 to 18 mm were available.

A total of 25 patients participated in the study. All had CTO of native coronary arteries older than 3 months.

Patients included in the TOSCA study, where CTOs were treated with BMS, were used as the control group for analysis of the 6-month in-stent late loss. There was a significant reduction of in-stent late loss compared with the TOSCA patients.

Six-month angiographic results showed no significant change in minimum luminal diameter from postprocedure to late follow-up. The in-stent binary restenosis rate was 0%, but the in-lesion binary restenosis rate was 8%, due to a dissection distal to the stent in one patient and large gap between two stents in another patient.

Only 18 patients pre-procedure, 13 patients postprocedure, and 17 patients at late follow-up underwent IVUS studies. No significant change in MLD postprocedure and at 6 months follow-up were noted.

The importance of the study is the use of IVUS to validate the angiographic data demonstrating significant inhibition of in-stent neointima formation.

Another study using paclitaxel-eluting stents was designed to evaluate the safety and effectiveness in patients with CTO with lesions of different lengths and morphologies. Additionally, whether the lesion in CTO should be covered with DES alone or with a combination of BMS and DES was assessed [33].

The patients were enrolled from February 2003 until August 2004. The study group comprised 82 patients and was compared to historically matched controls with BMS. The study group comprised patients treated with Taxus stents and included a subgroup of 21 patients, where in addition to the Taxus stent one or more BMSs were implanted for distal dissections or residual narrowings. This was considered the hybrid control group.

The clinical characteristics were similar for both groups and all stents were successfully implanted. There was no difference in in-hospital MACE. Angiographic follow-up demonstrated significantly lower-diameter stenosis in the Taxus group and in the Taxus hybrid group compared with controls. The incidence of late reocclusion in the Taxus group was 1.7% as compared to 21.7% in the BMS group ($p < 0.001$), and the target vessel failure was significantly lower at 1.7% compared to 55% in the BMS group ($p < 0.001$). The MACE rate at 6 months was 13.3% in the Taxus group versus 56.7% in the BMS group ($p < 0.001$). The MACE rate in the hybrid group was almost triple that of the Taxus group.

A recently published study compared sirolimus- and paclitaxel-eluting stents for the treatment of CTO [34]. The study included 136 patients who underwent PCI for CTO from March 2003 to December 2004. The procedural success rate was 98.1% in the SES group and 100% in the PES group. The restenosis rate after 6 months angiographic follow-up was significantly higher in the PES group (28.6% vs. 9.4%; $p = 0.020$). MACE-free survival rate was significantly higher in the SES group (95.8% vs. 85.8%; $p = 0.049$). These results indicate improved angiographic and clinical outcomes in CTO patients treated with SES when compared with PES.

PCI of CTO in SVG

PCI to occluded vein grafts is one of the most challenging procedures in interventional cardiology. In view of the completely different pathology in vein grafts with soft and friable tissue associated with large and bulky thrombi compared with atherosclerotic disease in native vessels, the optimal revascularization treatment still remains debatable.

Due to advances in technical skills and introduction of new devices such as distal protection devices, some centers have reached a higher technical success rate. The use of antiplatelet drugs associated with DES led to improved postprocedural outcomes and lower restenosis rates. Which revascularization strategy should be recommended to patients with CTO of SVG? Is it advisable to try to open the SVG occlusions or should we attempt to treat the native bypassed arteries?

Meliga and associates, in a retrospective study, tried to elucidate the question. All patients who underwent successful PCI for CTO and had previous CABG with SVG at their center were analyzed. Of this group 13 patients underwent PCI on the occluded graft and 11 patients underwent PCI of the native vessel that supplied the same territory. The median time from bypass surgery was 10 years. Distal embolic protection was used in 38.4% of cases. The patients with PCI to SVGs more frequently presented with acute coronary syndrome and triple-vessel disease, and received a slightly higher number of stents and with a larger reference vessel diameter. There was no difference in procedural and in-hospital outcomes including MACE. At 3-year follow-up, there was no difference in death rates, with 7.6% in the SVG group versus 9% in the native vessel group. No significant differences were noted with regard to MI (0 in both groups), re-CABG (0 in both groups), and MACE (2 patients [15.3 %] in the SVG group and 2 patients [18.1%] in the native group) [35].

This study, although retrospective, demonstrates that in patients with occluded SVGs, reopening of the graft or of the native vessel is feasible and that DES is a safe option that carries a good long-term outcome.

New Devices for CTO Revascularization

Several devices have been developed in the last years. Some of them are in routine use but others are still under investigation [36].

Tornus
The Tornus specialty catheter, with its threaded stainless steel construction, enables the exchange and support required for treating chronically stenosed lesions. After a wire crosses the CTO and a balloon does not cross it, the Tornus device is advanced by counterclockwise rotations encroaching in the lesion. In some cases it can also be "screwed in" to a CTO to enable good backup and facilitate crossing of the guidewire. The Tornus can also

make a smooth channel, allowing for passage of low-profile balloon.

Safecross

Safecross uses radiofrequency energy to facilitate lesion crossing. It has high resolution and precise control of RF energy released at the distal tip of the wire. It uses optical coherence reflectometry, using light with very high resolution to determine morphology within the vessel, analogous to sound in ultrasound systems. It still has several limitations, in particular that it is not very steerable; therefore it is used predominantly to break through the fibrous cap.

Laser

The laser technique has several limitations and its future is uncertain. Directability of the device is still a main concern, particularly as it relies on imprecise steering of the wire. The wire is also easily deflected by tough material within the vessel. Because the laser ablates only in the forward direction, it becomes more difficult to manipulate the wire through the laser-created channel.

Frontrunner

The Frontrunner device is designed to create intra-luminal blunt microdissection to create a channel through the occlusion to facilitate wire placement and enable penetration of the fibrous cap. It has jaws on the distal end of the catheter designed to separate tissue planes within the CTO. Although the device was designed for peripheral vessels, it has been used in two pilot trials with reasonable results, achieving recanalization in 43% to 77% of patients [37,38].

Vibration and Ultrasound: Crosser Catheter

The Crosser catheter delivers vibrational energy through a nitinol-core wire catheter with stainless steel tip to power through lesions. The European clinical experience reports a success rate of 67% in previously guidewire-failed CTOs (MACE rate 2.8%). Two other studies in the United States, the Factor and the Patriot studies, reported a success rate of 61% and 78%, respectively, with low MACE rate and no clinical perforations.

Other Recently Developed Devices Not in Clinical Use: Biological Approach

The main extracellular component of a plaque is collagen. Investigators have induced collagen degradation with metalloproteinases in animal models (rabbits), infusing collagenase through a wire port and allowing diffusion through the occlusion. When attempting again 72 hours later, they succeeded in crossing the lesion in many other cases (twofold increase).

Technical Considerations

Before approaching treatment of CTO it is crucial to obtain a proper and diagnostic angiography and document the length of the lesion and the presence of collaterals. It is essential to document and evaluate the collaterals distal to the lesion in order to assess the length of the occluded segment and the location of the run-off. The lesion should never be crossed without knowing the direction of the vessel. It is therefore recommended to document the presence and direction of the collaterals by performing a contralateral injection via a diagnostic catheter introduced through a radial approach or through a contralateral groin if necessary.

Another important point is the selection of the guiding catheter, which has to provide enough support to enable the crossing of the lesion with a balloon or with a stent.

In the left coronary artery, one of the most used guiding catheters is the extra back-up and in the right coronary artery the Amplatz left or right catheter. Several technique have been described in order to improve wire support [39,40].

Anchor Wire Technique

In the presence of a reasonably sized side branch proximal to the CTO (eg, first diagonal branch for mid-LAD occlusion), a stiff support wire can be introduced into the diagonal branch to help to fix the catheter in a stable position.

Anchor Balloon Technique

In the anchor balloon technique the operator introduces a wire with a balloon into a side branch proximal to the CTO. After inflating the balloon with low pressure, the guiding catheter can be anchored deeply over the balloon catheter shaft.

Parallel Wire Technique

In some cases a wire that has been advanced into a wrong plane (subintima) can be used as a marker while a second wire is used in order to enter the correct plane.

One of the modifications of this technique is the "seesaw wiring method," where the parallel wires are used using two support catheters (over the wire balloon or transit catheter (Cordis, Johnson & Johnson). This enables alternate use of the wires, alternating their roles as marking wire and advancing wire through the CTO.

Reentry: The Star Technique

The star technique, described by Colombo and coworkers, uses the "re-entry" subintimal tracking approach. As in peripheral artery disease, a hydrophilic wire with a J-configuration is advanced and pushed through the intimal dissection plane. Distal to the CTO the J tip is directed towards the true lumen in an attempt to reenter the true lumen [40]. Obviously the procedure involves a high risk of perforation but in several cases it succeeded to recanalize the CTO.

Which Guidewire Should Be Used?

Several types of guidewires have been developed in the recent years with different degrees of stiffness and with or without hydrophilic coating [39]. The two group of wires use in CTO are polymer-coated and coil wires.

The polymer-coated wires have hydrophilic coating that lowers friction, which helps to handle the wire in the vessel lumen.

The coil wires have good torquability and allow very good pushability. Both wires have a higher risk of perforations and dissection. These wires should therefore be used after trying conventional wires and preferably by experienced operators.

The most commonly used tapered-tip wires are Confienza 0.014-0.009" and Crossit 0.014-0.010". There are also stiffer coil wires such as Crossit 300-400 and Miracle 9, 12 g.

As a general rule the operator should always start with a soft tip wire and change to stiffer wires if necessary.

Over-the-Wire Support System

An over-the-wire support system may be very helpful in many cases in order to facilitate wire exchange, improve the torque control of the guidewire, and reduce also the friction between the guidewire and the vessel wall. For that purpose it is possible to use a small-diameter balloon (1.5–2 mm) or infusion catheters such as Transit (Cordis, USA) or Excelsior (Boston Scientific).

Future Trends

The introduction of new guidewires in the last few years, the development of new devices and techniques, and improving operator experience all enable more and more difficult patients to be tackled with improving results. More studies are required to evaluate results in different groups and indications for PCI in CTO.

References

1. Stone GW, Kandzari DE, Mehran R, *et al.* Percutaneous recanalization of chronically occluded coronary arteries: a consensus document: part I. *Circulation.* 2005;112:2364–2372.
2. Werner GS, Emig U, Mutschke O, Schwarz G, Bahrmann P, Figulla HR. Regression of collateral function after recanalization of chronic total coronary occlusions: a serial assessment by intracoronary pressure and Doppler recordings. *Circulation.* 2003;108:2877–2882.
3. Tamai H, Berger PB, Tsuchikane E, *et al.* Frequency and time course of reocclusion and restenosis in coronary artery occlusions after balloon angioplasty versus Wiktor stent implantation: results from the Mayo-Japan Investigation for Chronic Total Occlusion (MAJIC) trial. *Am Heart J.* 2004;147:E9.

4. Zidar FJ, Kaplan BM, O'Neill WW, *et al.* Prospective, randomized trial of prolonged intracoronary urokinase infusion for chronic total occlusions in native coronary arteries. *J Am Coll Cardiol.* 1996;27:1406–1412.

5. Anderson HV, Shaw RE, Brindis RG, *et al.* A contemporary overview of percutaneous coronary interventions. The American College of Cardiology-National Cardiovascular Data Registry (ACC-NCDR). *J Am Coll Cardiol.* 2002;39:1096–1103.

6. Williams DO, Holubkov R, Yeh W, *et al.* Percutaneous coronary intervention in the current era compared with 1985-1986: the National Heart, Lung, and Blood Institute Registries. *Circulation.* 2000;102: p2945–2951.

7. He ZX, Mahmarian JJ, Verani MS. Myocardial perfusion in patients with total occlusion of a single coronary artery with and without collateral circulation. *J Nucl Cardiol.* 2001;8:452–457.

8. Stone GW, Grines CL, Cox DA, *et al.* Comparison of angioplasty with stenting, with or without abciximab, in acute myocardial infarction. *N Engl J Med.* 2002;346:957–966.

9. Srivatsa SS, Edwards WD, Boos CM, *et al.* Histologic correlates of angiographic chronic total coronary artery occlusions: influence of occlusion duration on neovascular channel patterns and intimal plaque composition. *J Am Coll Cardiol.* 1997;29:955–963.

10. Katsuragawa M, Fujiwara H, Miyamae M, Sasayama S. Histologic studies in percutaneous transluminal coronary angioplasty for chronic total occlusion: comparison of tapering and abrupt types of occlusion and short and long occluded segments. *J Am Coll Cardiol.* 1993;21:604–611.

11. Meier B. Chronic total occlusion. In: Topol EJ. *Textbook of Interventional Cardiology*. 2nd ed. Philadelphia: Saunders; 1994:318–338.

12. Suero JA, Marso SP, Jones PG, *et al.* Procedural outcomes and long-term survival among patients undergoing percutaneous coronary intervention of a chronic total occlusion in native coronary arteries: a 20-year experience. *J Am Coll Cardiol.* 2001;38:409–414.

13. Ramanathan K, Gao M, Nogareda G, *et al.* Successful percutaneous recanalization of a non-acute occluded coronary artery predicts clinical outcomes and survival. *Circulation.* 2001;104:415.

14. Olivari Z, Rubartelli P, Piscione F, *et al.* Immediate results and one-year clinical outcome after percutaneous coronary interventions in chronic total occlusions: data from a multicenter, prospective, observational study (TOAST-GISE). *J Am Coll Cardiol.* 2003;41:1672–1678.

15. Aziz S, Stables RH, Grayson AD, Perry RA, Ramsdale DR. Percutaneous coronary intervention for chronic total occlusions: improved survival for patients with successful revascularization compared to a failed procedure. *Catheter Cardiovasc Interv.* 2007;70:15–20.

16. Sirnes PA, Myreng Y, Molstad P, Bonarjee V, Golf S. Improvement in left ventricular ejection fraction and wall motion after successful recanalization of chronic coronary occlusions. *Eur Heart J.* 1998;19: 273–281.

17. Baks T, van Geuns RJ, *et al.* Prediction of left ventricular function after drug-eluting stent implantation for chronic total coronary occlusions. *J Am Coll Cardiol.* 2006;47:721–725.

18. Hochman JS, Lamas GA, Buller CE, *et al.* Coronary intervention for persistent occlusion after myocardial infarction. *N Engl J Med.* 2006;355:2395–2407.

19. Delacretaz E, Meier B. Therapeutic strategy with total coronary artery occlusions. *Am J Cardiol.* 1997;79:185–187.

20. Cohen HA, Williams DO, Holmes DR Jr., *et al.* Impact of age on procedural and 1-year outcome in percutaneous transluminal coronary angioplasty: a report from the NHLBI Dynamic Registry. *Am Heart J.* 146:513–519.

21. Srinivas VS, Brooks MM, Detre KM, *et al.* Contemporary percutaneous coronary intervention versus balloon angioplasty for multivessel coronary artery disease: a comparison of the National Heart, Lung and Blood Institute Dynamic Registry and the Bypass Angioplasty Revascularization Investigation (BARI) study. *Circulation.* 2002;106:1627–1633.

22. Safian RD, McCabe CH, Sipperly ME, McKay RG, Baim DS. Initial success and long-term follow-up of percutaneous transluminal coronary angioplasty in chronic total occlusions versus conventional stenoses. *Am J Cardiol.* 1988;61:23G–28G.

23. Mauser M, Ennker J, Fleischmann D. Dissection of the sinus valsalvae aortae as a complication of coronary angioplasty. *Z Kardiol.* 1999;88:1023–1027.

24. Bell MR, Berger PB, Menke KK, Holmes DR Jr. Balloon angioplasty of chronic total coronary artery occlusions: what does it cost in radiation exposure, time, and materials? *Cathet Cardiovasc Diagn.* 1992;25:10–15.

25. Kahn JK, Rutherford BD, McConahay DR, *et al.* High-dose contrast agent administration during complex coronary angioplasty. *Am Heart J.* 1990;120:533–536.

26. Kawakami T, Saito R, Miyazaki S. Chronic radiodermatitis following repeated percutaneous

transluminal coronary angioplasty. *Br J Dermatol.* 1999;141:150–153.

27. Prasad A, Rihal CS, Lennon RJ, Wiste HJ, Singh M, Holmes DR Jr. Trends in outcomes after percutaneous coronary intervention for chronic total occlusions: a 25-year experience from the Mayo Clinic. *J Am Coll Cardiol.* 2007;49:1611–1618.

28. Rosenmann D, Meerkin D, Almagor Y. Retrograde dilatation of chronic total occlusions via collateral vessel in three patients. *Catheter Cardiovasc Interv. 2006;* 67:250–253.

29. Saito S. Different strategies of retrograde approach in coronary angioplasty for chronic total occlusion. *Catheter Cardiovasc Interv.* 2008;71:8–19.

30. Ozawa N. A new understanding of chronic total occlusion from a novel PCI technique that involves a retrograde approach to the right coronary artery via a septal branch and passing of the guidewire to a guiding catheter on the other side of the lesion. *Catheter Cardiovasc Interv.* 2006;68:907–913.

31. Migliorini A, Moschi G, Vergara R, Parodi G, Carrabba N, Antoniucci D. Drug-eluting stent-supported percutaneous coronary intervention for chronic total coronary occlusion. *Catheter Cardiovasc Interv.* 2006;67:344–348.

32. Lotan C, Almagor Y, Kuiper K, Suttorp MJ, Wijns W. Sirolimus-eluting stent in chronic total occlusion: the SICTO study. *J Interv Cardiol.* 2006;19:307–312.

33. Werner GS, Schwarz G, Prochnau D, *et al.* Paclitaxel-eluting stents for the treatment of chronic total coronary occlusions: a strategy of extensive lesion coverage with drug-eluting stents. *Catheter Cardiovasc Interv.* 2006;67:1–9.

34. Jang JS, Hong MK, Lee CW, *et al.* Comparison between sirolimus- and Paclitaxel-eluting stents for the treatment of chronic total occlusions. *J Invasive Cardiol.* 2006;18:205–208.

35. Meliga E, Garcia-Garcia HM, Kukreja N, *et al.* Chronic total occlusion treatment in post-CABG patients: saphenous vein graft versus native vessel recanalization-long-term follow-up in the drug-eluting stent era. *Catheter Cardiovasc Interv.* 2007;70:21–25.

36. Harrington M. New devices for CTO revascularization. *J Interv Cardiol.* 2007;20:402–405.

37. Loli A, Liu R, Pershad A. Immediate- and short-term outcome following recanalization of long chronic total occlusions (> 50 mm) of native coronary arteries with the Frontrunner catheter. *J Invasive Cardiol.* 2006;18:283–285.

38. Orlic D, Stankovic G, Sangiorgi G, *et al.* Preliminary experience with the Frontrunner coronary catheter: novel device dedicated to mechanical revascularization of chronic total occlusions. *Catheter Cardiovasc Interv.* 2005;64:146–152.

39. Weisz G, Moses JW. New percutaneous approaches for chronic total occlusion of coronary arteries. *Expert Rev Cardiovasc Ther.* 2007;5:231–241.

40. Colombo A, Mikhail GW, Michev I, *et al.* Treating chronic total occlusions using subintimal tracking and reentry: the STAR technique. *Catheter Cardiovasc Interv.* 2005;64:407–411.

CHAPTER 4

Nonrevascularization Therapy

Jean-Paul Schmid

Cardiology, Swiss Cardiovascular Center Bern, University Hospital Bern, Bern, Switzerland

---

Chapter Overview

- The volume of patients with chronic refractory angina pectoris without option for revascularization is estimated to be between 2.5% and 5% of coronary angiography procedures.
- Alternative nonrevascularization strategies in the treatment of refractory angina pectoris can be categorized into approaches acting on strategies to stimulate neovascularization, neural transmission of pain sensation, or redistribution of blood flow.
- Low-energy shock-wave therapy induces neovascularization by the up-regulation of angiogenic markers, including vessel endothelial growth factor (VEGF), endothelial nitric oxide synthase (eNOS) expression, and endothelial cell proliferation.
- Proved clinical effects of myocardial shock-wave therapy are a decrease in symptoms, improved myocardial perfusion, and a positive remodelling after acute myocardial infarction.
- Spinal cord stimulation is the most effective adjunct therapy of nervous system modulation, exerting beneficial effects on the severity of anginal complaints and the perceived quality of life.
- The percutaneous transvenous implantation of a "coronary sinus reducer" in patients with refractory angina was found to be safe and feasible. Its clinical applicability, however, remains to be shown.

Despite increasing number of coronary interventions over recent years, there is still a considerable number of patients suffering from chronic refractory angina pectoris. The volume of no-option patients is estimated to be between 2.5% and 5% of coronary angiography procedures [1,2]. This group of patients includes those with angina despite optimal medical therapy, those who may not have been offered percutaneous coronary intervention (PCI) or coronary artery bypass surgery (CABG) because of severe diffuse coronary artery disease (CAD), and those who continue to experience severe angina after CABG, PCI, or both.

A considerable number of therapeutic strategies have been investigated to treat severe chronic angina, approaching the problem from different pathophysiologic angles. The different interventions can be categorized into approaches acting on strategies to stimulate neovascularization, neural transmission of pain sensation, or redistribution of blood flow. In this chapter new developments in each of these categories are presented.

Shock-Wave Therapy

High-energy extracorporeal shock-wave therapy has been used to fragmentize kidney stones for over 30 years. A shock wave (SW) is a longitudinal acoustic wave, emitted as a single pressure pulse with a short needle-like positive spike < 1 µs in duration and up to 100 MPa in amplitude, followed by a tensile part of several microseconds with lower

Current Best Practice in Interventional Cardiology. Edited by B Meier. © 2010 Blackwell Publishing.

amplitude. SW are known to exert the "cavitation effect," a micrometer-sized violent collapse of bubbles inside and outside the cells [3], and have recently been demonstrated to induce localized stress on cell membranes that resembles shear stress [4].

Different distinct vascular effects of low-energy SW therapy have been described in various experimental settings. Wang and associates [5] were the first to show SW-induced neovascularization in a tendon–bone junction of a rabbit model, confirmed by the presence of angiogenic markers, including vessel endothelial growth factor (VEGF), endothelial nitric oxide synthase (eNOS) expression, and endothelial cell proliferation. These data were confirmed by Gutersohn and associates [6], who showed that SW up-regulate vascular endothelial growth factor m-RNA in human umbilical vascular endothelial cells. Furthermore, non-enzymatic NO production by SW treatment of an L-arginine–containing solution has been reported by Gotte and colleagues [7].

If SW-induced angiogenesis could be reproduced in vivo, it would provide a unique opportunity to develop a new angiogenic therapy that would not require invasive procedures such as open-chest surgery or catheter intervention. In recent years, several studies have now evaluated the effect of cardiac SW therapy in animal models and humans.

Shock-Wave Therapy in a Model of Chronic Ischemia

Nishida and associates [8] were the first to report about a myocardial application of SW. In a porcine model of chronic myocardial ischemia, they evaluated the effect of SW in ischemia-induced myocardial dysfunction. Domestic pigs were anesthetized for implantation of an ameroid constrictor around the circumflex coronary artery (LCx) to gradually induce a total occlusion of the artery in 4 weeks without causing myocardial infarction. SW therapy was applied at an energy of 0.09 mJ/mm^2 to 9 spots in the ischemic region (200 shots/spot) with the guidance of an echocardiogram equipped within a specially designed SW generator (Storz Medical AG; Fig. 4.1). The SW treatment was performed under anesthesia (n = 8) 4 weeks after the implantation of an ameroid constrictor, 3 times within 1 week for 4 weeks, whereas animals in the control group (n = 8) received the same anesthesia procedures but without SW treatment.

Four weeks after ameroid implantation, coronary angiography demonstrated a total occlusion of the LCx, which was perfused via collateral vessels with severe delay in both, the control and the SW group. At 8 weeks after ameroid implantation (4 weeks after SW therapy), the SW group, but not the control group, had a marked development of coronary collateral vessels in the ischemic LCx region, an increased Rentrop score, and an increased number of visible coronary arteries in the region. Similarly, at 4 weeks, ventriculography demonstrated an impaired left ventricular ejection fraction in both groups, whereas at 8 weeks, left ventricular ejection fraction was normalized in the SW group but remained impaired in the control group.

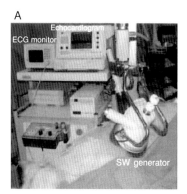

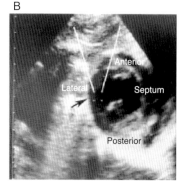

Figure 4.1 Extracorporeal cardiac shock-wave (SW) therapy in a pig (Reproduced with permission from [8]). **A.** The machine is equipped with a SW generator and in-line echocardiography. The SW generator is attached to the chest wall when used. **B.** The SW pulse is easily focused on the ischemic myocardium under the guidance of echocardiography (*black arrow*).

Myocardial Shock-Wave Therapy in Humans

The first report about myocardial shock-wave therapy in humans was published by Fukomoto and coworkers [9]. They applied SW in patients with severe CAD in order to test their effect on myocardial ischemia. Selected patients had stable chronic angina pectoris with evidence of myocardial ischemia despite adequate medication but without indication for PCI or CABG because of diffuse distal coronary artery narrowing. Nine patients with severe CAD were enrolled for cardiac SW therapy and followed for 1 year.

Patients were treated three times a week with 200 shots/spot at 0.09 mJ/mm^2 for a total of 20 to 40 spots. Thereafter patients were controlled at 1, 3, 6, and 12 months. When it was seen that additional improvement could be expected with further SW therapy on the basis of the results at 1 and 3 months, the treatment was repeated up to three series.

Cardiac SW therapy significantly improved symptoms as evaluated by the Canadian Cardiovascular Society (CCS) class score and the use of nitroglycerin, and tended to do so for 6-minute walking distance and treadmill test duration. Importantly, the SW therapy improved myocardial perfusion as evaluated by dipyridamole stress thallium scintigraphy only in the ischemic myocardium where SW was applied. Indeed, when the anteroseptal area was treated with SW, myocardial perfusion was improved only in the treated area, and when subsequently the lateral area was treated, myocardial perfusion was improved only in that area. The anti-ischemic effects of SW therapy were noted as early as 3 months after the therapy and persisted for 12 months. These clinical benefits of SW in patients with chronic refractory angina pectoris were subsequently confirmed by Khattab and colleagues [10].

Myocardial Shock-Wave Therapy and Left Ventricular Remodelling

An important further step in the evaluation of SW therapy on the induction of angiogenesis and improved myocardial perfusion and function was made by Uwatoku and associates [11]. They examined the impact of SW therapy on left ventricular

(LV) remodeling in the border zone of infarcted myocardium and, if it occurred, the appropriate timing for SW therapy after acute myocardial infarction (AMI).

In a total of 20 domestic male pigs, the proximal segment of the LCx was ligated and stripped to create AMI. Coronary angiography was performed and LV volume and myocardial blood flow (mL/min/g) of the LV wall in the infarcted area, the border zone, and the remote normal area was calculated with colored microspheres.

Low-energy cardiac SW were applied to the border zone around the infarcted myocardium. LV wall motion was assessed by echocardiography both before and after creating the infarction.

Two treatment protocols were performed. The first was the early treatment protocol. SW therapy was started 3 days after AMI and performed at days 3, 6, and 9, whereas the control group underwent the same procedures but without SW treatment (n = 5 each). In all animals, angiography, echocardiographic studies, and measurement of regional myocardial blood flow were performed at baseline and 4 weeks after AMI. In the second treatment protocol, the late treatment protocol, SW therapy was started 4 weeks after AMI and performed at days 28, 31, and 34, with a control group (n = 5 each). Angiography, echocardiographic studies, and measurement of regional myocardial blood flow were performed at baseline and 4 and 8 weeks after AMI.

The study showed that SW therapy improved LV remodeling after AMI in pigs when the therapy was started in the early phase, but not in the chronic phase of the disorder (Fig. 4.2). No procedural complications or adverse effects with SW therapy were noted.

In response to acute ischemia, the expression of multiple angiogenic factors and the mobilization of endothelial progenitor cells (EPCs) are enhanced [12]. Interestingly, in a model of hind-limb ischemia it has been shown that preconditioning of the target tissue with low-dose energy shock-wave therapy may enhance the recruitment of progenitor cells to non-ischemic tissue [13]. As the mobilized progenitor cells play an important role in the healing process after AMI [14], SW-induced

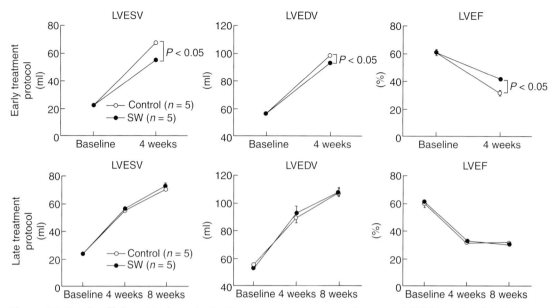

Figure 4.2 Results of left ventriculography for the inhibitory effects of the cardiac shock-wave (SW) therapy on the development of left ventricular (LV) remodeling after AMI. The inhibitory effects of the SW therapy were noted in the early treatment protocol (*upper panel*) but not in the late treatment protocol (*lower panel*). Results are expressed as mean ± SEM (n = 5 each). (AMI, acute myocardial infarction; Control, control group without the SW therapy; LVEDV, LV end-diastolic volume; LVEF, LV ejection fraction; LVESV, LV end-systolic volume; SW, SW group) (Reproduced with permission from [11]).

angiogenesis is expected to be more effective when the SW therapy is started in the earlier phase. As shown in the late treatment protocol in this study, once LV remodeling is established after AMI, the SW therapy may not be so effective at improving LV remodeling.

The way by which SW therapy can reduce LV remodelling may be explained by different mechanisms. SW therapy up-regulates the expression of VEGF with a resultant increase in the capillary density and regional myocardial blood flow in ischemic myocardium[8]. VEGF is known to induce angiogenesis by activating mobilization and homing of EPCs from the bone marrow to ischemic tissue [15]. In this study, SW therapy increased capillary density and regional myocardial blood flow in the border zone of the infarcted myocardium. These results suggest that SW-induced angiogenesis may contribute to salvaging myocardium in the border zone and therefore improves LV remodeling. Furthermore, endogenous angiogenic systems, such as the eNOS, may also be involved in the beneficial effects of SW therapy. Indeed, it has been reported that SW up-regulates the expression of eNOS in vascular endothelial cells in vitro [6] and that eNOS gene delivery attenuates LV remodeling after AMI in rats in vivo [16]. Last but not least, SDF-1 seems to be essential for the retention of proangiogenic stem cells in peripheral organs, although the up-regulation of VEGF is sufficient to mobilize stem or progenitor cells from the bone marrow to the systemic circulation [17]. Therefore, SW therapy possibly enhances the incorporation of circulating EPCs by repeatedly pronouncing the expression of SDF-1 in the border zone of the infarcted heart, a mechanism that has been suggested recently by Aicher and colleagues [13].

Shock-Wave Activation of Cultured Progenitors and Precursors of Cardiac Cells

In a very recent study, Nurzynska and associates [18] tested whether the application of SW could have positive effects on an endothelial cell population and cardiac primitive early committed cells. They established a method of isolating and expanding the cells from human biopsy specimens. The quantification of cardiac primitive cells of cardiomyocyte, smooth muscle, and endothelial lineage obtained from normal hearts and hearts with postischemic cardiomyopathy was performed in vitro on both the SW-treated and untreated cells, as was the analysis of the expression of proteins characteristic for the committed cardiac cells and their mRNA.

Cardiac primitive cells were isolated from bioptic fragments of normal and pathologic human hearts (patients who have died from noncardiovascular disease and patients with terminal ischemic cardiomyopathy). The cells were subjected to 800 impulses of SW at an energy flux density of 0.1 mJ/mm^2. After the treatment, the cells were cultured for 7 days before being analyzed. An identical number of cells was cultured at the same time and served as a control.

The treatment of adherent cells was favorable for the study of biological activity and differentiation of primitive cells, making it possible to preserve intercellular contacts, as well as contacts with the extracellular matrix and outside–inside signaling. The study confirmed that SW treatment can have a positive effect on the proliferation and differentiation of endothelial cells, with an increase in the number of mature endothelial cells as well as endothelial cells involved in neoangiogenesis. At the same time, SW improved the number of primitive cardiomyocytes and smooth muscle cells without any significant pro-apoptotic effect, apparently decreasing the fibroblast growth rate.

The expression of mRNA and proteins characteristic of cardiac muscle cells always increased after cell exposure to SW. In most cases, these changes were more prominent in the normal heart cells than in those taken from pathologic hearts. However, the untreated cells from pathologic hearts showed a higher expression of proteins compared with the untreated cells from normal hearts, indicating that the former are activated during the progression of a disease in response to chronic pathologic conditions.

Spinal Cord Stimulation

Spinal cord neuromodulation owes its origin to the gate theory of pain proposed by Melzack and Wall [19]. On the basis of this theory, it was predicted that stimulation of visceral afferent nerves would reduce or block the transmission of pain-related signals relaying through the spinal cord.

In the late 1960s, modulation of the nervous system to obtain a reduction in pain in ischemic cardiovascular disease was introduced [20]. Among the available adjunct therapies, spinal cord stimulation (SCS) turned out to be the most effective. Both observational and randomized studies on SCS have demonstrated beneficial effects, expressed in a reduction in severity of angina complaints, the number of short-acting nitrates, and perceived quality of life (QoL) [21], in conjunction with an improvement in exercise capacity [22–24]. In approximately 80% of patients, the beneficial effects of SCS lasted for at least 1 year, and in nearly 60% of these patients improvements in exercise capacity and QoL were reported for up to 5 years [25].

There have been concerns with regard to the safety of SCS, as it might deprive the patient of an important angina "warning signal." However, the fear of a potential increase in adverse myocardial events turned out to be unjustified. Rather than abolishing anginal pain, SCS enhances the angina threshold, and pain perception during acute myocardal infarction is intact. Prospective studies also did not show an adverse effect on mortality [24,26].

In addition to analgesic achievements, SCS employs anti-ischemic effects. Both open and randomized studies have demonstrated that the reduction in anginal pain during SCS enables the patient to prolong exercise without aggravating myocardial ischemia. Furthermore, the anti-ischemic effects of SCS have been demonstrated by a reduction in ST segment depression on ECG recordings during exercise stress testing [23,27] and ambulatory ECG monitoring [22,23]. The rise in the anginal threshold is thought to be related to a redistribution of coronary blood flow from myocardial regions with a normal perfusion in favor of regions with impaired myocardial perfusion [28,29].

Pain transmitted from the heart during an episode of angina begins in the adventitia of the coronary arteries and the myocardium. These pain afferents, along with sympathetic nerve branches, transmit to the upper four thoracic parasympathetic ganglia. The pain afferents continue until they reach the segments in the spinal cord. During angina, the activated fibers stimulate the sympathetic afferent fibers that enter the T1-T6 spinal cord segments.

SCS is performed by placing a lead in the epidural space at the level of C7 through T1 and surgically implanting a pacemaker-sized generator in the left lower abdominal area. Patients receive 1 hour of stimulation per day and can activate the device with a hand-held magnet to treat breakthrough pain. The beneficial effects of the technique on angina are explained by its suppression of the capacity of intrinsic cardiac neurons to generate activity during myocardial ischemia, or its resolution of sympathetic activity, leading to improved myocardial blood flow.

The main reported adverse reactions were epidural hematoma and infection, occurring in about 1% of patients. In addition, SCS may interfere with the function of pacemakers and implantable defibrillators.

First Placebo-Controlled Randomized Trial of Thoracic Spinal Cord Stimulation in Patients with Refractory Angina Pectoris

The lack of placebo-controlled trials has represented a major shortcoming of SCS in refractory angina pectoris so far. The reason for this was because SCS is generally performed with stimulation intensity that causes a prickling sensation in the corresponding dermatome. It has consequently not proved possible to blind a patient to active treatment. The effect of thoracic SCS at a stimulation intensity below the sensory threshold had never been tested in a clinical setting, because it was thought to be ineffective. In contrast, animal studies have revealed that SCS at intensities below motor threshold produced cutaneous vasodilatation [30], and Gherardini and associates [31] demonstrated an improved survival of a groin flap in a rat model with low-intensity stimulation (70% of motor threshold) compared to high-intensity stimulation (90% of motor threshold). In a report from a single patient, a peripheral vasodilator response was also described by stimulation with an intensity unable to evoke paraesthesia [32]. Eddicks and coworkers [33] therefore designed a study to test whether a stimulation at an intensity below the sensory threshold could induce a therapeutic effect in comparison to stimulation intensity near 0 V (control) in patients with refractory angina. To be classified as a responder, patients had to show a reduction in the number of angina episodes by at least 50%.

Subthreshold output was defined as 85% (range, 2.1–4 V) of the minimum stimulation output (voltage) causing paraesthesia. The lowest output programmable while the neurostimulator was still fully functional (0.1 V) was selected as the maximum output in the control phase. This output is thought to have no effect on the neuronal system.

Patients were randomized into four consecutive treatment arms (intraindividual crossover), each lasting for 4 weeks, with various stimulation timing and output parameters: stimulation 3 × 2 hr/day with conventional output (phase A), 24 hr/day with conventional output (phase B), 3 × 2 hr/day with subthreshold output (phase C), and 24 hr/day with 0.1 V output (phase D). Functional status, evaluated by the 6-minute walk test (6-MWT), and QoL were assessed at the end of each 4-week treatment period.

The primary end point was total walking distance in the 6-MWT; secondary end points were time to angina (during 6-MWT), number of angina attacks, nitrate usage, CCS class, QoL, and premature termination of a study phase owing to intolerable symptoms.

In treatment phases A to C, walking distance in the 6-MWT did not differ significantly. By contrast, stimulation with 0.1 V was inferior compared to stimulation with conventional output, or to stimulation just below the output inducing paraesthesia. There was significant worsening of CCS class and angina frequency in phase D compared with phases A to C, and 3 patients in phase D (placebo) prematurely terminated this part of the study owing to intolerable angina symptoms, whereas no patients prematurely terminated phases A to C (subthreshold stimulation). In phases A to C, compared with phase D, there were significant improvements in two parameters (angina severity and angina frequency) of the Seattle Angina Questionnaire (SAQ) and the EuroQol Visual Analog Scale.

This first randomized placebo-controlled trial of SCS in patients with refractory angina pectoris revealed the possibility of improvement in functional status and in QoL, as well as of reduction in angina frequency in phases with conventional or subthreshold stimulation, in comparison to a low-output (placebo) phase. A placebo effect as the only mechanism of action therefore seems unlikely.

Neurostimulation in Patients with Refractory Chest Pain and Normal Coronary Arteries

In 10% to 20% of patients with typical chest pain, angiography reveals normal coronary arteries (cardiac syndrome X, CSX) [34]. The pathophysiology of this syndrome of chest pain with normal coronary arteries has not yet been clarified, but an abnormal cardiac pain perception has been reported [35], as well as evidence of endothelial dysfunction [36]. De Vries and colleagues [37] started a study to define the influence of long-term neurostimulation on QoL, the effect on use of medication, occurrence of angina pectoris-like chest pain, exercise capacity, and treatment satisfaction in patients with CSX. Only patients showing a benefit from neurostimulation were followed.

Initially all patients received transcutaneous electrical nerve stimulation (TENS), for a trial period of 2 weeks. Treatment was continued if pain was relieved at least 50%. Thirteen patients stopped using TENS despite efficacy, due to side effects such as the ortho-ergic skin reaction. These patients were offered an implantable neurostimulator (ie, SCS), which was implanted in 8 of the 13 patients; the efficacy of the results was comparable to TENS. Three patients refused SCS implantations and 2 patients did not experience chest pain anymore.

Hospital records were used to evaluate the data for adverse effects. A stimulation protocol of 3 times an hour was advised, and patients were free to stimulate whenever they experienced chest pain. Since there is no evidence that either the underlying mechanisms of action or the outcomes between TENS and SCS differ, the two groups were considered to be equal.

Of 36 patients with typical CSX with beneficial results, 24 patients were finally studied. Twelve patients were lost to follow-up. The SAQ was used to assess the health-related QoL, both at baseline (retrospectively) and at follow-up. Frequency of chest pain attacks, short-acting nitroglycerin consumption, and walking distance were noted at baseline and follow-up.

After 5 years of neurostimulation, chest pain was reduced in 57% of the patients and a 30% increase in exercise capacity was observed. Orthoergic skin reaction developed in 13 of the 24 patients with TENS, after a mean period of more than 1 year. Three patients were able to stop anti-anginal medication. The SAQ showed the greatest improvement for the activities that are most limiting like walking uphill, gardening, or lifting heavy objects. No difference between TENS or SCS was noted.

This study showed that neurostimulation is effective in CSX, that SCS and TENS provide comparable results on efficacy as measured by the SAQ, and that SCS is an alternative to TENS in case of skin irritation.

The long-term effect of patients with CSX treated by spinal cord stimulation was investigated by Sgueglia et al.[38] in a prospective, long-term comparison between patients with CSX who underwent spinal cord stimulation (SCS group) and a group of CSX patients eligible for SCS because of refractory angina episodes but who refused this form of treatment (controls).

A total of 30 consecutive patients (8 men, 22 women, mean age 60.9 ± 8.6 years) were proposed to undergo SCS device implantation. Of those, 9 refused the treatment and formed the control group. Of the 21 patients who underwent SCS, 1 successively refused definitive neurostimulator implantation because of ineffectiveness of SCS during the trial period with the temporary device. The SCS device was removed in another patient 12 months after the definitive implantation owing to loss of effectiveness. Thus, the SCS group included 19 patients with complete long-term follow-up.

Patients were followed up for a median period of 36 (range, 15–82) months. At the follow-up visit, the frequency of angina ($p = 0.005$) and the use of short-acting nitrates ($p = 0.028$) were significantly lower in the SCS group than in controls, as a result of a significant improvement in the SCS group. Of note, angina at rest was reported by all controls but only by 21% of patients with SCS ($p = 0.001$). All SAQ scores and EuroQoL Visual Analogue Scale-assessed QoL were significantly higher in the SCS group than in controls, due to a significant improvement of scores in the SCS group ($p < 0.001$ for all scales), whereas no significant changes were observed in controls.

Patients in the SCS group showed less exercise-induced angina and > 1 mm ST-segment depression than controls, although the differences did not achieve statistical significance. Yet time and rate-pressure product at angina, at 1-mm ST-segment depression and at peak exercise, were significantly better at follow-up in the SCS group than in controls, as a result of a significant improvement in the SCS group but not in controls.

This prospective study showed that the early beneficial effects of SCS in patients with CSX and angina episodes refractory to maximal multidrug treatment are maintained at 3-year follow-up. It was the first study to show long-term efficacy of SCS in patients with CSX afflicted by severe anginal symptoms using a controlled protocol.

Spinal Cord Stimulation for Refractory Angina and Concomitant Internal Cardioverter Defibrillator

Until now, the implantation of a device for SCS has been considered relatively contraindicated in patients who carry a pacemaker (PM) or an automatic implantable cardiac defibrillator (ICD) due to the concern of possible interferences or missensed electrical activity leading to inappropriate ICD shocks. So far, only one case of SCS in a patient previously implanted with an ICD has been described, but in that one, the lead was placed at the Th 11 level, in order to treat severe limb ischemia, thus quite far from the ICD detection field. Furthermore, the SCS was programmed in the unipolar configuration that was the most suitable for that particular patient, so that ICD/SCS compatibility was assessed in this configuration too. Usually in patients suffering from refractory angina, the stimulation configuration of choice is the bipolar one, because it allows a great number of stimulation options and interferes less with ICDs or pacemakers. Ferrero and associates [39] reported about a patient previously implanted with an ICD and treated with SCS because of his suffering from refractory angina.

The real-time IEGM showed no sensed artefact due to the concomitant SCS even at the highest tolerated output energy level (4.5-V amplitude/450-μs impulse duration, and 80-Hz rate), and the induced ventricular fibrillation was properly detected and treated by the ICD. This case therefore provided further evidence of the safety of combined use of SCS with a lead placed at the cervical level and ICD with the precaution of thorough intraoperative and careful follow-up tests.

Coronary Sinus Restriction

The Coronary Sinus (CS) Reducer (Neovasc Medical, Or Yehuda, Israel) is a stainless steel balloon-expandable stent specially designed to establish a narrowing of the coronary sinus, which is the final pathway of the cardiac venous drainage, and to increase coronary venous pressure (Fig. 4.3). The Reducer is implanted by a percutaneous transvenous approach. The aim of this procedure in patients with CAD and refractory angina who are not candidates for conventional revascularization procedures, is to elevate CS pressure and to enhance perfusion to ischemic territories of the myocardium to improve their symptoms.

Elevated coronary venous pressure achieved by narrowing of the CS as a therapeutic approach was first described and used by Beck and Leighninger in 1955 in patients with disabling angina [40,41]. Elevating CS pressure using intermittent CS occlusion and pressure-controlled intermittent CS occlusion have been described to be effective in salvaging ischemic myocardium in several experimental models of coronary artery occlusion [42,43]. However,

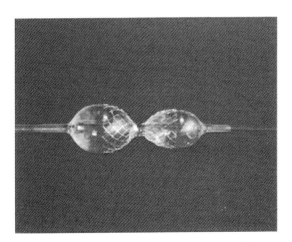 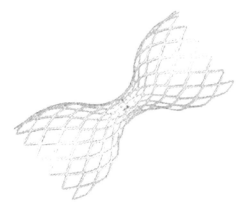

Figure 4.3 Coronary Sinus Reducer stent: a stainless steel balloon-expandable stent designed to establish narrowing of the coronary sinus. **Left.** The Reducer stent on the inflated designated balloon. The diameter at its midportion is 3 mm, and it can reach a diameter of 7.0 to 13.0 mm at both ends using inflation pressure of 2 to 4 bars. **Right.** The Reducer stent. In case it is necessary to remove the narrowing from the coronary sinus, balloon inflation to a pressure of 8 bars will completely open the Reducer, which will then attain a tubular shape (Reproduced with permission from [48]).

the modes of action of these interventions remain speculative. The CS pressure elevation enhances coronary collateral flow and reduces subendocardial ischemia, with a positive correlation between the elevated CS pressure and the changes in collateral blood flow from nonischemic to ischemic territories of the myocardium [44]. Clinical application of CS interventions during the early reperfusion period has shown improvement in regional myocardial function and salvaging of ischemic myocardium, especially by limiting the infarct from its border [45–47].

Banai and associates [48] published the first-in-man study in a multicenter, nonrandomized, open-label prospective study that evaluated the safety and feasibility of the CS Reducer. Patients were included if they had a history of CAD with refractory angina (CCS class II to IV) despite optimal medical therapy, objective evidence of reversible myocardial ischemia, and an ejection fraction > 30%. All patients were considered unacceptable candidates for PCI or CABG.

The primary end point in this study was the absence of any major adverse cardiac events related to the procedure during 6 months of follow-up. An adverse event was defined as death, myocardial infarction, perforation of the CS, CS occlusion, or

need for urgent dilatation of the Reducer. The secondary end point was successful delivery and deployment of the Reducer in the CS, as assessed by angiogram and/or by computed tomographic (CT) angiography.

Under fluoroscopic guidance, a preshaped guiding sheath was introduced into the CS through a right internal jugular vein. After CS pressure was recorded, angiography was performed (Fig. 4.4). The dimensions of the proximal segment of the CS were measured using quantitative coronary angiography. The optimal site for implantation was chosen according to the vessel diameters and to avoid side branch bifurcation. The Reducer, crimped on a balloon, was then inserted over the wire into the CS, positioned at the desired site, and implanted by inflating the balloon. Postimplantation angiography was performed to ensure appropriate implantation, patency, and appropriate reduction of the lumen's diameter, and to ensure lack of migration of the Reducer, thrombosis within the Reducer or the CS, and perforation or dissection of the CS (Fig. 4.5).

A single Reducer was implanted in the CS of 15 patients at three medical centers. All had proven CAD, evidence of reversible myocardial ischemia, and all suffered from refractory angina. All

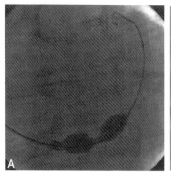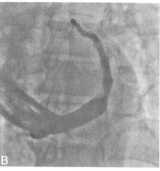

Figure 4.4 Implantation of the Coronary Sinus Reducer stent in human coronary sinus. **A.** Contrast-filled inflated balloon at the time of implantation of the Reducer stent in human coronary sinus, introduced into the CS through the right internal jugular vein. **B.** Retrograde angiography of the coronary sinus after implantation of the Reducer (Reproduced with permission from [48]).

implantation procedures were completed successfully and patients were discharged from hospital 1 to 2 days later without clinical complications. No major adverse cardiac events had occurred during the periprocedural period or during the follow-up period of 10 to 12 months. In 12 patients, CT angiography was performed. All Reducers were patent, well positioned, and located at the exact site of deployment with no evidence of migration.

Angina score improved significantly 6 months after implantation. The CCS class was lower after 6 months in 12 of the 14 patients and remained constant in 2. Most patients reported improvement in QoL and reduction in anginal symptoms only several weeks after implantation of the Reducer.

Of the 11 patients in whom electrocardiographic tracings at baseline and at the 6-month stress test were of good technical quality, transient ST-segment depression was documented during the baseline exercise stress test in 9. At 6-month follow-up, ST-segment depression was lower in 6 of these 9 patients, and was no longer present in 2 of the 6. One patient had a higher ST-segment depression at 6 months. In 9 of the 11 patients, exercise duration and peak heart rate increased at the 6-month follow-up stress test compared with baseline. For the whole group, the average double product and exercise duration were unchanged 6 months after implantation compared with baseline.

In 13 of the 14 patients, dobutamine echocardiography data were of good technical quality. In 8 of these 13 patients there was a medically significant improvement (a change of 1 score or more in at least 2 segments) when the stress images at baseline and 6 months were compared. The average score of all 18 segments was lower at 6 months.

In 10 patients SPECT images were of good technical quality at baseline and 6 months. In 4 of

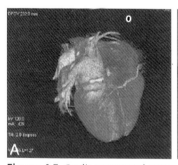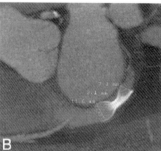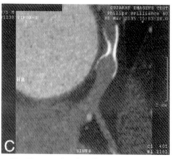

Figure 4.5 Cardiac computed tomographic angiography of human hearts after implantation of the coronary sinus reducer stent. **A.** Three-dimensional reconstruction of the posterior aspect of the heart. The Reducer stent implanted at the proximal segment of the coronary sinus is clearly seen. **B, C.** Longitudinal section of the coronary sinus. The proximal and distal diameters of the Reducer perfectly match the funnel-shaped coronary sinus (Reproduced with permission from [48]).

the 10 patients there was a medically significant reduction in the extent and/or severity of my-ocardial ischemia as measured by the total score. Among the remaining 6 patients, the SPECT images were unchanged in 5 and worsened in 1 patient at 6 months. The average score for the group was 12.6 at baseline and 9.6 at 6 months.

In this first human experience with the implan-tation of CS Reducer, no adverse events occurred during up to 12 months of follow-up, suggesting that the implantation of the Reducer is feasible and safe.

Few pathophysiologic mechanisms are proposed to explain the anti-ischemic effects of elevated CS pressure: first, the opening of pre-existing collateral vessels between normally perfused and ischemic segments of the myocardium; and second, rever-sal of the endocardial/epicardial blood flow ratio in favor of the endocardium with an increase in en-docardial blood flow [49]. In the long run, the po-tential for formation of new blood vessels also has been suggested.

Significant stenosis of an epicardial coronary artery is associated with decreased myocardial per-fusion and activation of compensatory mechanisms to overcome this limitation. Distal vessels dilate, and pre-existing collateral connections are opened and develop over time into significant vessels that transmit blood from normally perfused territories to ischemic regions. New coronary collaterals de-velop over time as well. Previous studies with an increase in CS pressure have shown clearly that the coronary collateral circulation is enhanced in a significant way by this intervention. Fur-thermore, the subendocardium is more vulnerable to ischemic damage than the midmyocardium or subepicardium.

Epicardial coronary stenoses are associated with reduction in the subendocardial-to-subepicardial flow ratio. This mechanism, which has been demonstrated in multiple experiments, is explained by the high intramyocardial forces acting on vessels in the subendocardium. This high intramyocardial force does not enable the vasodilatory response of the vascular system to fully compensate for the de-crease in coronary perfusion caused by the stenosis. The CS Reducer, by increasing backpressure into the precapillary arteriolar system, should facilitate dilatation of the constricted subendocardial capil-laries. Any change in the diameter of these vessels will be more pronounced than the changes tak-ing place in the already dilated vessels in the epi-cardial territory, thereby facilitating the directional changes in flow toward the subendocardial seg-ments [44,46,50]. Improved capillary perfusion in the subendocardium of the ischemic territory will improve contractility and increased oxygen con-sumption [51].

In this open-label, multicenter, nonrandomized, prospective study, the use of percutaneous transve-nous implantation of the CS Reducer in patients with refractory angina was found to be safe and fea-sible, which supports further evaluation of the CS Reducer in a randomized placebo-controlled trial, as an alternative tool for treating patients with re-fractory angina who are not candidates for or are at high risk for revascularization.

References

1. Mannheimer C, Camici P, Chester MR, *et al.* The prob-lem of chronic refractory angina; report from the ESC Joint Study Group on the Treatment of Refractory Angina. *Eur Heart J.* 2002;23:355–370.

2. Mukherjee D, Bhatt DL, Roe MT, Patel V, Ellis SG. Direct myocardial revascularization and angiogenesis—how many patients might be eli-gible? *Am J Cardiol.* 1999;84:598–600.

3. Apfel RE. Acoustic cavitation: a possible consequence of biomedical uses of ultrasound. *Br J Cancer Suppl.* 1982;5:140–146.

4. Maisonhaute E, Prado C, White PC, Compton RG. Surface acoustic cavitation understood via nanosec-ond electrochemistry. Part III: shear stress in ultra-sonic cleaning. *Ultrason Sonochem.* 2002;9:297–303.

5. Wang CJ, Wang FS, Yang KD, *et al.* Shock wave therapy induces neovascularization at the tendon-bone junction. A study in rabbits. *J Orthop Res.* 2003;21:984–989.

6. Gutersohn A, Gaspari G. Shock waves upregulate vascular endothelial growth factor m-RNA in hu-man umbilical vascular endothelial cells. *Circulation.* 2000;102(suppl):18.

7. Gotte G, Amelio E, Russo S, Marlinghaus E, Musci G, Suzuki H. Short-time non-enzymatic nitric oxide

synthesis from L-arginine and hydrogen peroxide induced by shock waves treatment. *FEBS Lett.* 2002;520:153–155.

8. Nishida T, Shimokawa H, Oi K, *et al.* Extracorporeal cardiac shock wave therapy markedly ameliorates ischemia-induced myocardial dysfunction in pigs in vivo. *Circulation.* 2004;110:3055–3061.

9. Fukumoto Y, Ito A, Uwatoku T, *et al.* Extracorporeal cardiac shock wave therapy ameliorates myocardial ischemia in patients with severe coronary artery disease. *Coron Artery Dis.* 2006;17:63–70.

10. Khattab AA, Brodersen B, Schuermann-Kuchenbrandt D, *et al.* Extracorporeal cardiac shock wave therapy: first experience in the everyday practice for treatment of chronic refractory angina pectoris. *Int J Cardiol.* 2007;121:84–85.

11. Uwatoku T, Ito K, Abe K, *et al.* Extracorporeal cardiac shock wave therapy improves left ventricular remodeling after acute myocardial infarction in pigs. *Coron Artery Dis.* 2007;18:397–404.

12. Massa M, Rosti V, Ferrario M, *et al.* Increased circulating hematopoietic and endothelial progenitor cells in the early phase of acute myocardial infarction. *Blood.* 2005;105:199–206.

13. Aicher A, Heeschen C, Sasaki K, *et al.* Low-energy shock wave for enhancing recruitment of endothelial progenitor cells: a new modality to increase efficacy of cell therapy in chronic hind limb ischemia. *Circulation.* 2006;114:2823–2830.

14. Minatoguchi S, Takemura G, Chen XH, *et al.* Acceleration of the healing process and myocardial regeneration may be important as a mechanism of improvement of cardiac function and remodeling by postinfarction granulocyte colony-stimulating factor treatment. *Circulation.* 2004;109: 2572–2580.

15. Grunewald M, Avraham I, Dor Y, *et al.* VEGF-induced adult neovascularization: recruitment, retention, and role of accessory cells. *Cell.* 2006;124: 175–189.

16. Smith RS Jr., Agata J, Xia CF, Chao L, Chao J. Human endothelial nitric oxide synthase gene delivery protects against cardiac remodeling and reduces oxidative stress after myocardial infarction. *Life Sci.* 2005;76:2457–2471.

17. Askari AT, Unzek S, Popovic ZB, *et al.* Effect of stromal-cell-derived factor 1 on stem-cell homing and tissue regeneration in ischaemic cardiomyopathy. *Lancet.* 2003;362:697–703.

18. Nurzynska D, Di Meglio F, Castaldo C, *et al.* Shock waves activate in vitro cultured progenitors and precursors of cardiac cell lineages from the human heart. *Ultrasound Med Biol.* 2008;34:334–342.

19. Melzack R, Wall P. Pain mechanisms: A new theory. *Science.* 1965;150:971–997.

20. Braunwald E, Epstein SE, Glick G, Wechsler AS, Braunwald NS. Relief of angina pectoris by electrical stimulation of the carotid-sinus nerves. *N Engl J Med.* 1967;277:1278–1283.

21. Vulnink NCC, Overgaauw DM, Jessurun GAJ, *et al.* The effects of spinal cord stimulation on quality of life in patients wirh therapeutically refractory angina pectoris. *Neuromodulaton.* 1999;2:29–36.

22. de Jongste MJ, Hautvast RW, Hillege HL, Lie KI. Efficacy of spinal cord stimulation as adjuvant therapy for intractable angina pectoris: a prospective, randomized clinical study. Working Group on Neurocardiology. *J Am Coll Cardiol.* 1994;23:1592–1597.

23. Hautvast RW, DeJongste MJ, Staal MJ, van Gilst WH, Lie KI. Spinal cord stimulation in chronic intractable angina pectoris: a randomized, controlled efficacy study. *Am Heart J.* 1998;136:1114–1120.

24. Mannheimer C, Eliasson T, Augustinsson LE, *et al.* Electrical stimulation versus coronary artery bypass surgery in severe angina pectoris: the ESBY study. *Circulation.* 1998;97:1157–1163.

25. Bagger JP, Jensen BS, Johannsen G. Long-term outcome of spinal cord electrical stimulation in patients with refractory chest pain. *Clin Cardiol.* 1998;21:286–288.

26. TenVaarwerk IA, Jessurun GA, DeJongste MJ, *et al.* Clinical outcome of patients treated with spinal cord stimulation for therapeutically refractory angina pectoris. The Working Group on Neurocardiology. *Heart.* 1999;82:82–88.

27. Mannheimer C, Augustinsson LE, Carlsson CA, Manhem K, Wilhelmsson C. Epidural spinal electrical stimulation in severe angina pectoris. *Br Heart J.* 1988;59:56-61.

28. Hautvast RW, Blanksma PK, DeJongste MJ, *et al.* Effect of spinal cord stimulation on myocardial blood flow assessed by positron emission tomography in patients with refractory angina pectoris. *Am J Cardiol.* 1996;77:462–467.

29. Diedrichs H, Zobel C, Theissen P, *et al.* Symptomatic relief precedes improvement of myocardial blood flow in patients under spinal cord stimulation. *Curr Control Trials Cardiovasc Med.* 2005;6:7.

30. Tanaka S, Barron KW, Chandler MJ, Linderoth B, Foreman RD. Low intensity spinal cord stimulation may induce cutaneous vasodilation via CGRP release. *Brain Res.* 2001;896:183–187.

31. Gherardini G, Lundeberg T, Cui JG, Eriksson SV, Trubek S, Linderoth B. Spinal cord stimulation improves survival in ischemic skin flaps: an experimental study of the possible mediation by calcitonin gene-related peptide. *Plast Reconstr Surg.* 1999;103:1221–1228.

32. Linderoth B. Spinal cord stimulation in ischemia and ischemic pain. In: Horsch S, Claeys L, eds. *Spinal Cord Stimulation: An Innovative Method in the Treatment of PVD and Angina.* Heidelberg: Steinkopff; 1995:19–35.

33. Eddicks S, Maier-Hauff K, Schenk M, Muller A, Baumann G, Theres H. Thoracic spinal cord stimulation improves functional status and relieves symptoms in patients with refractory angina pectoris: the first placebo-controlled randomised study. *Heart.* 2007;93:585–590.

34. Phibbs B, Fleming T, Ewy GA, et al. Frequency of normal coronary arteriograms in three academic medical centers and one community hospital. *Am J Cardiol.* 1988;62:472–474.

35. Chauhan A, Mullins PA, Thuraisingham SI, Taylor G, Petch MC, Schofield PM. Abnormal cardiac pain perception in syndrome X. *J Am Coll Cardiol.* 1994;24:329–335.

36. Sanderson JE, Woo KS, Chung HK, Chan WW, Tse LK, White HD. The effect of transcutaneous electrical nerve stimulation on coronary and systemic haemodynamics in syndrome X. *Coron Artery Dis.* 1996;7:547–552.

37. de Vries J, Anthonio RL, Dejongste MJ, et al. The effect of electrical neurostimulation on collateral perfusion during acute coronary occlusion. *BMC Cardiovasc Disord.* 2007;7:18.

38. Sgueglia GA, Sestito A, Spinelli A, et al. Long-term follow-up of patients with cardiac syndrome X treated by spinal cord stimulation. *Heart.* 2007;93:591–597.

39. Ferrero P, Grimaldi R, Massa R, et al. Spinal cord stimulation for refractory angina in a patient implanted with a cardioverter defibrillator. *Pacing Clin Electrophysiol.* 2007;30:143–146.

40. Beck CS, Leighninger DS. Scientific basis for the surgical treatment of coronary artery disease. *JAMA.* 1955;159:1264–1271.

41. Wising PJ. The Beck-I operation for angina pectoris: medical aspects. *Acta Med Scand.* 1963;174:93–98.

42. Aldea GS, Zhang X, Rivers S, Shemin RJ. Salvage of ischemic myocardium with simplified and even delayed coronary sinus retroperfusion. *Ann Thorac Surg.* 1996;62:9–15.

43. Ikeoka K, Nakagawa Y, Kawashima S, Fujitani K, Iwasaki T. Effects of intermittent coronary sinus occlusion on experimental myocardial infarction and reperfusion hemorrhage. *Jpn Circ J.* 1990;54:1258–1273.

44. Sato M, Saito T, Mitsugi M, et al. Effects of cardiac contraction and coronary sinus pressure elevation on collateral circulation. *Am J Physiol.* 1996;271:H1433–H1440.

45. Syeda B, Schukro C, Heinze G, et al. The salvage potential of coronary sinus interventions: meta-analysis and pathophysiologic consequences. *J Thorac Cardiovasc Surg.* 2004;127:1703–1712.

46. Mohl W, Glogar DH, Mayr H, et al. Reduction of infarct size induced by pressure-controlled intermittent coronary sinus occlusion. *Am J Cardiol.* 1984;53:923–928.

47. Mohl W, Kajgana I, Bergmeister H, Rattay F. Intermittent pressure elevation of the coronary venous system as a method to protect ischemic myocardium. *Interact Cardiovasc Thorac Surg.* 2005;4:66–69.

48. Banai S, Ben Muvhar S, Parikh KH, et al. Coronary sinus reducer stent for the treatment of chronic refractory angina pectoris: a prospective, open-label, multicenter, safety feasibility first-in-man study. *J Am Coll Cardiol.* 2007;49:1783–1789.

49. Ido A, Hasebe N, Matsuhashi H, Kikuchi K. Coronary sinus occlusion enhances coronary collateral flow and reduces subendocardial ischemia. *Am J Physiol Heart Circ Physiol.* 2001;280:H1361–H1367.

50. Rouleau JR, White M. Effects of coronary sinus pressure elevation on coronary blood flow distribution in dogs with normal preload. *Can J Physiol Pharmacol.* 1985;63:787–797.

51. Dijkman MA, Heslinga JW, Sipkema P, Westerhof N. Perfusion-induced changes in cardiac contractility depend on capillary perfusion. *Am J Physiol.* 1998;274:H405–H410.

PART II
Noncoronary Interventions

CHAPTER 5

Transcatheter Aortic Valve Implantation

Helene Eltchaninoff and Alain Cribier
Department of Cardiology, Hospital Charles Nicolle, University of Rouen, Rouen, France

---

Chapter Overview

- Surgical aortic valve replacement (AVR) is the gold standard therapy for symptomatic patients with severe aortic stenosis.
- About one-third of patients cannot be operated upon because of associated comorbidities.
- The first case of percutaneous aortic valve replacement was performed by Cribier on April 16, 2002 in Rouen, France.
- Percutaneous aortic valve replacement is an alternative to surgical AVR in patients at too high a risk or who are contraindicated for conventional surgery.
- Two models are currently commercialized in Europe: the balloon-expandable Edwards–Sapien bioprosthesis and the self-expandable Medtronic CoreValve.
- The Edwards–Sapien bioprosthesis can be implanted using either a transfemoral or transapical approach
- A large, randomized multicenter study (PARTNER-US) is ongoing in the United States comparing the Edwards–Sapien bioprosthesis to surgical AVR in high-risk patients and to medical treatment alone in patients contraindicated for AVR.

For patients with symptomatic aortic stenosis (AS), aortic valve replacement (AVR) has been proven to improve survival. However, the risks of open heart surgery prompted Cribier to develop alternative therapies, including balloon aortic valvuloplasty (BAV) [1] in 1985 and percutaneous heart valve (PHV) in 2002 [2]. Indeed, as described in the EuroHeart Survey on valvular disease [3], patients with valvular heart disease are often undertreated. Approximately one-third of symptomatic patients with severe AS do not undergo surgical treatment as a consequence of their age or the presence of left ventricular dysfunction or comorbidities.

In our center, the concept of catheter-based valve replacement emerged during the early 1990s as a potential therapy for patients with nonsurgical calcific AS, and as a possible solution to rule out valvular restenosis after BAV, which was a major issue. In 1994, we confirmed the ability to anchor a balloon-expandable stent in the calcified and fibrotic aortic annulus of human cadavers with aortic stenosis. These experiments also provided the initial data regarding optimal stent length and diameter. Five years later, with the creation of PVT (Percutaneous Valve Technologies, Fort Lee, New Jersey), prototypes of PHV were developed and tested in a sheep model [4].

The first human percutaneous aortic valve implant was performed by our group in April 2002 [2] using a bovine bioprosthesis in a

Current Best Practice in Interventional Cardiology. Edited by B Meier. © 2010 Blackwell Publishing,

balloon-expandable stainless steel stent. Initial series of human implantations for compassionate use followed and were serially reported [5–7]. Following the acquisition of PVT by Edwards LifeSciences in 2004, further modifications of the valve (Cribier–Edwards and Edwards–Sapien Percutaneous Heart Valve) and its implantation instruments preceded multicenter clinical trials in Europe and in the United States [8].

In 2004, another valve device was developed, the CoreValve PHV, a self-expanding porcine bioprosthesis mounted in a nitinol stent [9]. The two systems (the Edwards–Sapien, Edwards Lifesciences Inc.; and the CoreValve Revalving System, Medtronic Inc.) have CE mark approval and are in widespread use in Europe and elsewhere. This article will provide an overview on these two commercially available systems. Several valve prototypes are under evaluation in different stages of development.

Edwards–Sapien (Previously Cribier–Edwards) Prosthesis

First in man percutaneous aortic valve implantation was performed in Rouen, France on April 16, 2002 by Cribier and his team. The procedure was done using an antegrade (venous) approach since the patient had severe occlusive peripheral vascular disease and no suitable arterial access. Following this first successful case, two feasibility trials were conducted in our center [5,6]: the REVIVE and the RECAST studies including 36 compassionate patients. These early trials were determinant to demonstrate the feasibility of the technique and showed the optimal function of the PHV leading to impressive hemodynamic and clinical improvement.

Since then, there have been numerous refinements in the device and instruments. With ongoing experience, several changes have also been introduced in the implantation protocols. Currently the valve is placed through a retrograde arterial approach or through a transapical minimally invasive surgical approach.

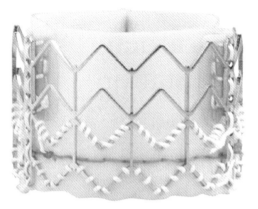

Figure 5.1 Cribier–Edwards bioprosthesis. Side view of the stented valve (exit to the top).

Percutaneous Valve and Delivery Systems

The Edwards valve delivery system consists of the bioprosthetic valve (Fig. 5.1), balloon catheter, retroflex catheter, and crimping tool.

The Valve

The currently used Edwards–Sapien valve is a trileaflet valve composed of three equal sections of bovine pericardium integrated into a stainless steel balloon-expandable stent frame. This second-generation valve has replaced the previous model (Cribier–Edwards valve), an equine pericardium bioprosthesis. A fabric cuff is sewn onto the frame, covering one-half of the stent, which is oriented towards the left ventricle when deployed. The original stent measured 14.5 mm in length and was designed for a maximal expansion of 23 mm diameter. Due to the variability of aortic annulus size, a larger stent with a 26-mm diameter and a 16-mm length was introduced. This valve is intended to be implanted in the subcoronary position, using the native calcific valve to anchor the stent. Bench testing has established a durability > 10 years.

Balloon Catheter

To deliver and deploy the PHV, an Edwards balloon catheter is used.

Crimping Tool

A unique crimping device is used to symmetrically compress the PHV from its expanded size to its minimal delivery profile. Today, the 23-mm PHV is compatible with a 22F sheath, and the 26-mm PHV with a 24F sheath.

Retroflex Catheter

The retroflex catheter was introduced in 2005 to facilitate the retrograde delivery of the PHV. Its tip changes direction when activated by rotation of an external hub incorporated into the handle. The PHV assembly protrudes distally, and is not covered by the guide catheter. The guide catheter is then used to direct the Retroflex catheter–PHV assembly through the arterial system, around the aortic arch, and across the aortic valve. This provides a less traumatic passage of the PHV through a tortuous and diseased aorta. There is also improved ability to center and push the PHV assembly across the calcified and stenotic native valve. This system also allows precise positioning of the PHV at the aortic annulus.

Technical Aspects for PHV Implantation Using the Edwards–Sapien Valve

The techniques that will be described below include the antegrade transseptal approach, the retrograde arterial approach, and the transapical approach that we have used at our center.

Baseline Measurements and Premedication

Baseline transthoracic echocardiography (TTE), right and left heart catheterization, left ventriculography, supra-aortic angiography, and coronary angiography are obtained prior to the planned PHV. This is necessary to determine the severity of the AS, the diameter of the aortic annulus, left ventricular function, associated coronary artery disease, and visualize the amount and distribution of valvular calcification. Supra-aortic angiography is performed to establish the optimal projection for PHV deployment. This view (generally slight LAO and slight cranial) should profile the aortic valve and its annulus as well as demonstrate the coronary ostia clearly. A frame is stored for display on an adjacent monitor screen during the PHV implant. Aortography with angiography of the iliac and femoral arteries prior to the procedure, CT scan (Fig. 5.2), or MR angiography of the aorta and pelvic vessels are nec-

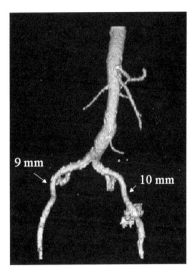

Figure 5.2 CT scan demonstrating large femoroiliac vessels.

essary to plan the strategy for a retrograde femoral artery approach or antegrade transapical approach.

Acetylsalicylic acid 160 mg and clopidogrel 300 mg are given orally at least 24 hours prior to the procedure. Antibiotic prophylaxis is administered prior to and up to 48 hours after the procedure. Clopidogrel (75 mg/day) is continued for 1 month, and acetylsalicylic acid (160 mg/day) indefinitely.

Predilatation of the Native Valve

Common to each technique is BAV prior to PHV deployment to prepare the native aortic valve and to facilitate its crossing. This is achieved using a 20-or 23-mm diameter balloon (depending on the final valve size of 23 or 26 mm) and rapid ventricular pacing (RVP). RVP pacing, developed by Cribier for optimal PHV delivery, has been described for several years and is routinely used for BAV. A pacemaker lead is positioned in the right ventricle and used to pace the heart at 180 to 220 beats per minute. RVP will immediately lead to a drop in aortic blood pressure below 60 mm Hg and a decrease in cardiac output, allowing balloon stabilization across the aortic valve. A brief period of RVP (< 10 sec) is sufficient to inflate and deflate the balloon. Return to pre-BAV aortic pressure after RVP is mandatory before performing an additional balloon inflation.

Antegrade Transseptal Approach

Technical steps related to the antegrade transseptal approach have been described earlier [5,6,8] and will not be detailed here. This approach was used per protocol in 85% of patients included in the feasibility trials I-REVIVE and RECAST and has not been used in the recent multicenter trials.

The advantage of the antegrade approach is that it is truly percutaneous and performed under local anesthesia. This technique avoids the potential complications related to small-caliber diffusely diseased tortuous iliac and femoral arteries encountered in the elderly. The PHV assembly is positioned and deployed in the direction of blood flow across the surface of the valve, which is usually less diseased, resulting in smoother passage and greater stability. Failure to cross the native aortic valve using the antegrade approach was never experienced. Although the interatrial septum is crossed with a large-profile device, problems with residual shunting were not encountered.

This approach is technically demanding and more complicated than the retrograde approach. The antegrade technique requires a significant learning curve, limiting its widespread use. Because of the complexity of the antegrade approach, and the hemodynamic instability that can arise from interference or injury to the mitral valve if the guidewire is not handled properly, there was renewed emphasis on refining the retrograde approach. However, the technique might revive in the future as offering a solution to patients with contraindications to both retrograde and transapical approaches.

Retrograde Approach

The retrograde approach is the most frequently used in the trials since 2005. It was facilitated by the development of a specific catheter, the Retroflex catheter described previously.

Femoral Puncture, Retrograde Crossing of Aortic Valve, Predilation of Valve and Femoral Artery

At our center, the procedure is performed under local anesthesia and mild sedation (midazolam and nalbuphine) after surgical cut-down of the common femoral artery. In the vast majority of centers, the procedure is done under general anesthesia and the femoral artery is either exposed surgically or punctured percutaneously.

After retrograde catheterization of the aortic valve (in the 40-degree left anterior oblique (LAO) projection in our center, using an Amplatz left catheter), the straight-tip 0.35-inch guidewire is exchanged for an extra stiff guidewire (Cook), and predilation of the aortic valve is done as described previously. The femoral artery is then predilated with a series of dilators of increasing size (18F, 20F, and 22F) in order to facilitate entry of the 22 F or 24F sheath. The sheath is carefully advanced if necessary under x-ray visualization and placed above the renal arteries. The procedure should be aborted in case of excessive difficulties to advance the sheath.

PHV Delivery and Deployment

The PHV is advanced over the extra stiff guidewire in AP view. When reaching the aortic arch, the projection is moved to 40-degree LAO view and the Retroflex is rotated in order to limit the friction of the device against the wall of the arch. Final projection is then selected (usually 10-15 LAO and 10-15 cranial), and the Retroflex is fully rotated and placed across the native aortic valve. It is then retrieved by 3 to 4 cm and the PHV is deployed using RVP (Figs. 5.3 and 5.4). Postimplantation hemodynamic and angiographic measurements are performed with special attention to the supra-aortic angiogram to assess any paravalvular leak (Fig. 5.5). Arterial sheath is carefully retrieved and arterial access is managed by surgical repair in the catheterization laboratory or Perclose suture [10]. A final adominal aortogram is obtained to ensure the absence of vascular complications.

The retrograde approach's main advantage relies on its similarities to routine BAV, a familiar technique for the interventional cardiologist. Its main limitations center at the present time on the arterial sheath size required for device insertion. Valve positioning is another key point. It is now clear that the proximal part of the stent has to be placed

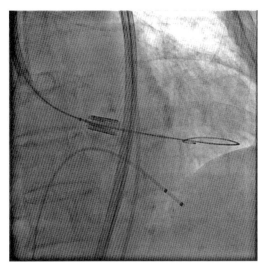

Figure 5.3 The Cribier–Edwards valve has been advanced over a wire entering the femoral artery and is positioned at the level of the native valve's calcifications.

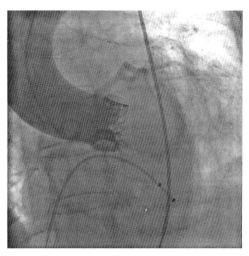

Figure 5.5 A supra-aortic angiogram is performed after percutaneous heart valve delivery to assess the degree of paravalvular leak (no regurgitation in this case).

on the proximal calcifications of the valve after having selected the optimal projection (Figs. 5.3–5.5). Optimal projection is that showing the aortic valve perpendicular to the screen, that is, showing only two cusps and not three. This requisite is crucial for optimal PHV positioning.

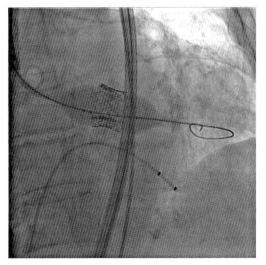

Figure 5.4 The Cribier–Edwards valve is delivered by balloon inflation under rapid pacing.

Clinical Experience with the Cribier PVT/Edwards Bioprosthesis

Following the report of our first PHV implant [2], initial patient series were selected on a compassionate basis after being formally declined for valve replacement by two independent cardiac surgeons. They were part of either the I-REVIVE trial (using either the antegrade or retrograde approach) or the RECAST trial (using solely the antegrade approach) [5,6]. Following these two feasibility trials conducted solely in our center in Rouen, patients were included in the multicenter European trial REVIVE (Registry of EndoVascular Implantation of Valves in Europe) in 2006 to 2007. The 1-year follow-up of this study is now completed and will soon be reported. The multicenter European PARTNER trial, evaluating both transfemoral and transapical implantations in a high-risk population, was partially presented at the TCT meeting in 2008 by Lefevre. Parallel to these studies in Europe, the REVIVAL II (tri-centric U.S. trial) and the Easy Access Canadian trial of Webb in Vancouver were conducted. Results of these series will be detailed below.

Feasibility Studies I—REVIVE and RECAST

The initial results of this "first in man" series of patients have been published and will not be detailed here [5]. In summary, these studies demonstrated the feasibility of the technique. Despite compassionate use in 36 patients, the implantation success rate was high (85%) and hemodynamic results were remarkable. Final AVA increased from 0.60 ± 0.11 cm^2 to 1.70 ± 0.10 cm^2 ($p < 0.0001$), and residual gradient was negligible (< 10 mm Hg). There was no coronary obstruction. Close clinical and echocardiographic follow-up did not show any valve dysfunction or secondary valve migration. One patient is alive 5 years after implantation with perfectly stable clinical and echocardiographic results. A second patient reached 4.5 years with similar results.

Retrograde Arterial Approach Studies

To enhance the effectiveness of the retrograde approach, a lower-profile system was needed with better ability to traverse the vascular system and aortic arch, as well as to overcome wire bias and resistance to crossing the native valve. Furthermore, because of the concern of PHV migration and paravalvular leaks, a larger-diameter PHV was designed and produced. These two major advances led to the revival of the retrograde arterial transfemoral approach. For regulatory reasons, these technological advances could not be used in France before 2006 and were evaluated initially by Webb and associates in Canada [11,12]. The technique was also evaluated in the United States in 55 patients in 3 centers included in the REVIVAL II trial.

Data on this retrograde transfemoral approach are growing, with more than 2000 patients implanted as of October 2008. After a preliminary series of 18 patients [11], Webb and coworkers reported in 2007 the updated series on 50 patients [12]. The procedural success rate was 86% and the 30-day mortality was 12%. Their data also showed improvement following a learning curve of 25 procedures. Final valve area increased from 0.6 ± 0.2 cm^2 to 1.7 ± 0.4 cm^2. Clinical and hemodynamic improvement was maintained at 1 year. The multicenter REVIVE trial in Europe/Canada (96 patients implanted) and the REVIVAL II trial in the United States (55 patients) are completed and were aimed at assessing the acute and 1-year results using this new technology. The results have been presented (S. Kodali, oral communication, TCT meeting 2008). Implantation success rate was 88% among 161 patients (83.5 ± 5.9 years). Thirty-day mortality was 8% in the REVIVAL II trial and 12% in the European REVIVE trial. One-year mortality was 27% among the overall group. Following the REVIVE trial in Europe, the PARTNER trial was conducted, evaluating the technique in a comparable high-risk population and using both the arterial transfemoral and the transapical approach. Preliminary results have been presented at the TCT meeting.

In September 2007, the Edwards–Sapien valve received the CE mark in the European Community, prompting diffusion of the technique and its utilization out of research protocol for high-risk individuals. Reported data of patients who underwent transcatheter valve placement in the European postmarketing SOURCE Registry (n = 598 patients) reveal a 95% success rate (TCT meeting, 2008). Thirty-day survival was 94%. Valve implantation was aborted in 2% due to failed arterial access and inability to cross the aortic valve. Intraprocedural death was 0.3%, cerebrovascular events 3%, and vascular complications 7%. These vascular complications increase mortality, suggesting the crucial role of careful patients selection for this approach.

Further improvements are on the way. In order to facilitate advancement of the PHV assembly up to and then across the stenotic aortic valve, a new delivery system (Harmony, Edwards Lifesciences, Irvine, CA) has been developed and is under investigation in Canada. A new-generation valve with a cobalt-chromium stent platform will decrease the device's profile by 4 to 5F, allowing a fully percutaneous procedure. This new valve is currently under clinical investigation in Vancouver.

The Transapical Approach

The transapical approach for PHV implantation has now been used since 2005 [13–16]. This approach offers the unique alternative therapy to patients with poor vascular access and impossibility of transfemoral Edwards valve implantation. The same Edwards PHV and its delivery catheter are introduced under direct vision into the left ventricle via a small left lateral thoracotomy, preferably in a hybrid operative suite. After ventricular puncture, a guidewire is used to cross the aortic valve under fluoroscopic guidance, and the rest of the procedure follows the same steps involved in valve preparation and deployment as described earlier for the retrograde technique. The introduction of the valve catheter requires the Ascendra Transapical Delivery System (Edwards Lifescience, Irvine, CA).

This technique obviates the concerns of vascular access in the presence of small-caliber vessels and/or vascular occlusive disease. It potentially reduces the risk of stroke related to passage of a stiff device through a diseased and tortuous aorta, as shown in a recently published series by Walther and associates [16]. Patients with a "porcelain aorta," previous cardiac surgery, or mediastinal radiation may be suitable for this approach. Currently, general anesthesia and mechanical ventilation are required, limiting the applicability in patients with chronic lung disease or other disorders that would contraindicate general anesthesia. The earliest and largest experience come from Leipzig [13]. Data on 59 patients from four centers were published in 2008 [16], followed by the results of the TRAVERCE Trial presented at the TCT meeting (preliminary results). Included were 168 patients from three centers in Germany (Heart Center, Leipzig, 116 patients; University Clinic, Frankfurt, 16 patients) and Austria (Medical University, Vienna, 36 patients). There was no intraprocedural death, and 12 patients (7%) were converted to open AVR for malposition, valve migration, or aortic insufficiency. The 12-month survival was 65%. Results of the transapical arm of the European PARTNER trial (67 patients; mean Logistic EuroScore: 34%; 9 centers) were also presented recently. The implant success rate was as high as 96%. The overall 6-month survival was 56% in comparison to 70% in TRAVERCE and 76% in the Leipzig series. Differences in outcomes have been reported, reflecting the complexity of the technique and importance of appropriate patient selection. Patients who require the transapical approach have a higher incidence of peripheral vascular disease, which is also associated with poorer long-term outcome.

The need for randomized trials that compare devices with surgery is clear. In this regard, the North American PARTNER (Placement of AoRTic traNscathetER) trial will be a landmark development in the emerging field of transcatheter valve therapies. This trial (Edwards–Sapien PHV) is currently enrolling patients in the United States and Canada. The primary end point is 1-year mortality. The trial includes patients with severe symptomatic AS who are poor surgical candidates and has two treatment arms: (1) an arm powered for noninferiority analysis compares traditional AVR to transcatheter AVR in patients with elevated surgical risk (STS score > 10%), while (2) a superiority analysis will be applied to the arm that compares medical treatment and balloon aortic valvuloplasty to transcatheter AVR. Results of this trial will determine the diffusion of transcatheter AVR, and will help establish conditions for future use.

In the future, the interventional cardiologist will have several technical alternatives to ensure the procedural success of PHV implantation, depending on various anatomic and clinical features.

Future Strategies

Pulmonary Valve and Degenerated Bioprosthetic Valve

Placement of PHV technology in the pulmonary position has been reported in animals [17]. Human implantation has been reported in an adolescent boy who had a prior Ross procedure with subsequent replacement with a homograft in the pulmonary position [18]. When the homograft became stenotic, the patient had stenting of the pulmonary valve followed by deployment of the Cribier–Edwards valve with a successful result.

Balloon valvuloplasty has been carried out for stenotic bioprosthetic valves in the aortic, tricuspid, or mitral positions [19–22]. Since the bioprosthetic "stent" can provide the means of anchoring the PHV, there is future potential for nonsurgical management of bioprosthetic valve failure with this balloon-expandable device [23]. A surgical valve-in-valve procedure has been performed in a patient with a failed bioprosthetic mitral valve, suggesting the feasibility of this approach [24].

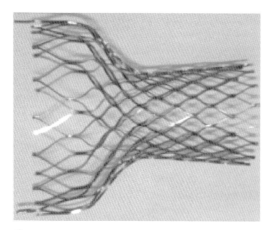

Figure 5.6 CoreValve side view of the self-expanding stented valve (exit to the left).

Medtronic Corevalve Revalving System

The second available PHV is the Medtronic CoreValve Revalving System first implanted in humans in 2004 [9], 2 years after the first human implantation with the Cribier–Edwards bioprosthesis.

Percutaneous Valve and Delivery Systems

The Medtronic CoreValve PHV is a self-expanding nitinol-stented porcine valve (Fig. 5.6), which is being developed for the treatment of aortic regurgitation and AS. The CoreValve prosthesis consists of a trileaflet bioprosthetic porcine pericardial tissue valve, which is mounted and sutured in a self-expanding nitinol stent frame. The lower portion of the prosthesis has high radial force to expand and exclude the calcified leaflets and to avoid recoil. The middle portion is constrained to avoid the coronary arteries, whereas the upper portion is flared to center and fix the stent frame firmly in the ascending aorta and to provide longitudinal stability and coaxial positioning. The prosthesis is sized according to the LVOT diameter. The system has the advantage of being self-centering and partially repositionable. The device was initially available on a 24F platform and was placed with extracorporeal circulation requiring full anesthesia and surgical cut-

down for valve placement. A second-generation 21F valve followed, which has since been replaced by an 18F device that makes it a truly percutaneous procedure. With generation three (18F), there are two different device sizes available for different annulus dimensions: the 26-mm prosthesis for aortic valve annulus sizes from 20 to 24 mm, and the 29-mm prosthesis for aortic valve annulus sizes from 24 to 27 mm.

Technical Aspects for PHV Implantation Using the Medtronic CoreValve Revalving System

Pretreatment includes acetylsalicylic acid (100 mg/day, indefinitely) and clopidogrel (600 mg loading dose followed by 75 mg/day for 6 to 12 months) orally at least 1 day before the procedure. In the initial series with 25F, 21F, and the beginning of 18F, the procedure was performed under general anesthesia; whereas later in the study local anesthesia with a mild systemic sedative/analgesic medication was sufficient. With the last 18F generation, the common femoral artery was the predominant access site with standard percutaneous access techniques and percutaneous closure using a preloaded Prostar XL suture device (Abbott Vascular, Abbott Park, Illinois).

As with the Edwards, the aortic valve is predilated. The prosthesis is then deployed and implanted within the aortic annulus over a stiff guidewire (Fig. 5.7). Postdilatation of the CoreValve prosthesis is performed at the discretion of the operator depending on the perceived proper placement of the device and the degree of aortic regurgitation (Fig. 5.8). Patients are followed clinically and by echocardiography during hospital stay, at 30 days, and 6 and 12 months after device implantation.

Clinical Experience with the Medtronic CoreValve Revalving System

More than 2000 patients have been treated with this technique. Published data from the original cohort that utilized 24F and 21F systems described a population of 25 patients [25]. The third-generation device using a 18F system was quickly

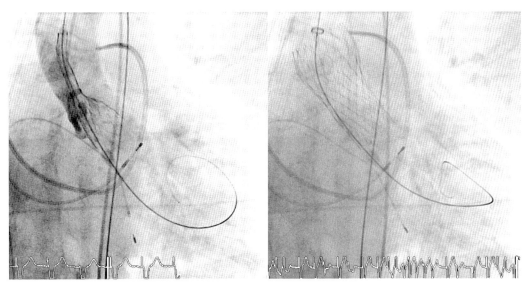

Figure 5.7 The CoreValve has been partially (*left panel*) and fully (*right panel*) deployed.

developed. The initial [26] immediate and midterm results with this device in 86 patients were promising, with a procedural success of 88% and a 30-day mortality of 12%. However, the risk of stroke (10%) and tamponade (7%) was non-negligible.

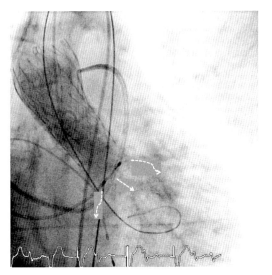

Figure 5.8 Moderate aortic regurgitation after CoreValve implantation (*arrows*) warranting final balloon dilatation

Patients included in the published registries had the following characteristics: (I) severe AS with a valve area < 1 cm^2, with or without aortic valve regurgitation and (1) age ≥ 80 years or a logistic EuroScore $\geq 20\%$ for the 25/21F group and age ≥ 75 years or logistic EuroScore $\geq 15\%$ for the 18F group, respectively; or (2) age ≥ 65 years with EuroScore $\geq 15\%$ and at least one of the following complicating criteria: cirrhosis of liver, pulmonary insufficiency (FEV < 1L), pulmonary hypertension (> 60 mm Hg), previous cardiac surgery, porcelain aorta, recurrent pulmonary embolus, or right ventricular insufficiency; (II) echocardiographic aortic valve annulus diameter ≥ 20 mm and ≤ 27 mm; and (III) diameter of the ascending aorta ≤ 45 mm at the sinotubular junction.

With the use of the 18F delivery system, circulatory support was no more used and the procedure became truly percutaneous without the need for surgical cutdown. CE mark was achieved in 2007, and since then a multicenter registry utilizing the 18F prosthesis has been created, encompassing currently over 2000 cases.

Recently, data on the largest single-center experience were published by Grube and associates [27] and showed a procedural success of 97% in a population of 136 patients with a logistic EuroScore of 23.1 ± 15.0% treated between 2005 and 2008. The femoral artery was the selected approach in 99% (all except 1 in the 18F group). An additional valve in valve placement was necessary in 3 patients (2.9%). There was no procedural death in the 18F group (102 patients). The procedural stroke rate was reduced to 2.9% compared with 10% and 4.2% in generation 1 (25F) and 2 (21F), respectively. There was no evidence of coronary occlusion with need for revascularization. Cardiac tamponade occurred in 2% of patients due to myocardial wire perforations using a very stiff wire, requiring open surgery with pericardial drainage. These 2 patients died. Overall 30-day mortality was 10%. The need for permanent pacemaker implantation after valve implantation, including both procedure-related atrioventricular blocks as well as medication-related bradycardias, was observed in 10% and 14% in generations 1 and 2, respectively, and 33% in the more recent 18F group. Hemodynamic results (postprocedural gradient: 8.1 ± 3.8 mm) remained stable over the 12-month follow-up period. Aortic regurgitation (always paravalvular) was more important before implantation in 26% of patients. There were only 2 cases of grade 3 regurgitation and no grade 4. Piazza and colleagues [28] recently reported similar 30-day results in a series of 646 patients included in the multicenter registry. Concerning the pacemaker implantation rate, Piazza and associates [29] reported a rate of 18% in their series of 40 consecutive patients in Rotterdam. This risk is lower with the Edwards system [6,30], with virtually no impact on the perivalvular anatomic structures. Sinahl and coworkers [30] reported a 6% rate of new and sustained complete AV block requiring permanent pacemakers. As illustrated by Piazza and associates [31], the close anatomic relationship between the aortic valvular complex and the branching AV bundle may provide an explanation for the observed increase in conductive disturbances observed after CoreValve implantation, the distal portion of which may protrude into the left ventricle by 5 to 10 mm.

At the present time, the two advantages of the CoreValve bioprosthesis include a smaller sheath size and the ability to reposition the valve before full deployment.

Other Competing Technologies

More than 10 other models of percutaneous aortic valves are under development. The most advanced experiences have been obtained with the Direct Flow (Santa Rosa, CA) [32], the Lotus (Sadra Medical, Saratoga, CA) [33], the AorTx (Palo Alto, CA), and the Paniagua valve.. First human implantation of a Direct Flow valve was performed in October 2007, followed by a feasibility study (8 patients) reported in 2008 by Low and associates [32]. Two patients received open surgical valve implantation while 6 patients underwent percutaneous implantation. Procedural success was achieved in 7 out of the 8 patients, with a mean postimplantation gradient of 17.9 ± 9.1 mm Hg. There was 1 death and all other patients subsequently received open AVR with explantation of the Direct Flow valve. A multicenter feasibility study has been recently started in Europe with this model of valve. Three implantations of the Lotus aortic valve were reported in 2008 [33].

Current Indications and Patient Selection

Patient selection is crucial for transcatheter success. To be considered for PHV, patients must have severe symptomatic aortic stenosis and be judged at too high a risk for open AVR. In addition, PHV should be offered to patients who have a potential for functional improvement after valve replacement with life expectancy over 1 year concerning comorbidities. In addition to these prerequisites, anatomic criteria must be met: diameter of aortic annulus (for both systems) and diameter of the aortic arch (for CoreValve only). If all these criteria are present, vascular access has to be evaluated by angiography and/or CT scan. A minimal iliofemoral size > 6 mm is required for the CoreValve and > 7 mm for the 23-mm Edwards (> 8 for the 26-mm valve). When vascular access is poor (diameter < 6–7 mm, excessive tortuosities, massive or circular calcifications), the transapical approach is an alternative with the Edwards–Sapien system. Transiliac implantation using a Dacron tube can also be proposed for the Edwards valve. A subclavian access can be used for the Medtronic CoreValve system, which cannot be reverted on the carrier catheter.

Conclusions

Initially complex, the procedures of percutaneous valve implantation have become simpler with fast technological improvement. With the current devices used, the hemodynamic results are excellent, leading to dramatic patient functional improvement. Thirty-day perivalvular complications are still an issue, but these are steadily decreasing with improved screening and experience. The long-term outcome is encouraging; it takes years for definitive conclusions. No valvular bioprosthesis dysfunction was reported so far, but valve and platform durability need to be demonstrated. The results of the pivotal randomized PARTNER study (Edwards–Sapien prosthesis) in the United States should provide the required evidence-based verification that transcatheter valve implantation is at least comparable to surgery in this high-risk population. Until then, a careful commercialization process including training and postmarket surveillance is crucial to avoid uncontrolled expansion.

The future of this technology and its application is dependent on the continued collaboration between general internists, cardiologists, surgeons, engineers, and industry. Because there is a substantial learning curve with each of the techniques and for each device, there must be collaboration between cardiologists and cardiac surgeons in order to disseminate the necessary knowledge and skills. There is a fundamental knowledge, skill set, and clinical wisdom of general physicians, imagers, interventionalists, and surgeons that must be shared, coordinated, and synchronized to ensure successful outcomes and future development of the new techniques.

References

1. Cribier A, Savin T, Saoudi N, *et al.* Percutaneous transluminal valvuloplasty of acquired aortic stenosis in elderly patients: an alternative to valve replacement? *Lancet*. 1986;1:63–67.
2. Cribier A, Eltchaninoff H, Bash A, *et al.* Percutaneous transcatheter implantation of an aortic valve prosthesis for calcific aortic stenosis: first human case description. *Circulation*. 2002;106:3006–3008.
3. Iung B, Baron G, Butchart EG, *et al.* A prospective survey of patients with valvular heart disease in Europe: the Euro Heart Survey on Valvular Heart Disease. *Eur Heart J*. 2003;24:1231–1243.
4. Eltchaninoff H, Nusimovici-Avadis D, Babaliaros V, *et al.* Five month study of ercutaneous heart valves in the systemic circulation of sheep using a novel model of aortic insufficiency. *EuroIntervention*. 2006;1:438–444.
5. Cribier A, Eltchaninoff H, Tron C, *et al.* Early experience with percutaneous transcatheter implantation of heart valve prosthesis for the treatment of end-stage inoperable patients with calcific aortic stenosis. *J Am Coll Cardiol*. 2004;43:698–703.
6. Cribier A, Eltchaninoff H, Tron C, *et al.* Treatment of calcific aortic stenosis with the percutaneous heart valve. Mid-term follow-up from the initial feasibility studies: the French experience. *J Am Coll Cardiol*. 2006;47:1214–1223.
7. Bauer F, Eltchaninoff H, Tron C, *et al.* Acute improvement in global and regional left ventricular systolic function after percutaneous heart valve implantation in patients with symptomatic aortic stenosis. *Circulation*. 2004;110:1473–1476.
8. Eltchaninoff H, Tron C, Cribier A. Percutaneous imlantation of aortic valve prosthesis in patients with calcific aortic stenosis: technical aspects. *J Interv Cardiol*. 2003;16:515–521.
9. Grube E, Laborde JC, Zickermann B, *et al.* First report on a human percutaneous transluminal implantation of a self expanding valve prosthesis for interventional treatment of aortic valve stenosis. *Catheter Cardiovasc Interv*. 2005;66:465–469.
10. Kahlert P, Eggebrecht H, Erbel R, *et al.* A modified "preclosure" technique after percutaneous aortic valve replacement. *Catheter Cardiovasc Interv*. 2008;72:877–884.
11. Webb GW, Chandavimol M, Thompson CR, *et al.* Percutaneous aortic valve implantation retrograde from the femoral artery. *Circulation*. 2006;113:842–850.
12. Webb JG, Pasupati S, Humphries K, *et al.* Percutaneous transarterial aortic valve replacement in selected high risk patients with aortic stenosis. *Circulation*. 2007;116:755–763.

13. Walther T, Dewey T, Wimmer-Greinecker G, *et al.* Transapical approach for sutureless stent-fixed aortic valve implantation: experimental results. *Eur J Cardiothorac Surg.* 2006;29:703–708.

14. Ye J, Cheung A, Lichtenstein SV, *et al.* Transapical aortic valve implantation in humans. *J Thorac Cardiovasc Surg.* 2006;13:1194–1196.

15. Lichtenstein SV, Cheung A, Ye J, *et al.* Transapical transcatheter aortic valve implantation in humans. Initial clinical experience. *Circulation.* 2006; 114:591–596.

16. Walther T, Simon P, Dewey T, *et al.* Transapical minimally invasive aortic valve implantation. Multicenter experience. *Circulation.* 2007;116(suppl):I240.

17. Garay F, Cao Q-L, Olin J, *et al.* The Edwards-Cribier percutaneous heart valve in the pulmonic position: initial animal experience. *EuroIntervention.* 2006;1(suppl):A32–A35.

18. Garay F, Webb J, Hijazi Z. Percutaneous replacement of pulmonary valve using the Edwards-Cribier percutaneous heart valve: first report in a human patient. *Catheter Cardiovasc Interv.* 2006;67:659–662.

19. Calvo OL, Sobrino N, Gamallo C. Balloon percutaneous valvuloplasty for stenotic bioprosthetic valves in the mitral position. *Am J Cardiol.* 1987;60:736–737.

20. Fert F, Stecy PJ, Nachaime MS. Percutaneous balloon valvuloplasty for stenosis of a porcine bioprosthesis in the tricuspid valve position. *Am J Cardiol.* 1986;58:363–364.

21. Waller BF, McKay C, VanTassel J, *et al.* Catheter balloon valvuloplasty of stenotic porcine bioprosthetic valves. II. Mechanisms, complications, and recommendations for clinical use. *Clin Cardiol.* 1991;14:764–772.

22. Kirwan C, Richardson G, Rothman MT, *et al.* Is there a role for balloon-valvuloplasty in patients with stenotic bioprosthetic valves? *Catheter Cardiovasc Interv.* 2004;63:251–253.

23. Wenaweser P, Buellesfeld L, Gerckens U, Grube E. Percutaneous aortic valve replacement for severe aortic regurgitation in degenerated bioprosthesis: the first valve in valve procedure using the Corevalve revalving system. *Catheter Cardiovasc Interv.* 2007;70:760–764.

24. Tateishi M. Valve-in-valve replacement of primary tissue valve failure of bovine pericardial valve. *Kyobu Geka.* 2006;59:61–64.

25. Grube E, Laborde JC, Gerckens U, *et al.* Percutaneous implantation of the CoreValve self-expanding valve prosthesis in high risk patients with aortic valve disease. The Siegburg first-in-man study. *Circulation.* 2006;114:1616–1624.

26. Grube E, Schuler G, Buellesfeld L, *et al.* Percutaneous aortic valve replacement for severe aortic stenosis in high-risk patients using the second- and current third-generation self-expanding CoreValve prosthesis: device success and 30-day clinical outcome. *J Am Coll Cardiol.* 2007;50:69–76.

27. Grube E, Buellesfeld L, Mueller R, *et al.* Progress and current status of percutaneous aortic valve replacement: results of three device generations of the CoreValve Revalving system. *Circ Cardiovasc Intervent.* 2008;1:167–175

28. Piazza N, Grube E, Gerckens U, *et al.* Procedural and 30-day outcomes following transcatheter aortic valve implantation using the third generation (18 Fr CoreValve Revalving system): results from the multicentre, expanded evaluation registry 1-year following CE mark approval. *EuroIntervention.* 2008;4: 242–249.

29. Piazza N, Onuma Y, Jesserun E, *et al.* Early and persistent intraventricular conduction abnormalities and requirements for pacemaking after percutaneous replacement of the aortic valve. *J Am Coll Cardiol.* 2008;1:310–316.

30. Sinahl A, Altwegg L, Opasupati S, *et al.* Atrioventricular block after transcatheter balloon expandable aortic valve implantation. *J Am Coll Cardiol.* 2008;1:305–309.

31. Piazza N, de Jaegere P, Schultz, *et al.* Anatomy of the aortic valvar complex and its implications for transcatheter implantation of the aortic valve. *Circulation Intervent.* 2008;1:74–81.

32. Low RI, Bolling SF, Yeo KK, *et al.* Direct Flow Medical percutaneous aortic valve: proof of concept. *EuroIntervention.* 2008;4:256–261.

33. Buellesfeld L, Gerckens U, Grube E. Percutaneous implantation of the first repositionable aortic valve prosthesis in a patient with severe aortic stenosis. *Catheter Cardiovasc Diagn.* 2008;71:579–584.

CHAPTER 6

Patent Foramen Ovale Closure

Bernhard Meier

Cardiology, Swiss Cardiovascular Center Bern, University Hospital Bern, Bern, Switzerland

---

Chapter Overview

- A patent foramen ovale (PFO) is present in one-third to one-fourth of the population, decreasing with age.
- A PFO is a proven cause for systemic embolism (brain, eye, heart, kidney, etc).
- The risk of a PFO is small and dependent on PFO characteristics (opening width, atrial septal aneurysm, Eustachian valve, etc).
- A PFO may also be causally involved in a number of other problems (migraine, diving incidence, platypnea orthodeoxia, economy class stroke syndrome, sleep apnea, etc).
- Modern techniques allow reliable closure in an outpatient procedure with minimal risk.
- Observational proof of the benefit of PFO closure is abundant but not yet corroborated by randomized trials.

What is a Patent Foramen Ovale?

The patent foramen ovale (PFO) is a flap-like opening between the two atria of the heart (Fig. 6.1). This structure is essential during intrauterine life. The lungs are not yet functioning and collapsed, inducing a high resistance in the pulmonary circulation. This increases the right atrial pressure and the PFO stays constantly and maximally ajar. This affords the oxygenized blood from the placenta direct access to the left heart and the systemic circulation. After birth, the lungs unfold and the right atrial pressure falls below the left atrial pressure. The flap-valve consisting of the septum primum closes the PFO (the superior rim of the septum primum leans against the inferior rim of the septum secundum). Normally the two septa fuse permanently thereafter.

Prevalence of PFOs

The reported prevalence of PFOs depends on the methods of screening and the cohort examined. An autopsy study encompassing roughly 1000 cadavers deceased at any age and of any cause found an almost linear decrease of the prevalence of a PFO from 35% to 23% with increasing age [1]. This decrease was interpreted as evidence for continued closure of the PFO throughout the lifetime. What cannot be ruled out is a selective mortality of PFO carriers. They are, so to speak, weeded out. With transthoracic echocardiography, a rather poor tool to diagnose or exclude a PFO, the prevalence varies between 7% and 24% [2,3]. Transesophageal echocardiography is more uncomfortable for the patient but currently the only reliable technique to diagnose a PFO. Several respective studies indicated a prevalence of 20% to 40% [4–6]. Transcranial Doppler studies are based on the same principle as contrast echocardiography. Small bubbles are created by shaking air either into saline, blood, or a gel that does not pass the lung barrier. A bolus of this mixture is then injected into a vein at the end of a sustained (ideally 20 seconds

Current Best Practice in Interventional Cardiology. Edited by B Meier. © 2010 Blackwell Publishing.

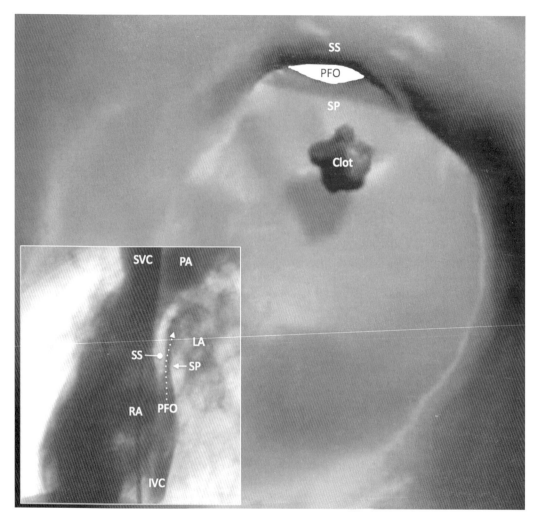

Figure 6.1 Interatrial septum seen from the right atrium (RA). The patent foramen ovale (PFO) is shown as a rent opened by a movement of the top rim of the septum primum (SP) into the left atrium (LA) away from the septum secundum (SS). This provides a passage from the RA to LA for contrast medium (insert showing a lateral x-ray picture of the heart) or clots. A left-to-right shunt will be prevented by the SP apposing the SS, thereby closing the PFO. (IVC, inferior vena cava; PA, pulmonary artery; SVC, superior vena cava.)

or more) Valsalva maneuver. At the release of such a Valsalva maneuver, both atria are volume depleted, and the venous blood from the extrathoracic space replenishes first the right atrium, hence pushing the PFO open. Absence of any contrast in the left atrium or the systemic circulation excludes a PFO with high specificity. Detecting bubbles within a few heartbeats (before the blood tsunami has passed the pulmonary circu-lation) either in the left atrium (echocardiography) or in one of the intracerebral arteries (transcranial Doppler technique) proves a right-to-left shunt but not necessarily a PFO. It is not clear why the only detection algorithm outside of the heart concentrates on the difficult-to-access intracerebral arteries. Any peripheral artery of small caliber would do, such as extracranial or digital arteries. In large-caliber arteries, bubbles passing by

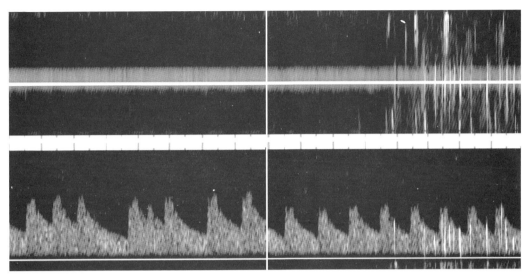

Figure 6.2 Power motion-mode transcranial Doppler bubble test after Valsalva. The picture in the left panel excludes a right-to-left shunt, the picture in the right panel proves it (arrival of high-intensity signals [HITs] in the middle cerebral artery, depicted by spikes and audible by crackles).

may be missed by the focused ultrasound. The criteria for documenting a right-to-left shunt by cranial Doppler examination have been defined in a consensus conference [7]. Figure 6.2 shows examples. The ultimate proof for a PFO can be provided by unequivocally documenting a Doppler passage or bubble shunt through the PFO by transesophageal echocardiography (Fig. 6.3).

Medical Interest in PFOs

The first description of the foramen ovale dates reportedly back to 1564, naming Leonardo Botallo, an Italian "surgeon," as author [8]. Julius Cohnheim, a German pathologist, first correlated a stroke to a PFO found at autopsy [9]. While the PFO continued to be mentioned occasionally

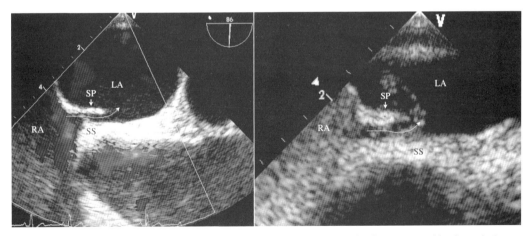

Figure 6.3 Transesophageal echocardiography. The left panel shows Doppler flow (*grey speckle*) through the rent between the right atrium (RA) and the left atrium (LA) and the right panel shows bubbles migrating through the PFO. The PFO channel is marked by a dashed arrow. (SP, septum primum; SS, septum secundum.)

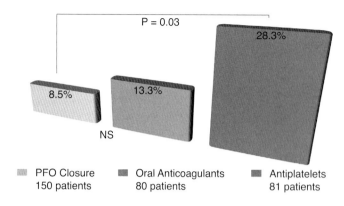

Figure 6.4 Recurrent death, stroke, or transient ischemic attack over 4 years in contemporary patients with an initial cerebral event and random treatment with PFO closure, oral anticoagulants, or antiplatelets (typically acetylsalicylic acid) [17].

as a possible cause of stroke [2,3,10], it moved to the front of the stage after an easy way of prevention (percutaneous PFO closure) was first reported [11]. Later reports tried to sort out what subtype of patients this treatment could and should be offered to [12–14]. More recently, interest has somewhat faded, with epidemiologic surveys failing to unequivocally document a causal relationship between the PFO and stroke [15,16]. Results of randomized trials for stroke prevention by device closure of the PFO may or may not rekindle the interest. A matched-control registry on about 350 patients treated with acetylsalicylic acid (about one-fourth), warfarin (about one-fourth), or device closure (about half) showed superior results with either device closure or warfarin compared to those achieved with acetylsalicylic acid at about 4 years (Fig. 6.4) [17]. This would suggest that the choice is between lifelong oral anticoagulation and device closure. A similar registry followed for 10 years showed device closure also superior to warfarin [18]. The currently running randomized trials (some still enrolling patients, some having closed enrollment but not completed following-up patients) may fail their defined end points. They were based on registry data indicating annual events of recurrent ischemic cerebral attacks under conservative therapy in 3% to 5% of patients. Fewer than 10% of patients evaluated with an index cerebral event and a PFO were randomized in these trials. This results in the fact that the low-risk patient-type dominates in the randomized cohorts. Hence, the overall incidence of events may be much smaller and the power calculations thus underestimated the number of patients or duration of follow-up necessary to show a true advantage of PFO closure over oral anticoagulation or antiplatelets (typically acetylsalicylic acid).

Clinical Assessment of PFO Risk

An important paper quantified the risk of having a recurrent ischemic event over 4 years as indifferent from a normal population in patients with an atrial septal aneurysm (ASA) without a PFO and patients with a PFO without an ASA (only 10 such patients included), but 3-fold increased in patients with both PFO and ASA [12]. A meta-analysis showed the prevalence of a PFO being 3-fold in patients with a prior stroke compared to controls, while the prevalence of a PFO and an ASA was 16-fold. Comparing cryptogenic stroke with controls, the respective prevalences were 5-fold and 24-fold, respectively [19]. The correlation was only significant for patients younger than 55 years. This is in stark contrast to the fact that venous thrombotic events (a prerequisite for paradoxical embolism, albeit not necessarily clinically apparent) are virtually absent in children and adolescents (so are embolic events ascribed to the PFO), rare during middle age, but steeply increasing in frequency after the age of 55 years [20]. It can be extrapolated that yearly 0.6% of octogenarians suffer from clinically apparent venous thrombotic events. More in keeping with these facts are data from a study of consecutive stroke patients (about 50% with an identified potential conventional cause such as atherosclerosis, prior myocardial infarction, or significant atrial arrhythmia) showing a positive association with the presence of a PFO also for the roughly two-thirds older than 55 years in addition to the one-third younger than 55 years.

In light of the increasing prevalence of venous thrombosis with age, the established and rather trivial increase of peripheral systemic embolism (14-fold increase) and mortality (2-fold increase) by the presence of a PFO in case of a clinically relevant pulmonary embolism [21] portends an ominous picture for the potential of a PFO to cause harm. This is corroborated by a large Danish database proving that the relative risk of myocardial infarction or stroke is significantly increased during and immediately after venous thromboembolism. The authors surprisingly failed to acknowledge the presence of a PFO to be expected in the usual percentage of these individuals as the most likely reason for it [22]. Moreover, the alarming increase of cerebral defects with increasing age in men and women demonstrable by magnetic resonance imaging can best be explained by the fact that a PFO is quite prevalent among the normal population [23]. Again, the authors failed to mention the causative role of the PFO for their findings while indicting a large number of much less likely mechanisms.

Among the large number of clinical situations possibly caused by a PFO (Table 6.1) [24], most attention was paid to the relationship between PFO and migraine apart from the stroke connection. Two issues explain the vested interest in the migraine–PFO connection. First, attenuation of migraine symptoms is appreciated by patients as an immediate subjective benefit. PFO closures for secondary prevention of systemic embolism lack that feature. Second, there is hope among physicians and device manufacturers alike that a significant benefit of PFO closure in migraineurs can be proved within a couple of years, because only a short follow-up is required. Proof of the prognostically important prevention of embolic events may take decades due to their scarcity.

Table 6.1 Ailments Causally Related to PFO

Anecdotally Proved
  Stroke
  Transient ischemic attack
  Myocardial infarction
  Embolic infarction of other organs
  Ischemia of legs or arms
  Economy class stroke syndrome
  Decompression illness in divers
  Platypnea orthodeoxia

Suggestive
  Sleep apnea syndrome
  Migraine with and without aura
  High-altitude pulmonary edema
  Excessive snoring
  Air or fat embolism during
    Major orthopedic surgery
    Brain surgery in sitting position

Percutaneous PFO Closure

Catheter-based percutaneous PFO closure derives from a technique for percutaneous atrial septal defect (ASD) closure described by King and Mills in 1974 [25]. It thus preceded percutaneous coronary angioplasty, which is generally considered the starting point in modern interventional cardiology. The potential of PFO closure to become as frequent or even more frequent than coronary angioplasty may prompt a historical milestone (launch of interventional cardiology) to someday shift from 1977 to 1974.

The kick-off for percutaneous closure of PFO rather than ASD dates back to 1992 and the publication of Bridges and colleagues [11]. Slowly, the medical community began to realize that PFO is a much more common blemish in adults than ASD, and that to close a PFO percutaneously is extremely straightforward in contrast to percutaneous closure of larger ASDs.

With the clinical introduction of the ingeniously conceived and biocompatibly manufactured dedicated Amplatzer PFO occluder in 1997, the procedure was definitely launched. Kurt Amplatz, a retired radiologist and one of the greatest inventors in invasive medicine, traveled with his first device

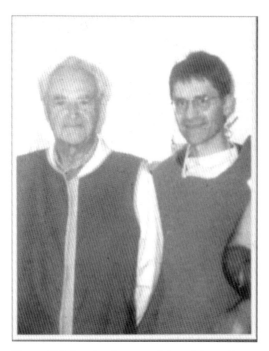

Figure 6.5 Kurt Amplatz, MD (*left*) and the author on the occasion of the world's first implantation of an Amplatzer PFO occluder in Switzerland on September 10, 1997.

Table 6.2 Frugal Technique of Amplatzer PFO Occlusion

Procedure
- No hospitalization required
- No echocardiographic guidance required
- Local anesthesia of groin
- Access preferably through right femoral vein (straight access to atrial septum)
- Heparin bolus of 5000 units
- Normal stiffness and length 0.035-inch guidewire for catheter access
- Crossing PFO with naked wire, wire directed by (multipurpose) catheter, or catheter directly
- No balloon gauging
- 9F sheath (fits all Amplatzer PFO occluder sizes)
- Right atrial hand injections of contrast medium for position control
- One shot of antibiotics (eg, cephalosporin) during the procedure

Follow-up
- 1 or 2 additional shots of antibiotics in the following hours
- Unrestricted physical activity after a few hours
- Acetylsalicylic acid (100 mg per day) for 5 months
- Clopidogrel (75 mg per day) for 1 month
- Prophylaxis against endocarditis for about 3 months
- Final TEE control at 6 months (1 month after stopping platelet inhibitors)

to Switzerland to perform the intervention together with the author (Fig. 6.5). His technique and others rapidly became routine in countries where closure devices were available and reimbursed.

Technique

It is commonly accepted that percutaneous PFO closure is the most simple interventional procedure in cardiology. There remain some controversies about how frugally it can be performed without compromising safety and results.

Table 6.2 summarizes the salient steps of the procedure. In about half of the cases, a curved U-tip guidewire will pass through the PFO without really looking for it. Using a straight guidewire increases that percentage, but makes moving up from the groin to the right atrium more tedious. In case several passages of the U-tip wire through the right atrium fail to find the PFO, the attempt is repeated after introducing a curved catheter (multipurpose shape suited best) just below the diaphragm pointing medially. This directs the guidewire path more ideally towards the atrial septum. Straightening the tip of the guidewire, or replacing a curved wire with a straight guidewire, again increases the chance of passing the PFO in case of a tiny rent.

Should this still not allow passage, the tip of the catheter is pushed upwards stroking the atrial septum and immediately torqued left or right, if it gets caught by a bulge in the septum, which usually is the fleshy lower rim of the septum secundum. Figure 6.6 shows a PFO that could only be passed using catheter and guidewire expertly and jointly. In cases where a TEE has clearly shown bubbles passing through a gap between septum primum and septum secundum (Fig. 6.7), technical success

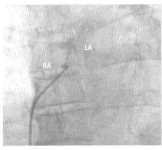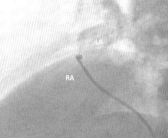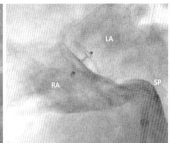

Figure 6.6 Difficult to canulate PFO. The tip of the catheter pinpoints it in an antero-posterior projection (*left panel*) and a left-anterior-oblique projection (*center panel*). The PFO was passed with a straight wire after which an Amplatzer 25-mm PFO occluder could be easily implanted (*right panel*). The aneurysmatic shape of the septum primum (SP) is apparent during final dye injection (right panel). (LA, left atrium; RA, right atrium; SP, septum primum; SS, septum secundum.)

including safe placement of an Amplatzer PFO occluder can virtually be guaranteed.

Once a wire is across the PFO, the device is prepared before a sheath is introduced to restrict indwelling time of the sheath to a minimum. Care is taken not to tighten the connecting screw on the pusher cable too much on the device. This avoids the otherwise not infrequent problem that upon attempt to release the device, the device rotates with the pusher cable rather than severing from it. If that

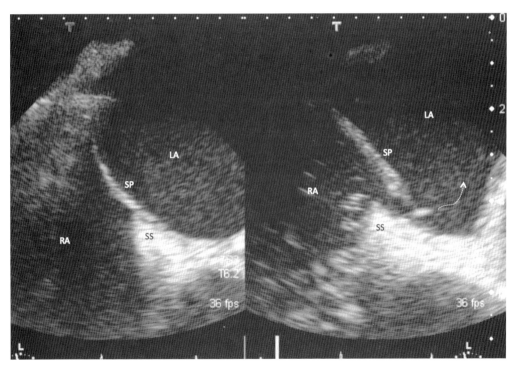

Figure 6.7 Transesophageal echocardiography before (*left panel*) and during (*right panel*) bubble contrasting. A single bubble is caught migrating through the PFO rent (*arrow* indicating its path). This already proves the PFO and guarantees technical success of closure. (LA, left atrium; RA, right atrium; SP, septum primum; SS, septum secundum.)

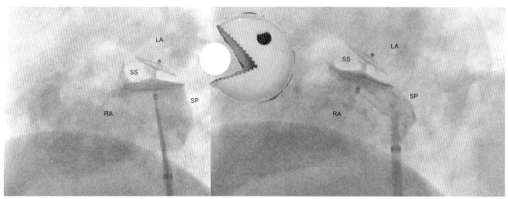

Figure 6.8 Fluoroscopy assessment of correct position before (*left panel*) and after (*right panel*) release of the occluder from the pusher cable. The projection is chosen so that the two device disks are shown in perfect profile without any overlap. A small injection of contrast medium through the sheath delineates the septum secundum (SS) as a white speckle into which the left (cranial) half of the device seems to bite. This invites the allusion to the arcade figure Pacman biting into a white dot. The PFO channel itself is seen as an oblique tunnel between the device disks. The septum primum (SP) is a thin membrane emerging from the right (caudal) side of the device. (LA, left atrium; RA, right atrium.)

occurs, it can be partially retracted into the sheath to increase friction and allow the screw to come off. A jerk while starting to unscrew may also help, not unlike the jerk used to loosen a wheel nut of a car.

To assure correct position before and after release, echocardiography is not required. Figure 6.8 shows that the so-called Pacman sign can be well demonstrated by fluoroscopy using the correct projection and a small amount of contrast medium. Occasionally a device proves too small and has to be exchanged before release from the pusher (Fig. 6.9).

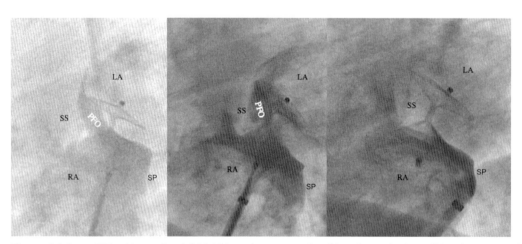

Figure 6.9 Large PFO with associated ASA (thin and pliable septum primum), requiring substitution of a 35-mm Amplatzer occluder (right disk 35 mm, left disk 25 mm) for the initially planned 25-mm Amplatzer occluder (right disk 25m, left disk 18 mm). The left disk did not reach the top of the PFO arch (*left panel*). It was replaced by a larger device, still barely covering the PFO (*central panel*) but showing an angiographically complete closure after release from the pusher cable (*right panel*). (LA, left atrium; RA, right atrium; SP, septum primum; SS, septum secundum.)

As the procedure only implies a venous puncture, the patient can put his or her finger on the puncture site while the operator is removing the sheath at the end of the intervention. The patient can then walk out of the catheterization laboratory. The venous pressure in a supine position is less than 10 mm Hg. When getting up, it climbs to about 50 mm Hg (dependent on the height of the patient, ie, the weight of the blood column from the top of the head to the groin). This means that the finger pressure on the puncture site has to be increased while the patient is erect but can be light while lying down. After an hour or two, the venous puncture should be healed and from then on, any type of physical exercise is allowed. There is no need to refrain from moving, coughing, or even straining. The device sits firmly in the septum and the septum moves vigorously and constantly, anyhow, irrespective of what the individual is doing.

Complications

Using the safest device, the Amplatzer PFO occluder, complications are extremely rare. The only significant complication occurring in our last 1000 consecutive PFO closures with this device were arteriovenous fistulae at the groin, occurring in less than 1%. In addition, more than half of our patients underwent concomitant coronary angiography requiring an additional arterial puncture, so that the incidence of this problem is bound to be even rarer if PFO closure is perfomed or analyzed separately. Table 6.3 provides a list of potential or reported complications of device-based PFO closure [26,27]. The report of an incidence of aortic regurgitation following PFO device closure in about 10% [27] appears odd considering the fact that we have never observed it in over 1000 TEE follow-up examinations.

Results

The literature abounds with single-center and multicenter data describing excellent outcome after PFO closure for prevention of recurrence of cere-

Table 6.3 Potential Complications of PFO Closure (Ranked per Frequency)

- Residual shunts (rather an imperfection than a complication)
- Atrial palpitation (about 20% early on, rare later)
- Arteriovenous fistula at puncture site
- New onset of migraine (significantly less frequent than improvement of migraine)
- Device embolization (risk dependent on device brand and size used)
- Thrombotic material on device (risk dependent on device brand used)
- Atrial fibrillation (practically only in elderly patients)
- Free atrial wall erosion (4 per 100,000 cases reported with Amplatzer PFO occluder)
- Compromise of valves (reported in 1 paper but unconfirmed) [27]

bral attacks. However, considering the benign natural course under warfarin, acetylsalicylic acid, or no treatment, this does not yet prove that that the PFO should be closed. The report coming closest to a randomized trial suggests that warfarin is the better treatment than acetylsalicylic acid, and device closure parallels if not outdoes warfarin (Fig. 6.4) [17].

It can be surmised that the protective effect will materialize sooner or later in the light of the safety of the current technique (particularly using the Amplatzer occluder), the uncontested hazard of the PFO to do evil, and the long life expectancy of typical patients undergoing PFO closure. However, this may take decades and the benefit is difficult to document, because events not taking place can only be indirectly proved by counting events in control groups of randomized trials. And then again, is it really ethical to keep patients in control arms of randomized trials for such a long time while the ones with device closure are having no problems from their trivial intervention and are being protected against paradoxical embolism for good? Admittedly, the complete closure rate being only 90% even with the best of devices, this protection is not 100% assured. Notwithstanding, even a residual shunt may mean a drastically reduced risk of paradoxical embolism, particularly if the shunt meanders through the device in a serpentine channel. In contrast to the straight shot a clot finds through a classical PFO, this is an unlikely path for particulate matter.

Of course, a complete protection against embolic events cannot even be guaranteed with complete closure of the PFO. There may be additional atrial shunts; typical are unrecognized small ASDs in an ASA. There is also the possibility that the closed PFO represented a small hole in one edge of the PFO mouth (imagine one edge of the mouth slightly open while the remainder of the mouth is shut). In such a situation there may well coexist a small opening in the opposite edge of the PFO mouth. Such a situation represents in a way two PFOs (Fig. 6.10).

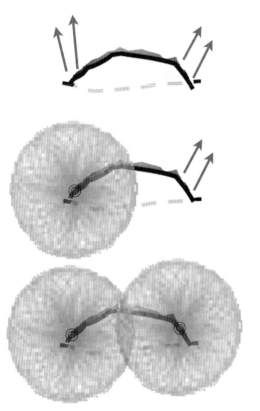

Figure 6.10 "Double" PFO. The mouth of the PFO is fused centrally but leaves two openings in its edges (*top panel*). Initial implantation of one PFO occluder leaves behind a residual shunt through the opposite edge (*central panel*). A second device is required to completely occlude this "double" PFO (*bottom panel*).

Moreover, emboli may cross via alternate pathways from the pulmonary into the systemic circulation (pulmonary fistulae). Finally, the entire venous bed of the pulmonary circulation remains a potential source of systemic emboli, although it is hardly mentioned as such and has remained one of the few remaining black boxes of the human body.

Outlook

PFO closure still leads a Cinderella-like life 35 years after it has been proved doable, 17 years after it has been called mandated at least in some patients, and 12 years after it has found an almost infallible technical solution with the Amplatzer PFO occluder.

The trick of using the quality-of-life issue of migraine to put the foot in the door and find a generally approved indication for PFO closure has failed so far. This is mostly due to the fact that the first respective randomized trial was planned with an unreasonable primary end point (cure of migraine in at least half of the patients), performed with a rather poor device, providing a low closure rate, and being fraught with a non-negligible percentage of implantation problems [28]. The fact that in the small group of about 70 patients being observed conservatively, 1 patient suffered a stroke during the short follow-up period, should compellingly point to why the PFO should really be closed (prevention of stroke). Having said that, the medical literature does not allow anecdotal evidence in potentially important matters.

The various randomized trials looking at PFO closure for stroke prevention have been running for as long as 9 years and have enrolled over 1000 patients. Nonetheless, premature analysis of the outcome may result in failing the somewhat overly ambitious end points. The control patients as well as the treated patients are typically at the low end of the risk strata (concerning number of prior events, association of aggravating factors such as ASA, Eustachian valve [29], or Valsalva-prone professions or hobbies). Hence, events may be absent entirely during the follow-up period or are at least extremely rare.

Should the idea of having a low threshold for PFO closure after an initial event or even performing it as primary prevention in high-risk individuals (eg, large PFO with an ASA) be permanently or at least for a significant amount of time abandoned because of these trials [8], this would mean that thousands of easily preventable strokes, myocardial infarctions, and other events will continue to happen and we should feel responsible for them [30,31].

References

1. Hagen PT, Scholz DG, Edwards WD. Incidence and size of patent foramen ovale during the first 10 decades of life: an autopsy study of 965 normal hearts. *Mayo Clin Proc.* 1984;59:17–20.

2. Lechat P, Mas JL, Lascault G, *et al.* Prevalence of patent foramen ovale in patients with stroke. *N Engl J Med.* 1988;318:1148–1152.

3. Webster MW, Chancellor AM, Smith HJ, *et al.* Patent foramen ovale in young stroke patients. *Lancet.* 1988;2:11–12.

4. Hausmann D, Mugge A, Becht I, Daniel WG. Diagnosis of patent foramen ovale by transesophageal echocardiography and association with cerebral and peripheral embolic events. *Am J Cardiol.* 1992;70:668–672.

5. Van Camp G, Schulze D, Cosyns B, Vandenbossche JL. Relation between patent foramen ovale and unexplained stroke. *Am J Cardiol.* 1993;71:596–598.

6. Meissner I, Whisnant JP, Khandheria BK, *et al.* Prevalence of potential risk factors for stroke assessed by transesophageal echocardiography and carotid ultrasonography: the SPARC study. Stroke Prevention: Assessment of Risk in a Community. *Mayo Clin Proc.* 1999;74:862–869.

7. Jauss M, Zanette E. Detection of right-to-left shunt with ultrasound contrast agent and transcranial Doppler sonography. *Cerebrovasc Dis.* 2000;10:490–496.

8. Messe SR, Kasner SE. Is closure recommended for patent foramen ovale and cryptogenic stroke? Patent foramen ovale in cryptogenic stroke: not to close. *Circulation.* 2008;118:1999–2004.

9. Cohnheim J. *Thrombose und Embolie: Vorlesung über allgemeine Pathologie.* Berlin: Hirschwald; 1877:134.

10. Loscalzo J. Paradoxical embolism: clinical presentation, diagnostic strategies, and therapeutic options. *Am Heart J.* 1986;112:141–145.

11. Bridges ND, Hellenbrand W, Latson L, Filiano J, Newburger JW, Lock JE. Transcatheter closure of patent foramen ovale after presumed paradoxical embolism. *Circulation.* 1992;86:1902–1908.

12. Mas JL, Arquizan C, Lamy C, *et al.* Recurrent cerebrovascular events associated with patent foramen ovale, atrial septal aneurysm, or both. *N Engl J Med.* 2001;345:1740–1746.

13. Homma S, Sacco RL, Di Tullio MR, Sciacca RR, Mohr JP. Effect of medical treatment in stroke patients with patent foramen ovale: patent foramen ovale in cryptogenic stroke study. *Circulation.* 2002;105:2625–2631.

14. Meier B, Lock JE. Contemporary management of patent foramen ovale. *Circulation.* 2003;107:5–9.

15. Di Tullio MR, Sacco RL, Sciacca RR, Jin Z, Homma S. Patent foramen ovale and the risk of ischemic stroke in a multiethnic population. *J Am Coll Cardiol.* 2007;49:797–802.

16. Serena J, Marti-Fabregas J, Santamarina E, *et al.* Recurrent stroke and massive right-to-left shunt. Results from the prospective Spanish multicenter (CODICIA) study. *Stroke.* 2008;39:3131–3136.

17. Windecker S, Wahl A, Nedeltchev K, *et al.* Comparison of medical treatment with percutaneous closure of patent foramen ovale in patients with cryptogenic stroke. *J Am Coll Cardiol.* 2004;44:750–758.

18. Schuchlenz HW, Weihs W, Berghold A, Lechner A, Schmidt R. Secondary prevention after cryptogenic cerebrovascular events in patients with patent foramen ovale. *Int J Cardiol.* 2005;101:77–82.

19. Overell JR, Bone I, Lees KR. Interatrial septal abnormalities and stroke: a meta-analysis of case-control studies. *Neurology.* 2000;55:1172–1179.

20. Anderson FA Jr., Wheeler HB, Goldberg RJ, *et al.* A population-based perspective of the hospital incidence and case-fatality rates of deep vein thrombosis and pulmonary embolism. *The Worcester DVT Study.* Arch Intern Med. 1991;151:933–938.

21. Konstantinides S, Geibel A, Kasper W, Olschewski M, Blumel L, Just H. Patent foramen ovale is an important predictor of adverse outcome in patients with major pulmonary embolism. *Circulation.* 1998;97:1946–1951.

22. Soerensen H, Horvath-Puho E, Pedersen L, Baron JA, Prandoni P. Venous thromboembolism and subsequent hospitalisation due to acute arterial cardiovascular events: a 20-year cohort study. *Lancet.* 2007;370:1773–1779.

23. Das RR, Seshadri S, Beiser AS, *et al.* Prevalence and correlates of silent cerebral infarcts in

the Framingham Offspring Study. *Stroke*. 2008;39: 2929–2935.

24. Meier B. Stroke and migraine: a cardiologist's headache. *Heart*. 2009;95:595–602.

25. King TD, Mills NL. Nonoperative closure of atrial septal defects. *Surgery*. 1974;75:383–388.

26. Kleber FX, Stretz A. Percutaneous closure of patent foramen ovale. *Swiss Med Wkly*. 2008;138:564–566.

27. Schoen SP, Boscheri A, Lange SA, *et al.* Incidence of aortic valve regurgitation and outcome after percutaneous closure of atrial septal defects and patent foramen ovale. *Heart.* 2008;94:844–847.

28. Dowson A, Mullen MJ, Peatfield R, *et al.* Migraine Intervention With STARFlex Technology (MIST) trial: a prospective, multicenter, double-blind, sham-controlled trial to evaluate the effectiveness of patent foramen ovale closure with STARFlex septal repair implant to resolve refractory migraine headache. *Circulation.* 2008;117:1397–1404.

29. Schuchlenz HW, Saurer G, Weihs W, Rehak P. Persisting eustachian valve in adults: relation to patent foramen ovale and cerebrovascular events. *J Am Soc Echocardiogr.* 2004;17:231–233.

30. Windecker S, Meier B. Is closure recommended for patent foramen ovale and cryptogenic stroke? Patent foramen ovale and cryptogenic stroke: to close or not to close? Closure: what else! *Circulation.* 2008;118:1989–1998.

31. Windecker S, Meier B. Is closure recommended for patent foramen ovale and cryptogenic stroke? Response to Messé SR and Kasner SE. *Circulation.* 2008;118:2004.

CHAPTER 7

Closure of Atrial and Ventricular Septal Defects in Adults

David Hildick-Smith

Sussex Cardiac Centre, Brighton and Sussex University Hospital NHS Trust, Brighton, UK

Chapter Overview

- Atrial septal defects > 8 mm diameter usually warrant closure now that procedural and long-term risks are low.
- A deficient anterosuperior rim is not a contraindication for closure.
- The Amplatzer device remains the most appropriate device for the majority of ASDs.
- VSD closure in adulthood is a low-volume specialist procedure.
- Postinfarction VSDs should be considered for interventional rather than surgical management if expertise is available, but not all cases are technically suitable.

Atrial Septal Defects

What Size Needs Closing?

Since percutaneous closure of an atrial septal defect (ASD) was first conceived, the available devices, equipment, and imaging techniques have improved to such an extent that the procedure can now be considered relatively routine in the majority of cases. As a result, the threshold at which ASD closure is considered has gradually come down. Historically, the traditional threshold for ASD closure was when the pulmonary to systemic shunt ratio was 2:1. This has now lessened to around 1.5:1, and indeed often the exact Qp:Qs is not measured.

In adult patients, the diagnosis of an atrial septal defect may be made due to investigation of lesion-specific symptoms; but just as often, because of the high-quality imaging techniques now available, the diagnosis is frequently "incidental." Patients who have an atrial septal defect $\geq$ 1 cm in diameter are certainly at risk of atrial fibrillation and right heart volume overload in the fullness of time and should have the defect closed [1]. Equally, patients who have a defect of 3 mm are not at risk of hemodynamic complications, so the only indication to close would be due to paradoxical embolism. Somewhere in the middle is a threshold at which it is reasonable to undertake ASD closure now that the procedure risks are relatively low and the long-term outlook postprocedure is good. Individual operators will have different thresholds, accounting for the fact that the smaller the defect, the easier the closure will be. But in general it is reasonable to consider percutaneous closure for ASDs > 6 to 8 mm.

What Age is Too Old?

Patients are never too old to be considered for ASD closure. Indeed, very good results can be achieved in this age group providing patient selection is good [2]. Clearly, however, the risks of the procedure rise with age and there is no need to consider an

Current Best Practice in Interventional Cardiology. Edited by B Meier. © 2010 Blackwell Publishing.

80-year-old man in whom an incidental 6-mm ASD has been found for ASD closure. Conversely, elderly patients with right heart failure who turn out to have a significant ASD can still be considered for ASD closure but have to be carefully managed. Such patients are often in a brittle state of hemodynamic balance, with moderately raised pulmonary artery pressures, and can be prone to acute pulmonary edema in the immediate postoperative period [3], such that they need to be managed on a high-dependency area during this time. As with most interventional procedures, however, although the elderly are at highest risk, they may also have the most to gain. Those who are beginning to decompensate due to right heart failure from an ASD can do extremely well following ASD closure.

What Size is Too Big?

The largest atrial septal defect closure device currently available (and unlikely to be exceeded) is the Amplatzer 42-mm device. With the additional wings on either side of the waist adding to a diameter of 56 mm, this would comfortably obliterate the entire atrial septum in the majority of adult patients. While it is possible to close defects of such size, and a number of cunning techniques have been described to achieve this aim, the question has to be asked whether it is wise to do so, and whether the risk of embolization or free wall erosion is greater with these large devices, which by necessity impinge on all rims of the atrial septum. For large ASDs a multidisciplinary approach is helpful so that echocardiographer, interventionist, and surgeon can decide on the best management for each individual patient.

When is Pulmonary Pressure Too High?

For many years, there was debate as to the relative contribution of atrial septal defects to the development of severe pulmonary hypertension. Fortunately the issue appears to have been resolved now by expert consensus—systemic pulmonary pressures do not occur in isolated atrial septal defects in the absence of either congenital pulmonary abnormalities or secondary pathologies. Patients who are born with both an atrial septal defect and abnormal

pulmonary vasculature may develop Eisenmenger syndrome. Patients do not develop systemic pulmonary pressures in adulthood as a result of an ASD in the absence of a second pathology such as primary pulmonary hypertension. Closing an ASD in the setting of systemic pulmonary pressures is extremely hazardous, as the right ventricle is likely to fail quickly without the relief afforded by the bidirectionality of interatrial shunting during the cardiac cycle.

However, patients with ASDs do gradually develop increasing pulmonary artery pressures due to hyperemic pulmonary flow over many years resulting in vessel wall hyperplasia and increased vascular resistance. Elderly patients in particular, therefore, may present on occasion with significant pulmonary hypertension (systolic pulmonary artery pressure > 60 mm Hg). Provided the pulmonary artery pressure is not more than two-thirds systemic, it is safe to close such ASDs, and indeed pulmonary artery pressure will fall following closure [4], with additional benefit to the patient in terms of symptom relief. Closure of ASDs in patients with pulmonary hypertension, however, may be associated also with the syndrome of brittle sudden-onset pulmonary edema, and therefore these patients have to be managed in a high dependency area postprocedure.

Anatomic Considerations

There are many types of ASDs, and only the secundum ASD is generally considered suitable for percutaneous closure. Fortunately for the interventionist, the others, such as the sinus venosus, coronary sinus, or ostium primum defects are not often encountered in adults. Anatomically, the key considerations, apart from the size of the defect discussed above, are the pulmonary venous drainage, proximity of the atrioventricular valves, the anterior superior aortic rim, and the posterior inferior rim. Of these, it is the anterior superior rim that causes the greatest concern, as it is often deficient (< 5 mm) and frequently appears absent altogether in some planes. Given the fears of erosion, a balance has to be struck between oversizing the device and risking erosion, versus undersizing the device and risking either embolization or the need to upsize the device

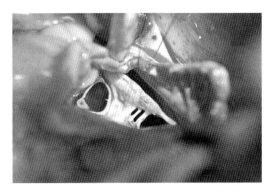

Figure 7.1 Operative view of ASD with multiple fenestrations.

at the time of implantation (an expensive eventuality unless the removed device be taken back as customary with manufacturers). As a general rule, there is a school of thought that suggests that unless you find yourself having to upsize at implantation in 10% of cases, you are probably routinely oversizing your ASD closures. This is a good rule of thumb.

Although the deficient aortic rim is much discussed, deficiency of the posteroinferior inferior vena cava rim is of greater concern. First, this is more difficult to diagnose, being less well visualized on transesophageal echocardiography (TEE) unless particular efforts are made, and is therefore sometimes overlooked. Second, in the absence of the inferior rim (in contrast to absence of the aortic rim), there is no associated structure to hang the device on, and therefore the risk of embolization is high. Intracardiac echocardiography may delineate the inferior rim better than TEE in some cases. Some atrial septal defects are multiple, in which case surgical closure may be required (Fig. 7.1).

The Procedure

The procedure is usually done under general anesthesia with TEE guidance, though increasingly intracardiac echocardiogarphy (ICE) is being used instead, under sedation (described later). Some operators have also done ASD closure under echocardiographic guidance, or fluoroscopy alone, but this is not advocated.

The relative merits of TEE and ICE are much discussed, and at the moment many operators are being seduced by the sophistication of ICE, without adequately considering its drawbacks. ICE allows the procedure to be done under local anesthesia with sedation and is very suited to PFO closure and straightforward small ASDs, but if the ASD is other than straightforward, the limitations of ICE in its current incarnation become apparent—first, the probe is not multiplane and therefore the optimal view for implantation may not be achieved, and second, the operator may have to switch between handling the ICE catheter and the implantation sheath at critical moments to try to obtain and hold the ideal view. An alternative strategy is to have an echocardiographer managing the ICE catheter, but this introduces additional logistical difficulties and does not solve the imaging problems. One area where ICE has the advantage is at the inferior margins of the ASD, which can sometimes be difficult to visualize with TEE, but until ICE catheters develop further, complex ASD closure is most flexibly done under general anesthesia with TEE control.

Who Should Do the Procedure?

As with all procedures, there is a correlation between volume and outcomes. As coronary intervention becomes devolved from surgical centers, adult cardiologists are taking an interest in PFO and ASD closure. ASD closure, however, is a specialist elective procedure and as such should be undertaken by high-volume operators where possible. The simple answer to the question is that the operator most skilled within a reasonable distance of the patient is the one to undertake the procedure. Pediatric interventional cardiologists are well placed to do this work in adult patients, but are not always available. Each country will find its own solutions, but certainly each large cardiothoracic center should have an operator experienced and skilled at ASD closure.

For those who wish to start ASD closure programes in adults there are certain core skills that are needed in addition to the implantation techniques. For example, the operator needs to be familiar with use of snares and retrieval sheaths so that they can deal effectively with embolization. A

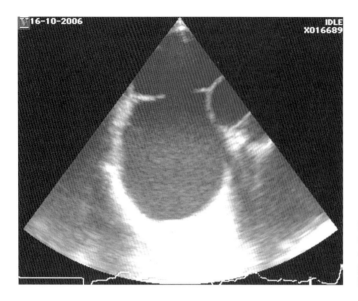

Figure 7.2 Two-dimensional transoesophageal midatrial view of an ostium secundum atrial setpal defect with good tissue margins both at the aortic and inferior rims.

minimum volume of 15 cases per year is probably needed to maintain skills. Preliminary experience with closure of patent foramen ovale should be a prerequisite.

Sizing the Defect

Accurate sizing of the defect is critical to a successful procedure. The echocardiographic images on TEE give multiple planes in which the defect can be measured. This can be done either using two-dimensional (Fig. 7.2) or, more recently, three-dimensional reconstruction (Fig. 7.3). This technology is rapidly developing and is set to revolutionize preprocedural and procedural assessment of the anatomy of the defect such that a true cir-cumferential image can be obtained rather than purely a cross-sectional image. Three-dimensional echocardiography is rapidly being introduced, but in the meantime, when using two-dimensional echocardiography, combining the caval view, four-chamber view, and short axis aortic view, the maximal diameter of the ASD can be measured. Balloon sizing of the defect should be undertaken, but gently. It is important not to stretch the defect, but it is equally important to "palpate" the edges of the defect to see if the rim is floppy or firm. On fluoroscopy, the balloon can be measured when the faintest waisting appears in the middle. However, an indentation has to occur on both sides, as the ballon may be leaning against the lower rim but

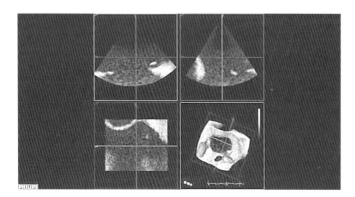

Figure 7.3 Three-dimensional reconstruction of an ostium secundum ASD. The top and bottom left pictures show the two-dimensional sections from which the three-dimensional image is reconstructed. The bottom right image shows the atrial septal defect itself.

not yet reaching the upper rim. The current optimal technique is using echocardiographic assessment of balloon inflation until color flow at the edges of the defect stops, and measuring the balloon diameter at this point. Correlation between the fluoroscopic and echocardiographic images is usually good. Some operators do not balloon size atrial septal defects but rely on the echo assessment alone. Usually this is reliable, but occasionally it is possible to be misled by unexpectedly floppy margins of the ASD.

Should Dual Defects Be Closed Together or at an Interval?

Dual atrial septal defects at the superior and inferior margins of the interatrial septum, usually associated with an aneurysm in addition, are not common, but occur frequently enough to present a therapeutic dilemma as to whether they should be closed at the same time or sequentially. Both options are reasonable. In general, the larger defect should be closed first if a sequential approach is to be used (though frequently flow through the smaller defect will augment following closure of the larger defect). The advantage of sequential closure is that the initial device is firmly fibrosed into place before the second device is placed. If a two-device simultaneous implantation technique is to be used, it is sensible to keep both devices attached to their delivery cables until both are in a position to be released, rather than releasing one device completely before attempting to place the other, which may increase the risk of embolization of the first.

Device Types

There is a great proliferation of interatrial septal closure devices. Most of these are designed for the PFO market in the expectation that this will outstrip the ASD market by a factor of ten to one in the fullness of time. The three devices in widest use in Europe for ASD closure are the Amplatzer, BioSTAR, and HELEX devices, from AGA, NMT, and Gore respectively. Other commercially available devices include the Cardia, Premere, and Occlutech. Each device has its merits and each its drawbacks.

The Amplatzer device has not changed significantly over the last 10 years, and remains the only device suitable for defects > 15 mm diameter. It is relatively straightforward to use and withstands multiple deployments if necessary. It has an excellent safety record, marred only by a relatively small number of cases of free wall erosion. Erosion (occuring usually where the device is pounding against the pulsating aorta) can cause immediate fatal tamponade, and therefore this complication is greatly feared. Cases of erosion appear fewer since the recommendation not to oversize was issued [5].

The BioSTAR is the first partially absorbable interatrial septal closure device, and as such is inherently attractive to patients and implanting physicians alike. More suited to PFO closure than ASD closure, the device can nonetheless be used in defects up to 15 mm in diameter with good results, using a device-to-defect ratio of 2:1.

The HELEX device is the softest closure device on the market. It is an elegant device that is intuitively more complicated for operators to grasp. It can be deployed and redeployed if necessary and has a negligible thrombus risk. It is suited to ASDs with a poor aortic rim to avoid the risk of erosion, and can be used in ASDs < 15 mm with a device-to-defect ratio of 2:1.

Management of Residual Shunts

Management of residual shunts is less of an issue than with PFO closure, in which a residual shunt leaves the patient still at risk of paradoxical embolism and is associated with a higher recurrence rate. In the setting of ASD closure, small residual shunts should be left alone as they will cause no hemodynamic compromise. Sometimes residual shunts are noted at follow-up due to additional unsuspected lesions. These should be assessed fully and a decision taken to close or not in their own right.

Erosion

Atrial wall erosions following implant of atrial septal occluders have been reported in a number of cases over the last 10 years [5]. Erosion can occur at the aorto-atrial continuity, the roof of the left or right atrium, or within the atrial septum itself. If the erosion is wholly intracardiac it may be asymptomatic, as in the case of an atrial septal marginal erosion, or can present subacutely with breathlessness. The most feared complication, however, is aortic erosion with resultant cardiac tamponade, which may be immediately fatal. Although such cases are numerically and proportionately few, they have concentrated the mind.

Anatomic examination of available postmortem specimens suggests that it may not be the flanges of the ASD occluder that cause the erosion—these are pushed away from the aorta with each cardiac contraction; rather, it may be the central waist of the device, which moves towards the aorta with each contraction, gradually abraiding and eventually eroding the vessel. As a result of these cases, an expert panel was convened that issued advice on sizing devices for closure, focusing on avoidance of oversizing. Since the issue of this guidance, cases of erosion have appeared fewer.

Angle of Implant

The angle at which atrial septal defect devices are implanted remains problematic. Given that the atrial septum may be almost parallel to the inferior vena cava, it is not surprising that this can cause difficulties, and a number of ingenious implantation techniques have been developed to try to get around this problem. Although sheaths have undergone redesign over the last few years, the problem remains and is overdue to be resolved.

Sheaths with a stronger braiding and more abrupt angulation would probably suffice; alternatively, adjustable sheaths as have been designed for other interventional procedures.

Ventricular Septal Defects

Percutaneous closure of a ventricular septal defect (VSD) is an uncommon and demanding procedure. Good knowledge of anatomic considerations is required, and good quality pre-procedure and per-procedure imaging is essential. The ideal team consists of a minimum of two implanting physicians, an echocardiographer, and an anesthetist, along with additional nursing, radiographic, and technical assistants, and is therefore resource-intense.

Perimembranous and muscular VSDs present electively and closure should be planned in a high-volume institution, though such a definition has to be made in the context of the low incidence of these lesions. Post-myocardial infarction defects exhibit most of the problems of the elective lesions, with added complexity. Other defects are unusual. One such, a VSD following mitral valve surgery, is shown in Fig. 7.4.

Who Needs a VSD Closed in Adulthood?

Closure of small congenital ventricular septal defects that are not causing any hemodynamic

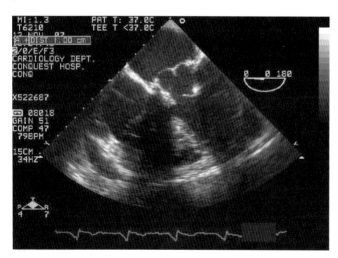

Figure 7.4 Ventricular septal defect of 1 cm diameter occurring following mitral valve replacement.

compromise is probably not warranted. Endocarditis occurs only rarely on VSDs, and therefore this alone does not constitute reason to close. Volume overload of the right ventricle and pulmonary circulation with Qp:Qs > 1.5 offers an indication to close, as does left ventricular dilatation due to volume loading. Patients with ventricular septal defects should be seen by an experienced interventionist to discuss device closure. Post-infarction VSDs are the exception to this rule. These should all be considered for interventional or surgical management as the patient will not otherwise survive.

Post-Myocardial Infarction VSD
Interventional management of post-infarction ventricular septal defect is one of the most demanding procedures in the repertoire of the interventional cardiologist. Not only is the concept of ventricular septal defect closure already technically challenging, requiring as it often does an arteriovenous circuit formation, but in addition to this the patients are often unwell and hemodynamically unstable, and the septal defect itself is typically necrotic and serpiginous. Nonetheless, interventional cardiologists have attempted to undertake these procedures chiefly because surgical results have remained disappointing.

Surgery for post-infarction VSD is most difficult in the acute phase, when the VSD may be enlarging and the tissues are friable. Inferior myocardial infarction defects have a worse outlook than anterior defects, both because the surgery is more technically challenging, dealing with a deeper and more posterior defect, and also because of the almost inevitable involvement of the right ventricle in the infarction zone.

Surgical or Interventional Management for Post-Infarction VSD?
This question will be resolved with a different outcome in different centers and depends on a multidisciplinary approach. Without either surgical or interventional management, the outlook for these patients is extremely bleak, with 95% mortality at 30 days. The remaining 5% subsequently also die from heart failure without intervention in the vast majority of cases, and the author has never seen a

long-term survivor of this condition who has not undergone either surgical or interventional management.

As a general rule, surgical management of inferior defects is disappointing, with a high preoperative mortality [6], while anterior defects may be more amenable to surgical closure. By contrast, interventional management of inferior defects may be successfully undertaken using a femorofemoral arteriovenous circuit, while anterior defects are often so anteroapical that there is very little septal tissue caudally on which to try to hook the device even when using a more appropriate jugulofemoral approach.

How to Image a Postinfarction VSD
Imaging the defect can be difficult because the patient is often unable to cooperate fully. Transthoracic echocardiography is usually the modality with which the diagnosis is made and may provide good images if the defect is inferoposterior or anteroapical. It cannot, however, usually delineate whether or not there are multiple tracks. TEE is therefore widely used in this situation to try to assess the defect in greater detail. However, while this modality may show an inferior or an anterior defect clearly, the anteroapical or truly apical VSDs may be poorly visualized, particularly with respect to the specific anatomic features such as multiplicity of defects, anatomy of funnel or aneurysmal defects, and degree of apical tissue remnant. Magnetic resonance imaging has been used successfully to clarify which defects may be suitable for device closure, and this is an area for further research.

Intra-Aortic Balloon Pump or Not?
A balloon pump is a double-edged sword in this situation. Once a balloon pump has been in situ > 48 hours, the risk of pump-associated vascular or infective complications rises appreciably. Many patients therefore succumb with complications likely related to balloon pumps while waiting for a definitive procedure. Our own practice in this situation is to try to resist the initial temptation to insert a balloon pump unless it is clear that the patient requires it for immediate stabilization. Once the balloon pump has been inserted, the clock is ticking,

and it is optimal to undertake a definitive procedure within 72 hours. If it is possible to delay balloon-pump insertion at the time of the development of the VSD, the pump may be inserted semi-electively 24 hours before interventional closure to improve procedural hemodynamics.

Timing of Procedure

Procedural mortality is lowest if the patient undergoes the interventional procedure several weeks after the initial development of the VSD, when the surrounding tissues have had a chance to fibrose and scar. By this stage however, 95% of patients with a post-MI VSD will have died waiting, so this approach (favored by some surgeons) is of little use to the patient. Interventional management within the first 24 hours after the VSD develops may be difficult both logistically and because the tissue margins are friable and the VSD may at this stage be still under development. A successful procedure may be done, only to find that a fresh extension of the VSD occurs subsequently and a further procedure is required.

The main determinants of an adverse outcome are the inflammatory indices, the size and contractility of the right ventricle, and the extent of renal dysfunction. All three of these factors must be observed on a daily basis in the patients, with intervention undertaken as soon as deterioration in any one of these parameters is seen. Some rare patients can wait for 2 to 3 weeks before undergoing percutaneous VSD closure, and of course these patients do the best, but most patients will require a procedure within 1 week of the diagnosis being made.

The Procedure

The essence of the procedure is the same irrespective of the indication, but for the post-infarct VSD, the stability of the patient and the sang-froid of the operator are at a premium. Ideally, the patient can be done under controlled remifentanyl anesthetic sedation, such that an anesthetist is in full control of the patient's analgesia and sedation, but the patient is not under general anesthetic with ventilation. However, if TEE is essential to be able to visualize the defect, general anesthesia is required. These procedures can be long, and the patient should therefore ideally be managed by a dedicated cardiac anesthetist through the periprocedural period.

Inferior defects are usually closed using two femoral sheaths for the arteriovenous rail, while anterior defects are approached from the right jugular vein to the right femoral artery. Occasionally, operators may choose to use a veno-venous loop via a transseptal puncture. Similarly, a direct perventricular approach may be used (see later).

The septal defect is crossed left to right using a Judkins catheter and a hydrophilic 0.035″ wire. The wire usually passes to the pulmonary artery and is snared here and exteriorized to the venous access point. Care needs to be taken to avoid damaging the tricuspid chordae. If the wire loop snags at the tricuspid level and resistance is encountered, it is imperative to recross the VSD and attempt to pass the hydrophilic wire up to the PA again with as cranial a passage as possible through the right ventricle to try to avoid the tricuspid chordae. Once a successful arteriovenous rail is created, the wire is snared and exchanged for a rope or noodle wire, which provides good support when straight but great flexibility at other times.

The defect may be balloon sized if necessary but usually the echocardiographic parameters are used to assess the appropriate size of Amplatzer device to use. Balloon sizing of post-infarct VSDs is to be avoided, as this may extend the defect. Using a "push-me-pull-you" kissing technique of catheters from both venous and arterial sides, the braided sheath is introduced from the venous side into the left ventricle and an appropriately sized device deployed to close the defect. One difficulty that can be encountered at this time is angulation of the device almost perpendicular to the line of the defect. This can often be solved by partial deployment of the waist of the device, or by upsizing the device and repeating this maneuver, but is not always amenable to this technique and occasionally an open or perventricular closure may be required instead. For elective closure, the device waist should match the defect size. For post-infarct VSDs, as the margins of the defect are necessarily infarcted and the tissue is friable, it is wise to take the largest post-infarction Amplatzer device that you think can be made to wedge comfortably in the defect. There is no hard and fast rule, but it is suggested to oversize the waist of the device by 6 to 8 mm in these cases. The largest device currently available is 24 mm and therefore post-infarct defects that measure more than 16 to 18 mm in diameter by echocardiography are unlikely to be successfully occluded with the current technology unless a large ASD closure device is used.

For apical defects, the right ventricular aspect of the device may not reform correctly if there is very little room in the RV tip. Reforming the disk with the help of active management of the cable may be helpful. Sometimes suboptimal RV disk formation has to be accepted, and in the context of a post-infarct VSD, this is not critical if the closure is proving effective. Unfortunately, a significant proportion of these defects are both serpiginous and multiple, and sometimes two or even three devices may be required to try to close a defect effectively. Generally with multiple devices, however, there is a law of diminishing returns (Fig. 7.5) [7].

Perventricular Closure

This hybrid approach has a number of features to recommend it. The disadvantage is that a median sternotomy is required, but the advantage is that there is no need for cardiopulmonary bypass and the defect can be approached at a favorable angle. If the defect appears to be inaccessible to closure percutaneously it may be possible to cross the defect directly from a right ventricular puncture under echocardiographic control and introduce an appropriately sized device down a short sheath. This procedure is in its infancy but may be a useful addition to pure percutaneous methods.

Who Should Do the Procedure?

Elective procedures should be done by operators with significant current experience, at centers with surgical support and a full inventory of equipment. The difficulties come with post-infarction VSDs that present indiscriminately to nonspecialist centers. If the joint opinion is that percutaneous closure is the preferred option, it is as often advisable to move the physicians rather than the patient. A "flying doctor" service for this scenario may well be the

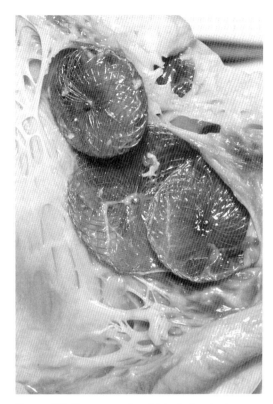

Figure 7.5 Placement of multiple devices in the interventricular septum of a patient with a post-infarction ventricular septal defect.

right approach, and in the UK we have been lucky to have Dr. Jo de Giovanni performing this function for some years with good success. The procedure needs two operators to manage the wires and catheters at each access site. At least one of the operators needs to be someone who closes VSDs on a regular basis and is fully versed in the use and management of snares and rail loops.

Postprocedure Complete Heart Block

There is concern about the incidence of complete heart block following perimembranous VSD device closure. Current data suggest that this may occur in more than 5% of cases, and may be a late development, with unpredictable sequelae in the community as a result. The incidence is higher than with surgical perimembranous VSD closure, and therefore some authorities still advocate a surgical approach for this lesion. Further data should clarify whether or not this is a major concern. For other VSDs, complete heart block is rare and is therefore not a consideration.

Management of Hemolysis

Hemolysis may complicate incomplete VSD closure, though it is uncommon. Patients should receive oral iron therapy, vitamin B_{12}, and folate, and transfusion as necessary.

If transfusion requirements are considerable, then consideration should be given to placing an extra device or performing surgical correction, but in general hemolysis will settle in due course, though this may take as long as 6 months.

Conclusions

Atrial and ventricular septal defect closures can be challenging procedures. Neither should be undertaken lightly, and both call for specific training and expertise, which takes time to accrue. Multidisciplinary teams are very important, particularly with regard to imaging and the relative merits of surgical and interventional treatment. Procedural techniques and device design are rapidly changing, such that an increasing array of defects can now be safely closed by percutaneous means.

References

1. Gatzoulis MA, Redington AN, Somerville J, Shore DF. Should atrial septal defects in adults be closed? *Ann Thorac Surg.* 1996;61:657–659.
2. Elshershari H, Cao QL, Hijazi ZM. Transcatheter device closure of atrial septal defects in patients older than 60 years of age: immediate and follow-up results. *J Invasive Cardiol.* 2008;20:173–176.
3. Schubert S, Peters B, Abdul-Khaliq H, Nagdyman N, Lange PE, Ewert P. Left ventricular conditioning in the elderly patient to prevent congestive heart failure after transcatheter closure of atrial septal defect. *Catheter Cardiovasc Interv.* 2005;64:333–337.
4. Balint OH, Samman A, Haberer K, *et al.* Outcomes in patients with significant pulmonary hypertension undergoing percutaneous atrial septal defect closure. *Heart.* 2008;94:1189–1193.
5. Amin Z, Hijazi ZM, Bass JL, Cheatham JP, Hellenbrand WE, Kleinman CS. Erosion of Amplatzer septal occluder device after closure of secundum atrial septal defects: review of registry of complications and recommendations to minimize future risk. *Catheter Cardiovasc Interv.* 2004;63:496–502.
6. Jones MT, Schofield PM, Dark JF, *et al.* Surgical repair of acquired ventricular septal defect. Determinants of early and late outcome. *J Thorac Cardiovasc Surg.* 1987;93:680–686.
7. Webb I, De Giovanni J, Hildick-Smith D. Multiple percutaneous VSD closures post-myocardial infarct. *Eur Heart J.* 2006;27:552.

CHAPTER 8
Carotid Artery Stenting

Paul Chiam,[1,2] Sriram Iyer,[1] Gary Roubin,[1] and Jiri Vitek[1]
[1]Department of Cardiac and Vascular Interventional Services, Lenox Hill Heart and Vascular
 Institute, New York, NY, USA
[2]Department of Cardiology, National Heart Center, Singapore

---

Chapter Overview

- Carotid stenting has to be performed with periprocedural stroke or death rates of $< 6\%$ and $< 3\%$, respectively, for symptomatic and asymptomatic patients.
- Appropriate patient and lesion selection is of paramount importance in any carotid stent procedure.
- Carotid stenting has been shown to be non-inferior to endarterectomy in symptomatic and asymptomatic patients who are at high surgical risk.
- Several carotid stent registries of high surgical risk patients demonstrate that carotid stenting can be performed with similar 1-year event rates as historical CEA control data.
- Carotid stenting did not prove non-inferiority compared to CEA in symptomatic patients at standard surgical risk.
- Octogenarians appear to experience elevated periprocedural event rates, as shown in several registries and in the lead-in phase of the CREST trial. More recent data from high-volume centers, however, demonstrate that carotid stenting can be performed in this elderly group with acceptable event rates.
- The ongoing CREST (symptomatic and asymptomatic at standard surgical risk), CAVATAS-2/ ICSS (symptomatic at standard surgical risk), and ACT1 and ACST-2 (asymptomatic at standard surgical risk) trials will provide important data in the near future.

Carotid stenting (CS) has rapidly evolved to become a widely utilized method of carotid artery revascularization. Collective experience with this technique has grown exponentially. Improved periprocedural outcomes have been achieved through technical and procedural innovations including improved devices, increased operator experience, understanding optimal technique, and understanding the importance of patient selection.

For CS to continue to develop, three important issues need to be addressed: (1) operator training,

(2) application of correct technique, and (3) importance of patient and lesion selection.

Historical Perspective

Results of several randomized trials published in the 1990s showed that carotid endarterectomy (CEA) was more effective than medical therapy in reducing the risk of stroke [1–5]. Thus, the American Heart Association (AHA) guidelines recommend CEA for symptomatic carotid stenosis $> 50\%$, and for asymptomatic carotid stenosis $> 60\%$ if these asymptomatic patients also have an expected life expectancy of 5 years, provided the periprocedural complication rates are less than

Current Best Practice in Interventional Cardiology. Edited by
B Meier. © 2010 Blackwell Publishing,

6% and 3%, respectively [6,7]. In particular, the ACST trial [5] demonstrated that asymptomatic patients, including women, derived benefit from CEA with the margin of benefit similar to the ACAS trial. Furthermore, medical management in ACST was better, with high proportions of patients on antiplatelet therapy, statins, and antihypertensive treatment.

During the late 1980s, several investigators began to apply the percutaneous approach to carotid revascularization [8,9]. Subsequently, in 1994, Roubin and coworkers reported the first rigorous prospective study of CS with independent neurology assessment [10]. Early results by this group and others [11] showed that CS was feasible and had acceptable complications rates despite the novel experience with this technique, use of primitive equipment, and lack of distal embolic protection devices (EPDs). In 2001, the first long-term (up to 5 years) follow-up of CS demonstrated that CS could be accomplished with acceptable complication rates and with durable results [12]. In addition, using transcranial Doppler (TCD), it was shown that microembolic signals (MES) were detected during every phase of CS and these MES were reduced with EPDs [13]. More recently, the clinical and anatomic markers of increased risk for CS have been identified [14].

Multicenter Clinical Trials

The first study to demonstrate equivalence of CS versus CEA was the CAVATAS trial, randomizing mostly symptomatic patients (90%) who were at standard surgical risk. The 30-day stroke or death rate (10% CS vs. 9.9% CEA) and 3-year ipsilateral stroke rate were not different [15]. The trial was criticized because event rates in the surgical arm were higher than expected; however, it must also be considered that the CS arm did not employ EPDs, and stents were used in only 26% (as they became available).

The SAPPHIRE trial [16]—a multicenter randomized trial of high surgical risk patients with either symptomatic > 50% carotid stenosis or asymp-

tomatic > 80% carotid stenosis—demonstrated that CS was non-inferior to CEA with myocardial infarction/stroke/death rates of 12.2% versus 20.1% respectively at 1 year, with clinical equipoise maintained at 3 years [17].

The CARESS trial, a multicenter, nonrandomized prospective comparative study of symptomatic and asymptomatic patients at high or low surgical risk, revealed no significant differences in the 30-day and 1-year stroke or death rates between CS and CEA (2.1% vs. 3.6% and 10.0% vs. 13.6%, respectively). Although the treatment was decided by the physicians, it reflects true clinical decision-making, suggesting that results of CS are comparable to CEA when appropriate case selection is made [18].

Recently, however, the EVA-3S and SPACE trials randomizing symptomatic patients at normal surgical risk showed that CS did not achieve parity with CEA [19,20]. Although 30-day ipsilateral stroke or death rates in the SPACE trial were similar (CS 6.84% vs. CEA 6.34%), CS was not proven non-inferior because of insufficient power, as the trial was terminated prematurely due to slow recruitment and lack of funding [19]. In the EVA-3S study, not only was non-inferiority not reached, CS performed worse with a higher 30-day stroke or death rate (9.6% vs. 3.9%, $p = 0.01$) [20]. Criticisms of the EVA-3S study were that embolic protection was not mandatory early in the trial, angiographic appearance of the lesion was not factored into patient selection, and the carotid interventionalists were inexperienced compared to the surgeons. Therefore, the results reinforce the important messages that distal EPDs must be considered an integral part of the procedure, and rigorous operator training and credentialing as well as patient selection are required.

Multicenter registries of CS (ARCHeR, CABERNET, CREATE, CAPTURE, BEACH, CASES-PMS, Pro-CAS, and ALKK), which enrolled symptomatic and asymptomatic patients mostly at high surgical risk, showed that the periprocedural stroke or death rates were between 2.8% and 6.9% [21–28]. These data show that acceptable adverse event rates have been achieved even as the procedure became more widely adopted. The recently reported 1-year results of the BEACH trial (symptomatic and asymptomatic high surgical risk patients) showed no difference in event rates between CS (8.9%) and that of CEA as predefined by FDA-approved objective performance criteria (12.6%) [26].

Indications and Contraindications of Carotid Stenting

The indications for carotid stenting are similar to those for CEA if the procedure can be accomplished with event rates within the AHA guidelines. Patients with increased surgical risk due to comorbidities such as severe cardiac or pulmonary disease; anatomic factors such as high lesions behind the mandible (C2 and above) or low lesions (necessitating thoracic exposure); or restenosis after previous CEA, contralateral ICA occlusion, and prior neck dissection/irradiation, may be more safely treated with CS.

With present-day devices and technologies, almost any carotid lesion can be stented. It is not, however, a question of an operator being able to access the lesion or eliminate the stenosis by placing a stent, but is absolutely related to the ability to perform these tasks safely with a low stroke/death rate. Thus, there are several situations that increase the likelihood of adverse events. The inability of the patient to tolerate dual antiplatelet agents, which are mandatory for at least 1 month post CS, inability to advance the EPD distal to the lesion and its deployment in a safe "landing" zone, inability to safely access the common carotid artery (CCA) (eg, severe CCA bifurcation stenosis/ECA occlusion with a type III arch), recent (< 14 days) moderate to large cerebral infarction, large thrombus burden, unfavorable arch anatomy, severe carotid artery tortuosity, heavy concentric lesion calcification, and the "string sign," are conditions that increase the risk of adverse events during CS (ie, relative contraindications). These patients may be more safely treated with CEA or medical therapy.

Role of Carotid Angiography in Patient Selection

Carotid angiography reconfirms the severity of ICA stenosis before stenting and also provides important information on carotid bifurcation level, presence of CCA stenosis, vascular tortuosity, vessel calcification, tandem lesions, intracranial stenoses, lesions characteristics such as presence of ulceration or thrombus, and cerebral collateral flow. Similar to guideline recommendations [29], we advocate that experienced operators study both carotid arteries, with optional angiographic imaging of a vertebral artery if that can be safely performed. One of the most important points to note is that the final decision to proceed with CS should be made after adequate carotid/cerebral angiograms have been performed, and sheath placed in the CCA. At least two views of the CCA bifurcation should be performed and the view with the most severe tortuosity used in decision-making and to guide the procedure. Often, certain anatomic findings (eg, vascular tortuosity, heavy concentric lesion calcification) that significantly increase stent risk are first detected during angiography, especially after sheath or guide placement. Depending on these findings, the decision to proceed with CS should be carefully reconsidered and the procedure terminated, if necessary.

Patient and Lesion Selection

As experience with CS has accumulated, clinical and anatomic markers for increased stroke risk during CS (high stent risk) have been identified [14]. These are age, reduced cerebral reserve, excessive vascular tortuosity, and heavy concentric lesion calcification (Table 8.1). Patients with any 2 or more of the 4 risk markers should be excluded from CS, since the risk of periprocedural stroke will be excessive. Alternative therapies, either medical or surgical, are thus recommended for these patients.

Excessive vascular tortuosity (Fig. 8.1) and heavy concentric lesion calcification (Fig. 8.2) increase stroke risk due to increased manipulation and procedural time [13,30], whereas reduced cerebral

Table 8.1 Markers of Increased Risk during Carotid Stenting

		Risk Factor	Features
Clinical	1.	Age ≥ 80 yrs	
	2.	Decreased cerebral reserve	Prior (remote) large stroke (> 1/3 middle cerebral artery territory infarction on CT brain)
			Multiple lacunar infarcts (diffuse lacunes associated with encephalomalacia and/or cerebral atrophy on CT brain)
			Intracranial microangiopathy (CT or MRI brain changes most prominent in the periventricular region)
			Dementia
Angiographic	3.	Excessive tortuosity	≥ 2 90-degree bends within 5 cm of the lesion (including the takeoff of the ICA from the CCA)
	4.	Heavy calcification	Concentric calcification; width ≥ 3 mm

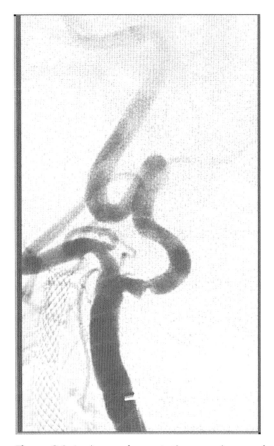

Figure 8.1 Angiogram demonstrating excessive vascular tortuotisy (≥ 2 90-degree bends within 5 cm of the lesion, including takeoff of the ICA).

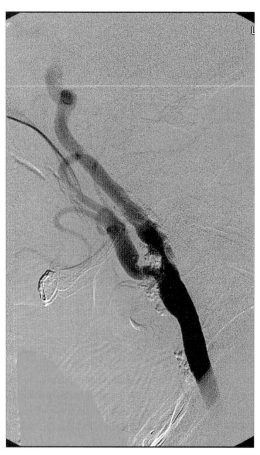

Figure 8.2 Angiogram demonstrating heavy concentric lesion calcification.

reserve decreases brain tolerance to further potential ischemic insult. It must be emphasized that even moderate vascular tortuosity can increase the complexity of the procedure, and presents a hazard for less experienced operators. Assessing vascular tortuosity in multiple views is essential to fully appreciate the challenge.

Age was demonstrated to be a predictor of adverse outcomes before [12] and even after the advent of EPDs [31,32]. The ongoing CREST trial lead-in phase showed that octogenarians had a significantly increased risk of adverse events (12.1% vs. 3.2% in non-octogenarians) not accounted for by other factors, and recruitment of these patients was stopped in the lead-in phase [31]. The SPACE trial documented a twofold increase in ipsilateral stroke/death among those > 75 years versus ≤ 75 years (11% vs. 5.9%) [19]. Possible reasons are that increased vascular tortuosity and vessel calcification are more common in elderly patients [33–35], and they are also more likely to have reduced cerebral reserve compared to a younger population.

Several investigators have, however, demonstrated that CS can be performed in the octogenarian group with low adverse event rates [34,36], raising the question whether age alone or patient selection and operator experience are the important factors. Recently, in the largest single-center series of CS in selected (using the above-mentioned criteria) elderly patients with independent neurology assessment, the authors demonstrated that CS can be performed with 30-day periprocedural event rates of 5.1% and 2.6% in the symptomatic and asymptomatic groups respectively [37], consistent with the AHA guidelines.

Therefore, CS and CEA should be viewed as complementary and not competitive revascularization options There will be patients who are at high surgical risk and more suitable for CS; conversely, there will be patients who are at increased stent risk and will be more suitable for CEA. Thus a new paradigm shift in patient selection is required, and must take into account the "stent risk" for the individual patient similar to considerations of high surgical risk in patients undergoing CEA (Fig. 8.3). Patients at increased risk for both procedures may be better and more safely treated with optimal medical therapy.

Expected Results with Experienced Operators and Appropriate Patient Selection

As with any interventional procedure, and even more so with CS, there is a steep learning curve. It has been demonstrated that increased operator experience leads to reduced complication rates [12], emphasizing the importance of thorough operator training on the technical and cognitive (patient selection) aspects of CS. It can be expected that event rates will meet the guidelines in ideal patient subsets performed by experienced operators. For example, the CREST lead-in phase reported 1.7% and 1.3% stroke or death rates for patients < 60 years and 60 to 69 years, respectively. Initial data from the ACT1 trial also showed a remarkably low 1.7% stroke or death rate for patients < 80 years (unpublished data). Guideline recommendations on operator training and credentialing have been detailed in a recent consensus statement of several of the involved professional societies [29].

Technical Considerations

Access for the procedure is usually via the femoral artery. Occasionally, in patients with severe peripheral vascular disease (PVD), the brachial or radial route can be used. Diagnostic cerebral angiography is routinely performed to confirm lesion severity and assess vascular tortuosity, vessel calcification, and intracranial collateral circulation. Dedicated neurovascular catheters (for example the Vitek catheter from Cook, Bloomington, IN) are used. Arch aortograms are not routinely performed in experienced centers since the operators are able to assess arch type based on the catheter configuration during diagnostic angiography and are able to access the CCA even with extended arches. For operators with lesser experience, arch angiograms are certainly useful to help guide decision-making and choice of equipment.

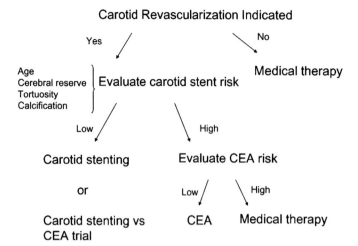

Figure 8.3 Clinical decision algorithm in the management of carotid artery stenosis.

All patients should be on dual antiplatelet therapy with acetylsalicylic acid and clopidogrel or ticlopidine. Strict adherence to this regimen has contributed towards the improved results seen with CS. Control of blood pressure (BP) must be meticulous. Anti-hypertensive medications are usually omitted on the morning of the procedure, as mild hypotension and bradycardia usually occur with balloon dilatation and stenting of the carotid bifurcation. Should BP remain > 160 to 180 mmHg systolic after stent implantation, rapidly performing postdilatation usually reduces BP expeditiously. Less commonly, control of BP with medication is required if it is still > 160 to 180 mm Hg systolic after postdilatation. It has been shown that strict BP control ≤ 140/90 mm Hg reduces the risk of hyperperfusion syndrome or cerebral hemorrhage [38]. Intravenous or intra-arterial nitroglycerin or IV labetalol can be used.

Sheaths are preferred over guide catheters as they have a less traumatic tip design, and also require a smaller arteriotomy in the vascular access site. Usually, 6F-sized sheaths are adequate for the vast majority of CS procedures. Occasionally for adverse arch anatomy or tortuous vessels, a 7F sheath may be required or an 8F guide with the appropriate curve can be utilized. The standard technique of placing the sheath in the common carotid artery (CCA) is most often used. This entails manipulating the diagnostic neurocatheter

into the external carotid artery (ECA) over a 0.038-inch Glidewire (Terumo, Tokyo, Japan) and then exchanging for a sheath over a stiff wire such as the Supracore wire (Abbott Vascular, Santa Clara, CA). Alternatively if the lesion involves the bifurcation of the CCA or if the ECA is occluded, the more advanced "telescopic" technique is employed. The 6F sheath is first placed in the descending thoracic aorta. A 125-cm 5F Vitek catheter with a 0.038-inch Glidewire or 0.035-inch Amplatz J stiff wire within are then advanced through the sheath and positioned in the CCA below the lesion. The sheath is then advanced to the CCA over the Vitek catheter and Glidewire/Amplatz wire. After sheath or guide placement, vascular tortuosity is reassessed. Occasionally, the vascular tortuosity significantly worsens and careful reconsideration is required to determine if CS should still proceed as the risk-benefit ratio may have altered.

Anticoagulation is administered once the sheath is in place with either weight-adjusted heparin or bivalirudin. Bivalirudin is a direct thrombin inhibitor and unlike heparin does not activate platelets. When used in percutaneous coronary intervention, it has been shown to produce the same efficacy as heparin and glycoprotein (GP) IIb/IIIa inhibitors combined but with less bleeding complications [39,40]. Limited data on bivalirudin use in peripheral vascular interventions show that its use appears safe [41,42]. GP IIb/IIIa inhibitors are not used due to higher risk of cerebral hemorrhage [43,44]. For these reasons, bilvalirudin alone is routinely used during the CS procedure in our institution. Care must be taken to avoid over-anticoagulation irrespective of regimen used, to reduce risk of cerebral hemorrhage. Atropine is administered before balloon pre-dilatation to reduce the incidence of severe bradycardia and hypotension, unless an elevated heart rate is present at the beginning of the procedure or if the lesion is a post-CEA restenosis [45].

After crossing the lesion with a filter wire—a separated wire/filter system (eg, the Bare wire system from Abbott Vascular, Santa Clara, CA) is preferred—the filter is deployed well distal to the lesion in a straight segment of the ICA. Deploying the filter around a bend may reduce its efficacy due to suboptimal apposition of the filter against the vessel wall. In the presence of a severe angulation distal to the filter, the risk of ICA dissection is increased as the filter may move during the procedure. In such situations, the procedure may be more safely performed with a proximal occlusion device or the patient considered for CEA.

In very severe stenosis, where difficulty crossing with the filter is anticipated, the "pre-pre-dilatation" technique is used. Any 0.014 wire, usually a hydrophilic wire such as the PT2 (Boston Scientific, Natuck, MA) is first advanced across the severe lesion and "pre-pre-dilatation" is performed with a small 2.0- to 2.5-mm balloon to facilitate advancement of the filter beyond the stenosis. This unprotected but controlled dilatation with a small balloon is preferable to multiple and prolonged attempts at passing the filter across the stenosis. Once the filter is deployed, gentle pre-dilatation is performed using a small balloon (3.0 – 3.5 mm) with a single inflation. The intent is to create a controlled dissection and "plastering" of plaque to facilitate stent placement and yet minimize plaque disruption from stent delivery.

Self-expandable nitinol stents are used almost exclusively, with stent design falling into two broad groups. The open-cell design (eg, Acculink, Abbott Vacular, Santa Clara, CA) is more flexible and trackable and conforms better to the vascular anatomy, especially if tortuous. Conversely, the closed cell design (eg, Xact stent, Abbott Vascular, Santa Clara, CA) is less flexible but theoretically would "entrap" atheromatous debris better and also cause less "hang-up" when retrieving the distal filter with the retrieval catheter. Cases where closed-cell stents cannot be placed due to tortuosity are exceedingly uncommon. In-vitro experimental work by Ohki showed that plaque prolapse through the stent struts was significantly less for closed-cell stents [46]. Clinical studies examining superiority of stent cell designs have yielded conflicting results, although it appears that symptomatic patients experience lower adverse event rates with the use of closed-cell stents [47–49]. For these reasons, the closed cell stent is preferred. Oversized straight 9- or 10-mm, or tapered 7- to 9-mm or 8- to 10-mm stents should be used to maximize plaque coverage by metal, and usually includes stenting a segment of the 9- to 10-mm distal CCA. It is advisable not to skimp on stent length since restenosis rates are low and stenting across the ECA, even if the ECA is "pinched" or even occluded, usually results in no sequelae. A 30- or 40-mm stent length is thus recommended for the vast majority of cases. When positioning the stent, it is important not to underestimate the "landing zone" length needing proximal to the filter. This is particularly critical if there is a sharp bend in the ICA distal to the filter, as inadvertent pushing and pulling on the filter may occur while attempting to position the stent, leading to dissection of the distal ICA (with possible catastrophic consequences). The stent should also be positioned well below a sharp bend; otherwise severe distal kinking of the ICA may result.

Postdilatation is performed with an undersized balloon (usually 5.0 mm diameter) with a single gentle inflation. The intention is to gently layer the stent onto the plaque, leaving the stent to slowly expand outward against the arterial wall. Our experience and that of others [50] indicates that this is the step most likely to cause clinically significant emboli. Aggressive postdilatation must be avoided to minimize dislodgement of plaque fragments that have prolapsed through the stent struts. Angioplasty in this setting should be used only to facilitate stent placement and not as a treatment in itself. Therefore, the previous term carotid angioplasty and stenting (CAS = carotid *angioplasty* and stenting) is better termed carotid stenting (CS) in light of this new understanding, emphasizing that stenting is the primary focus with balloon dilatation only facilitating the process.

Contrast injections are kept to a minimum throughout the intervention. This reduces risk of injecting microbubbles or microthrombi into the brain [51], and reduces risk of contrast-induced nephropathy in patients with chronic renal impairment. Balloon dilatation and stent placement can be performed accurately using bony landmarks. Residual stenoses up to 30%, residual ulcers, and mild to moderate distal vessel spasm are best left alone.

CS is now performed routinely with EPDs as studies have documented reduction in MES as well as adverse clinical events [13,52,53]. Filter dwell time is closely monitored and minimized. The CREATE registry showed that filter deployment duration was a predictor for adverse events [23]. Likely reasons are that increased filter deployment time is a surrogate for case complexity and that the longer the filter is deployed, the more the accumulation of fibrin and the filter itself may become a source of embolism. In the vast majority of CS procedures, a distal filter is used. Distal balloon occlusion protection with the Percusurge GuardWire system (Medtronic, Santa Rosa, CA) has the advantages of a lower profile, better trackability, and more complete emboli protection [54], although it is suitable only in patients with sufficient intracranial collateral circulation. With all distal protection devices, the initial wiring of the lesion is unprotected and has been shown to cause small amounts of microemboli [13]. Proximal protection devices, such as the Parodi Anti-Emboli System and MOMA device, have been developed to overcome this limitation [55–57]. Both systems work using balloon occlusion of proximal flow in the CCA and a second balloon occluding flow from the ECA before the lesion is crossed. An added advantage is that any 0.014-inch wire can be used. The Parodi system has an extra feature of creating a shunt and reversing blood flow in the ICA [55]. These systems are, however, more cumbersome to use, require a 9F sheath,

and like the distal balloon occlusion system, are not suitable for patients with contralateral ICA occlusion or "isolated hemisphere." To date they have not gained widespread usage. Regardless of system used, the procedure should be performed relatively fast by an operator facile in the technique. Average filter dwell time of < 9 minutes can be achieved even in the octogenarian population [37].

Causes of Stroke Prior to Treating the Lesion

Several factors are known to increase risk of periprocedural stroke before treatment of the lesion. Excessive manipulation in the aortic arch particularly with 8F guides, inadvertent placement of the 0.035-inch Supracore or Amplatz wire across the stenosis while attempting to access the CCA, and allowing the sheath to "snow plough" into a lesion extending into the CCA can occur even with experienced operators. Minimizing manipulations in the arch and paying careful attention to the wire and sheath tips can help to reduce or eliminate these complications.

Postprocedure Management

Patients are usually monitored closely in a dedicated unit for 4 to 6 hours. BP control is essential as either excessively low or elevated BP may have deleterious consequences. Simple hydration should not be overlooked as this not only reduces risk of contrast-induced nephropathy but is also beneficial for the relative hypotension that most patients experience post CS. Frequent neurologic assessments should be performed during the initial 24 hours and patients are usually discharged the next day following uncomplicated procedures. Dual antiplatelet therapy is continued for at least 4 weeks, and thereafter acetylsalicylic acid or clopidogrel is maintained lifelong. Doppler ultrasound should be performed at 1 month, serving as a baseline reference value for future follow-up.

Management of Hemodynamics
Hypotension and bradycardia usually occur after stenting and postdilatation due to stretching of

the baroreceptors, especially if the procedure involved the bulbous carotid, and is the commonest "complication" seen after CS. Usually it is transient and resolves with fluid bolus. More persistent or severe cases of hypotension can be rapidly reversed with small boluses of intravenous phenylephrine. Prophylactic atropine administration before balloon dilatation and stenting reduces bradycardia or hypotension [45]. Rarely, hypotension and bradycardia can persist for several days and intravenous pressors such as dopamine may be required. Early ambulation may reduce the frequency and severity of this phenomenon, and groin closure devices may provide an advantage in this aspect.

Hyperperfusion syndrome can occur after relief of a very severe stenosis especially if the periprocedural BP was elevated. The underlying process appears to be due to impaired cerebral autoregulation after prolonged and severe ICA stenosis. The classical symptom is headache. Nausea, vomiting, focal neurologic deficits, and seizures may also occur. A high index of suspicion for this complication should be entertained, especially if there was postprocedure hypertension. Brain CT may be normal or reveal vasogenic edema, and velocities in the ipsilateral middle cerebral artery may be elevated [58,59]. Treatment includes BP reduction with intravenous agents, withholding antiplatelet agents until symptom resolution, and close monitoring of neurologic status [60]. Stringent BP control pre- and post-CS has been shown to reduce the hyperperfusion syndrome and the risk of resultant cerebral hemorrhage [38].

Special Considerations

Advanced Techniques to Manage Unique Anatomy

In cases with very tortuous vascular anatomy, special measures to maintain stability of the system or to cross the lesion are required. Use of larger-sized sheaths or guides may help provide extra support. An extra 0.014-inch wire can also be placed in the ECA as a "buddy wire" to provide stability of the system. It must be considered however, that these maneuvers may increase risk of periprocedural adverse events.

Crossing a lesion in tortuous anatomy may be further aided by simple maneuvers, such as removing the patient's head restraint with neck extension and getting the patient to turn the head from side to side, which may help to reduce vascular tortuosity. Use of separated wire-filter systems such as the Emboshield filter (Abbott Vascular, Santa Clara, CA) or Spider filter (EV3, Plymouth, MN) may be helpful. Other options include using a hydrophilic 0.014-inch wire to cross the lesion to reduce tortuosity (buddy wire), and then pass the filter wire.

In very severely stenotic lesions, "pre-predilatation" with a small balloon may facilitate crossing of the filter.

Infrequently, the ICA take-off is severely angulated and the 0.014-inch filter wire does not negotiate the bend due to wire prolapse. A useful technique is to advance a 125-cm 5F JR4 or IMA catheter through the sheath or guide, positioning and directing the JR4 or IMA catheter towards the ICA ostium. This then facilitates passage of the 0.014-inch wire into the ICA and across the stenosis.

Carotid Stent Restenosis

Restenosis post-CS is uncommon, with most series documenting < 5% incidence [61–63], using a cut-off value of 80% and 50% for asymptomatic and symptomatic patients, respectively. Frequently, it is detected on Doppler ultrasound, since symptoms are uncommon. Restenosis seems to occur more frequently in those with smaller stent luminal diameter post-stenting [64], and in patients who undergo CS for post-CEA restenosis and post-radiation carotid stenosis [61]. Treatment with repeat balloon angioplasty, cutting balloon angioplasty, or restenting is usually effective [65].

Patients Undergoing Coronary Artery Bypass Surgery with Severe Carotid Stenosis

The incidence of coexisting carotid and coronary artery disease (CAD) ranges between 2% and 12% [66]. In patients with severe CAD and carotid stenosis, the risk of stroke during CABG (∼ 10%) is significantly higher than in patients without carotid disease [67]; and conversely, performing

CEA before CABG resulted in higher rates of MI (~ 11%) and death (~ 9%) [67]. The risks of MI (~ 5%)/stroke (~ 6%)/death (~ 6%) in performing CABG and CEA simultaneously are also elevated [68]. Recently, it has been shown that with current-day practice, performing CS prior to CABG resulted in a total MI/stroke/death rate of 6.7% [69]. In those who are suitable, staged CS followed by CABG may be a safer option.

Concurrent Medical Therapy

Medical therapy should be viewed as an integral part of carotid disease treatment *whether or not* CS is performed. Therefore CS should be viewed as an adjunct to optimal medical therapy, and that to accrue the greatest benefit from CS, concomitant optimal medical therapy is imperative. Antiplatelet therapy with acetylsalicylic acid or clopidogrel should be universal in patients with carotid disease. Short-term use of dual antiplatelet therapy in symptomatic carotid stenosis appears beneficial [70,71], although long-term use is not recommended as a previous study showed no significant reduction in stroke rate but increased major bleeding [72]. Dual antiplatelet therapy should also be used periprocedurally if not contraindicated whenever CS is performed.

The usual atherosclerotic risk factors should be assessed and treated. Hypertension is a strong risk factor for stroke. BP reduction lowers stroke risk, and use of angiotensin-converting enzme (ACE) inhibitors further reduces stroke risk over and above that attributable to BP lowering alone [73,74]. Lipid lowering therapy with statins helps plaque stabilization and may even promote plaque regression. A large randomized trial demonstrated reduction in stroke with aggressive lipid-lowering therapy with statins [75]. Aggressive use of statins before CS may possibly also reduce risk of embolization by stabilizing the plaque [76]. Smoking cessation should be advised at every opportunity. Glycemic control in diabetics is also important, although it has been shown that tight glycemic control reduces only microvascular but not macrovascular complications such as stroke [77]. Good glycemic control, however, improves lipid profile, which is important in these patients. Lifestyle changes should not be for-gotten as part of the general measures to reduce the atherosclerotic burden.

Future Directions

The optimal timing of CS in symptomatic patients is yet to be well defined. The risk-benefit ratio of revascularization is greatest in the early period after a transient ischemic attack or minor stroke and declines with time as demonstrated in the CEA studies, since the risk of stroke diminishes with time from the initial event [78]. Therefore, performing CS early after an event would theoretically yield the most protective benefit. However, anecdotal experience, now supported by published data, revealed that performing CS early (within 2 weeks) after an event resulted in higher adverse event rates than if CS was delayed [79].

For asymptomatic carotid stenoses, future studies will be needed to determine what clinical factors could predict subgroups most at risk of stroke and would hence derive the greatest benefit from CS. In this asymptomatic group, plaque imaging to detect the "vulnerable" plaque more likely to embolize could prove useful [80].

Technological advancements will result in decreased profile and increased maneuverability of devices, and in better EPDs and stents (especially closed cell), which may reduce complication rates and improve the safety of the procedure. In addition, rigorous operator training and further technique refinement will undoubtedly contribute towards reducing periprocedural events.

Ongoing trials will provide further data on the safety and efficacy of CS compared to CEA. The CREST trial will shed light on both symptomatic and asymptomatic patients with normal surgical risk, ICSS or CAVATAS-2 will randomize symptomatic patients at normal surgical risk, and ACT1 and ACST-2 will provide answers for asymptomatic patients at normal surgical risk.

The most important factor, however, that will further reduce periprocedural adverse events is that of careful patient selection. Akin to the concept of surgical risk, patients being considered for CS should be selected based on "stent risk" and greater efforts must be made to identify additional clinical or anatomic markers that increase the risk of CS.

Conflicts of Interest Disclosures

Dr. Sriram Iyer is a speaker for Abbott Vascular and Boston Scientific, receives royalties from Abbott Vascular and Boston Scientific, and has ownership interest in Boston Scientific. Dr. Gary Roubin is a consultant to Abbott Vascular, and receives royalties from Cook Inc. Drs. Paul Chiam and Jiri Vitek have no disclosures.

References

1. Beneficial effect of carotid endarterectomy in symptomatic patients with high-grade carotid stenosis. North American Symptomatic Carotid Endarterectomy Trial Collaborators. *N Engl J Med.* 1991;325:445–453.

2. Barnett HJ, Taylor DW, Eliasziw M, *et al.* Benefit of carotid endarterectomy in patients with symptomatic moderate or severe stenosis. North American Symptomatic Carotid Endarterectomy Trial Collaborators. *N Engl J Med.* 1998;339:1415–1425.

3. European Carotid Surgery Trialists Collaborative Group Medical Research Council European Carotid Surgery Trial. Randomised trial of endarterectomy for recently symptomatic carotid stenosis: final results of the MRC European Carotid Surgery Trial (ECST). *Lancet.* 1998;351:1379–1387.

4. Endarterectomy for asymptomatic carotid artery stenosis. Executive Committee for the Asymptomatic Carotid Atherosclerosis Study. *JAMA.* 1995;273:1421–1428.

5. Halliday A, Mansfield A, Marro J, *et al.* Prevention of disabling and fatal strokes by successful carotid endarterectomy in patients without recent neurological symptoms: randomised controlled trial. *Lancet.* 2004;363:1491–1502.

6. Biller J, Feinberg WM, Castaldo JE, *et al.* Guidelines for carotid endarterectomy: a statement for healthcare professionals from a Special Writing Group of the Stroke Council, American Heart Association. *Circulation.* 1998;97:501–509.

7. Sacco RL, Adams R, Albers G, *et al.* Guidelines for prevention of stroke in patients with ischemic stroke or transient ischemic attack: a statement for health-care professionals from the American Heart Association/American Stroke Association Council on Stroke: co-sponsored by the Council on Cardiovascular Radiology and Intervention: the American Academy of Neurology affirms the value of this guideline. *Stroke.* 2006;37:577–617.

8. Bockenheimer SA, Mathias K. Percutaneous transluminal angioplasty in arteriosclerotic internal carotid artery stenosis. *AJNR Am J Neuroradiol.* 1983;4:791–792.

9. Theron J, Raymond J, Casasco A, Courtheoux F. Percutaneous angioplasty of atherosclerotic and postsurgical stenosis of carotid arteries. *AJNR Am J Neuroradiol.* 1987;8:495–500.

10. Roubin GS, Yadav S, Iyer SS, Vitek J. Carotid stent-supported angioplasty: a neurovascular intervention to prevent stroke. *Am J Cardiol.* 1996;78:8–12.

11. Diethrich EB, Ndiaye M, Reid DB. Stenting in the carotid artery: initial experience in 110 patients. *J Endovasc Surg.* 1996;3:42–62.

12. Roubin GS, New G, Iyer SS, *et al.* Immediate and late clinical outcomes of carotid artery stenting in patients with symptomatic and asymptomatic carotid artery stenosis: a 5-year prospective analysis. *Circulation.* 2001;103:532–537.

13. Al-Mubarak N, Roubin GS, Vitek JJ, Iyer SS, New G, Leon MB. Effect of the distal-balloon protection system on microembolization during carotid stenting. *Circulation.* 2001;104:1999–2002.

14. Roubin GS, Iyer S, Halkin A, Vitek J, Brennan C. Realizing the potential of carotid artery stenting: proposed paradigms for patient selection and procedural technique. *Circulation.* 2006;113:2021–2030.

15. CAVATAS Investigators, Endovascular versus surgical treatment in patients with carotid stenosis in the Carotid and Vertebral Artery Transluminal Angioplasty Study (CAVATAS): a randomised trial. *Lancet.* 2001;357:1729–1737.

16. Yadav JS, Wholey MH, Kuntz RE, *et al.* Protected carotid-artery stenting versus endarterectomy in high-risk patients. *N Engl J Med.* 2004;351:1493–1501.

17. Gurm HS, Yadav JS, Fayad P, *et al.* Long-term results of carotid stenting versus endarterectomy in high-risk patients. *N Engl J Med.* 2008;358:1572–1579.

18. CaRESS Steering Committee. Carotid Revascularization Using Endarterectomy or Stenting Systems (CaRESS) phase I clinical trial: 1-year results. *J Vasc Surg.* 2005;42:213–219.

19. The SPACE Collaborative Group. 30 day results from the SPACE trial of stent-protected angioplasty versus carotid endarterectomy in symptomatic

patients: a randomised non-inferiority trial. *Lancet.* 2006;368:1239–1247.

20. Mas JL, Chatellier G, Beyssen B, *et al.* Endarterectomy versus stenting in patients with symptomatic severe carotid stenosis. *N Engl J Med.* 2006;355: 1660–1671.

21. Gray WA, Hopkins LN, Yadav S, *et al.* Protected carotid stenting in high-surgical-risk patients: the ARCHeR results. *J Vasc Surg.* 2006;44:258–268.

22. White CJ, Iyer SS, Hopkins LN, Katzen BT, Russell ME. Carotid stenting with distal protection in high surgical risk patients: the BEACH trial 30 day results. *Catheter Cardiovasc Interv.* 2006;67:503–512.

23. Safian RD, Bresnahan JF, Jaff MR, *et al.* Protected carotid stenting in high-risk patients with severe carotid artery stenosis. *J Am Coll Cardiol.* 2006;47:2384–2389.

24. Katzen BT, Criado FJ, Ramee SR, *et al.* Carotid artery stenting with emboli protection surveillance study: thirty-day results of the CASES-PMS study. *Catheter Cardiovasc Interv.* 2007;70:316–323.

25. Gray WA, Yadav JS, Verta P, *et al.* The CAPTURE registry: results of carotid stenting with embolic protection in the post approval setting. *Catheter Cardiovasc Interv.* 2007;69:341–348.

26. Iyer SS, White CJ, Hopkins LN, *et al.* Carotid artery revascularization in high-surgical-risk patients using the Carotid WALLSTENT and FilterWire EX/EZ: 1-year outcomes in the BEACH Pivotal Group. *J Am Coll Cardiol.* 2008;51:427–434.

27. Theiss W, Hermanek P, Mathias K, *et al.* Pro-CAS: a prospective registry of carotid angioplasty and stenting. *Stroke.* 2004;35:2134–2139.

28. Zahn R, Roth E, Ischinger T, *et al.* Carotid artery stenting in clinical practice results from the Carotid Artery Stenting (CAS)-registry of the Arbeitsgemeinschaft Leitende Kardiologische Krankenhausarzte (ALKK). *Z Kardiol.* 2005;94:163–172.

29. Bates ER, Babb JD, Casey DE, Jr., *et al.* ACCF/SCAI/SVMB/SIR/ASITN 2007 clinical expert consensus document on carotid stenting: a report of the American College of Cardiology Foundation Task Force on Clinical Expert Consensus Documents (ACCF/SCAI/SVMB/SIR/ASITN Clinical Expert Consensus Document Committee on Carotid Stenting). *J Am Coll Cardiol.* 2007;49:126–170.

30. Segal AZ, Abernethy WB, Palacios IF, BeLue R, Rordorf G. Stroke as a complication of cardiac catheterization: risk factors and clinical features. *Neurology.* 2001;56:975–977.

31. Hobson RW II, Howard VJ, Roubin GS, *et al.* Carotid artery stenting is associated with increased complications in octogenarians: 30-day stroke and death rates in the CREST lead-in phase. *J Vasc Surg.* 2004;40:1106–1111.

32. Gray WA, Yadav JS, Verta P, *et al.* The CAPTURE registry: predictors of outcomes in carotid artery stenting with embolic protection for high surgical risk patients in the early post-approval setting. *Catheter Cardiovasc Interv.* 2007;70:1025–1033.

33. Lin SC, Trocciola SM, Rhee J, *et al.* Analysis of anatomic factors and age in patients undergoing carotid angioplasty and stenting. *Ann Vasc Surg.* 2005;19:798–804.

34. Setacci C, de Donato G, Chisci E, *et al.* Is carotid artery stenting in octogenarians really dangerous? *J Endovasc Ther.* 2006;13:302–309.

35. Lam RC, Lin SC, DeRubertis B, Hynecek R, Kent KC, Faries PL. The impact of increasing age on anatomic factors affecting carotid angioplasty and stenting. *J Vasc Surg.* 2007;45:875–880.

36. Longo GM, Kibbe MR, Eskandari MK. Carotid artery stenting in octogenarians: is it too risky? *Ann Vasc Surg.* 2005;19:812–816.

37. Chiam PT, Roubin GS, Iyer SS, *et al.* Carotid artery stenting in elderly patients: importance of case selection. *Catheter Cardiovasc Interv.* 2008;72:318–324.

38. Abou-Chebl A, Reginelli J, Bajzer CT, Yadav JS. Intensive treatment of hypertension decreases the risk of hyperperfusion and intracerebral hemorrhage following carotid artery stenting. *Catheter Cardiovasc Interv.* 2007;69:690–696.

39. Lincoff AM, Bittl JA, Harrington RA, *et al.* Bivalirudin and provisional glycoprotein IIb/IIIa blockade compared with heparin and planned glycoprotein IIb/IIIa blockade during percutaneous coronary intervention: REPLACE-2 randomized trial. *JAMA.* 2003;289:853–863.

40. Stone GW, McLaurin BT, Cox DA, *et al.* Bivalirudin for patients with acute coronary syndromes. *N Engl J Med.* 2006;355:2203–2216.

41. Katzen BT, Ardid MI, MacLean AA, *et al.* Bivalirudin as an anticoagulation agent: safety and efficacy in peripheral interventions. *J Vasc Interv Radiol.* 2005;16:1183–1187; quiz 1187.

42. Bush RL, Lin PH, Mureebe L, Zhou W, Peden EK, Lumsden AB. Routine bivalirudin use in percutaneous carotid interventions. *J Endovasc Ther.* 2005;12:521–522.

43. Qureshi AI, Suri MF, Ali Z, *et al.* Carotid angioplasty and stent placement: a prospective analysis

of perioperative complications and impact of intravenously administered abciximab. *Neurosurgery.* 2002;50:466–473; discussion 473–5.

44. Qureshi AI, Saad M, Zaidat OO, *et al.* Intracerebral hemorrhages associated with neurointerventional procedures using a combination of antithrombotic agents including abciximab. *Stroke.* 2002;33:1916–1919.

45. Cayne NS, Faries PL, Trocciola SM, *et al.* Carotid angioplasty and stent-induced bradycardia and hypotension: Impact of prophylactic atropine administration and prior carotid endarterectomy. *J Vasc Surg.* 2005;41:956–961.

46. Ohki TV, Veith FJ. In-vitro models to analyse embolization during carotid stenting. In: Amor M, Bergeron P, Mathias K, Raithel D, Editors. *Carotid artery angioplasty and stenting.* Torino: Edizioni Minerva Medica; 2002: 178–186.

47. Schillinger M, Gschwendtner M, Reimers B, *et al.* Does carotid stent cell design matter? *Stroke.* 2008;39:905–909.

48. Hart JP, Peeters P, Verbist J, Deloose K, Bosiers M. Do device characteristics impact outcome in carotid artery stenting? *J Vasc Surg.* 2006;44:725–730; discussion 730–731.

49. Bosiers M, de Donato G, Deloose K, *et al.* Does free cell area influence the outcome in carotid artery stenting? *Eur J Vasc Endovasc Surg.* 2007;33:135–141; discussion 142–143.

50. Theron J. My history of carotid angioplasty and stenting. *J Invasive Cardiol.* 2008;20:E102–E108.

51. Markus H, Loh A, Israel D, Buckenham T, Clifton A, Brown MM. Microscopic air embolism during cerebral angiography and strategies for its avoidance. *Lancet.* 1993;341:784–787.

52. Kastrup A, Groschel K, Krapf H, Brehm BR, Dichgans J, Schulz JB. Early outcome of carotid angioplasty and stenting with and without cerebral protection devices: a systematic review of the literature. *Stroke.* 2003;34:813–819.

53. Zahn R, Mark B, Niedermaier N, *et al.* Embolic protection devices for carotid artery stenting: better results than stenting without protection? *Eur Heart J.* 2004;25:1550–1558.

54. Rubartelli P, Brusa G, Arrigo A, *et al.* Transcranial Doppler monitoring during stenting of the carotid bifurcation: evaluation of two different distal protection devices in preventing embolization. *J Endovasc Ther.* 2006;13:436–442.

55. Parodi JC, La Mura R, Ferreira LM, *et al.* Initial evaluation of carotid angioplasty and stenting with three different cerebral protection devices. *J Vasc Surg.* 2000;32:1127–1136.

56. Reimers B, Sievert H, Schuler GC, *et al.* Proximal endovascular flow blockage for cerebral protection during carotid artery stenting: results from a prospective multicenter registry. *J Endovasc Ther.* 2005;12:156–165.

57. Schmidt A, Diederich KW, Scheinert S, *et al.* Effect of two different neuroprotection systems on microembolization during carotid artery stenting. *J Am Coll Cardiol.* 2004;44:1966–1969.

58. Jansen C, Sprengers AM, Moll FL, *et al.* Prediction of intracerebral haemorrhage after carotid endarterectomy by clinical criteria and intraoperative transcranial Doppler monitoring: results of 233 operations. *Eur J Vasc Surg.* 1994;8:220–225.

59. Coutts SB, Hill MD, Hu WY. Hyperperfusion syndrome: toward a stricter definition. *Neurosurgery.* 2003;53:1053–1058; discussion 1058–1060.

60. Abou-Chebl A, Yadav JS, Reginelli JP, Bajzer C, Bhatt D, Krieger DW. Intracranial hemorrhage and hyperperfusion syndrome following carotid artery stenting: risk factors, prevention, and treatment. *J Am Coll Cardiol.* 2004;43:1596–1601.

61. Younis GA, Gupta K, Mortazavi A, *et al.* Predictors of carotid stent restenosis. *Catheter Cardiovasc Interv.* 2007;69:673–682.

62. Wholey MH, Al-Mubarek N, Wholey MH. Updated review of the global carotid artery stent registry. *Catheter Cardiovasc Interv.* 2003;60:259–266.

63. Levy EI, Hanel RA, Lau T, *et al.* Frequency and management of recurrent stenosis after carotid artery stent implantation. *J Neurosurg.* 2005;102:29–37.

64. Khan MA, Liu MW, Chio FL, Roubin GS, Iyer SS, Vitek JJ. Predictors of restenosis after successful carotid artery stenting. *Am J Cardiol.* 2003;92:895–897.

65. Reimers B, Tubler T, de Donato G, *et al.* Endovascular treatment of in-stent restenosis after carotid artery stenting: immediate and midterm results. *J Endovasc Ther.* 2006;13:429–435.

66. Huh J, Wall MJ Jr., Soltero ER. Treatment of combined coronary and carotid artery disease. *Curr Opin Cardiol.* 2003;18:447–453.

67. Moore WS, Barnett HJ, Beebe HG, *et al.* Guidelines for carotid endarterectomy. A multidisciplinary consensus statement from the Ad Hoc Committee, American Heart Association. *Circulation.* 1995;91:566–579.

68. Van Der Heyden J, Suttorp MJ, Bal ET, *et al.* Staged carotid angioplasty and stenting followed by cardiac surgery in patients with severe asymptomatic carotid

artery stenosis: early and long-term results. *Circulation.* 2007;116:2036–2042.

69. Markus HS, Droste DW, Kaps M, *et al.* Dual antiplatelet therapy with clopidogrel and aspirin in symptomatic carotid stenosis evaluated using doppler embolic signal detection: the Clopidogrel and Aspirin for Reduction of Emboli in Symptomatic Carotid Stenosis (CARESS) trial. *Circulation.* 2005;111:2233–2240.

70. Rothwell PM, Giles MF, Chandratheva A, *et al.* Effect of urgent treatment of transient ischaemic attack and minor stroke on early recurrent stroke (EXPRESS study): a prospective population-based sequential comparison. *Lancet.* 2007;370:1432–1442.

71. Diener HC, Bogousslavsky J, Brass LM, *et al.* Aspirin and clopidogrel compared with clopidogrel alone after recent ischaemic stroke or transient ischaemic attack in high-risk patients (MATCH): randomised, double-blind, placebo-controlled trial. *Lancet.* 2004;364:331–337.

72. Yusuf S, Sleight P, Pogue J, Bosch J, Davies R, Dagenais G. Effects of an angiotensin-converting-enzyme inhibitor, ramipril, on cardiovascular events in high-risk patients. The Heart Outcomes Prevention Evaluation Study Investigators. *N Engl J Med.* 2000;342:145–153.

73. PROGRESS Collaborative Group. Randomised trial of a perindopril-based blood-pressure-lowering regimen among 6,105 individuals with previous stroke or transient ischaemic attack. *Lancet.* 2001;358:1033–1041.

74. Collins R, Armitage J, Parish S, Sleight P, Peto R. Effects of cholesterol-lowering with simvastatin on stroke and other major vascular events in 20536 people with cerebrovascular disease or other high-risk conditions. *Lancet.* 2004;363:757–767.

75. Bicknell CD, Cowling MG, Clark MW, *et al.* Carotid angioplasty in a pulsatile flow model: factors affecting embolic potential. *Eur J Vasc Endovasc Surg.* 2003;26:22–31.

76. Intensive blood-glucose control with sulphonylureas or insulin compared with conventional treatment and risk of complications in patients with type 2 diabetes (UKPDS 33). UK Prospective Diabetes Study (UKPDS) Group. *Lancet.* 1998;352:837–853.

77. Rothwell PM, Eliasziw M, Gutnikov SA, Warlow CP, Barnett HJ. Endarterectomy for symptomatic carotid stenosis in relation to clinical subgroups and timing of surgery. *Lancet.* 2004;363:915–924.

78. Topakian R, Strasak AM, Sonnberger M, *et al.* Timing of stenting of symptomatic carotid stenosis is predictive of 30-day outcome. *Eur J Neurol.* 2007;14:672–678.

79. Mathiesen EB, Bonaa KH, Joakimsen O. Echolucent plaques are associated with high risk of ischemic cerebrovascular events in carotid stenosis: the tromso study. *Circulation.* 2001;103:2171–2175.

80. Diethrich EB, Margolis PM, Reid DB, *et al.* Virtual histology intravascular ultrasound assessment of carotid artery disease: the Carotid Artery Plaque Virtual Histology Evaluation (CAPITAL) study. *J Endovasc Ther.* 2007;14:676–686.

CHAPTER 9

Alcohol Ablation of Hypertrophic Cardiomyopathy

Otto M. Hess and Sven Streit

Cardiology, Swiss Cardiovascular Center, University Hospital, Bern, Switzerland

---

Chapter Overview

- Hypertrophic cardiomyopathy is characterized by asymmetric septal hypertrophy.
- About 25% to 30% of all patients present with outflow tract obstruction due to septal hypertrophy.
- Previous studies indicate an improvement in symptoms and clinical outcome after resection of the hypertrophied septum (surgical myectomy).
- New interventional techniques allow percutaneous ablation of septal hypertrophy by alcohol injection into the first to third septal branch (1–3 mL per branch).
- The technique is relatively safe, but transient or permanent atrioventricular block may occur in 10% to 15%.
- After alcohol ablation a significant reduction or complete elimination of the pressure gradient occurs in 70% to 80% of all patients at 6-month follow-up.
- Treatment recommendations suggest alcohol ablation as first-line therapy, which may be followed by surgical myectomy being reserved for cases with treatment failures or comorbidities (bypass surgery).

Clinical Picture of Hypertrophic Cardiomyopathy

Symptoms

Hypertrophic cardiomyopathy (HCM) is an autosomal dominant inherited disease with more than 250 mutations on more than a dozen genes [1]. A typical feature of HCM is an asymmetric hypertrophy of the ventricular septum with outflow tract obstruction (HOCM) in 25% to 30% of all patients. Under exercise the obstruction may occur in almost 70% of all patients due to sympathetic stimulation [2]. Management (Fig. 9.1) [3] of patients with hypertrophic cardiomyopathy is directed to alleviation of symptoms, prevention of complications (eg, atrial fibrillation), and reduction in sudden cardiac death [4].

Complications

Sudden death is one of the most important threats for patients with hypertrophic cardiomyopathy. Approximately 50% to 60% of all patients who die, die suddenly. Sudden death is usually assumed to be due to ventricular tachyarrhythmia [5], but hemodynamic factors and myocardial ischemia may also be causally involved. Risk stratification has been a major issue in patients with HOCM because of the albeit small risk of unexpected sudden cardiac death (SCD). Strategies to identify patients at risk for SCD have been manifold and the five most important risk factors are listed in Table 9.1 [6].

Syncope may occur in these patients either due to arrhythmia or a sudden increase in outflow

Current Best Practice in Interventional Cardiology. Edited by B Meier. © 2010 Blackwell Publishing.

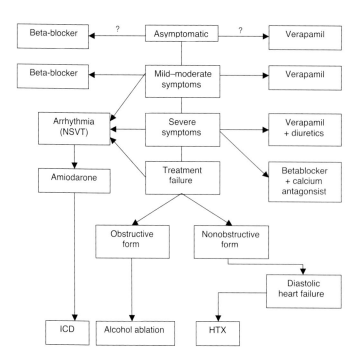

Figure 9.1 Treatment strategy in hypertrophic cardiomyopathy. (ICD, implantable cardioverter defibrillator; NSVT, nonsustained ventricular tachycardia; HTX, heart transplantation.) (From Hess OM. Risk stratification in hypertrophic cardiomyopathy: fact or fiction? *J Am Coll Cardiol.* 2003;42:880–881.)

tract obstruction. Rapid changes in body position or strenuous exercise may lead to an increase in outflow tract obstruction, either due to a decrease in venous return with a decrease in cardiac volumes and an increase in outflow tract obstruction, or due to an increase in cardiac contractility with hypercontraction of the left ventricle and elimination of left ventricular (LV) cavity (drop in cardiac output). Strenuous exercise or competitive sports should be avoided in patients with HOCM because of the risk of sudden death. Typically, sudden death occurs during or just after strenuous physical exercise. Atrial fibrillation as a cause of diastolic dysfunction with increased filling pressure and dilata-

tion of the atria should be pharmacologically or electrically converted because of the hemodynamic consequences of the loss of atrial contraction on cardiac output. If sinus rhythm cannot be restored, oral anticoagulation is mandatory when no contraindications exist. Infective endocarditis may occur in about 5% of HCM patients, and antibiotic prophylaxis is indicated. Infection typically occurs on the aortic or mitral valve or on the septal contact site of the anterior mitral leaflet.

Prognosis and Outcome

The clinical course in HOCM is variable and may remain stable over many years in many patients.

- Non-sustained ventricular tachycardia
- Abnormal exercise blood pressure response
- Family history of premature sudden death
- Unexplained syncope
- Severe left ventricular hypertrophy (septal thickness >30 mm).

Reproduced with permission from Elliott PM, Gimeno JR, Tome MT, et al. Left ventricular outflow tract obstruction and sudden death risk in patients with hypertrophic cardiomyopathy. *Eur Heart J.* 2006;27:1933–1941.

Table 9.1 Risk Factors for Sudden Cardiac Death [6]

Annual mortality rates have been reported to range between 2% and 3% but may be higher in children [7,8]. Clinical deterioration is often slow but clinical symptoms are poorly related to the severity of outflow tract obstruction. Generally, symptoms increase with age. However, larger randomized clinical trials are still missing. This may be either due to the relative low prevalence and the large variability of the disease with nonobstructive and obstructive forms as well as symptomatic and asymptomatic patients. There is an urgent need for randomized multicenter treatment trials.

Therapeutic Strategies in Hypertrophic Cardiomyopathy

Medical Versus Interventional Therapy

Asymptomatic patients with mild LV hypertrophy do probably not need drug therapy, whereas asymptomatic patients with severe LV hypertrophy should be treated with verapamil or diltiazem to improve relaxation and diastolic filling, thereby lowering diastolic filling pressure.

Treatment is indicated when the patient becomes symptomatic or LV hypertrophy is severe. Refractoriness to medical therapy usually indicates progression of the disease. At this point the use of more aggressive therapies such as alcohol ablation of the septum or surgical septal myectomy are indicated. Double-chamber pacing for symptomatic relief and reduction of outflow tract obstruction has been used previously but is not recommended at present for general use. Patients with severe LV hypertrophy, recurrent syncopes, sustained and nonsustained ventricular tachyarrhythmia (NSVT), a history of familial sudden cardiac death, and a genetic phenotype for an increased risk of premature death should be treated with an implantable cardioverter-defribrillator (Fig. 9.1) [3]. In particular, patients age < 30 years have an increased risk for sudden cardiac death if NSVT occurs [5].

Surgery Versus Alcohol Ablation

In 1995, Sigwart [9] introduced a new catheter-based nonsurgical reduction therapy of the inter-

ventricular septum by infusion of small amounts of pure alcohol into the first or second septal branch of the left anterior decending coronary artery (LAD). After early scepticism, this percutaneous treatment strategy has led to a new treatment option without the need for opening the chest and ascending aorta for removal of the excessive myocardium in the left ventricular outflow tract [3].

This technique has gained great popularity in the past few years and seen rapid expansion [10]. Many centers have adopted this technique as a first line treatment of patients with HOCM. The surgical treatment has been reserved for patients with comorbidities such as organic mitral regurgitation or severe coronary artery disease requiring coronary bypass grafting [11]. Simultaneous treatment of coronary artery disease by percutaneous interventions with stent implantation and alcohol ablation of the septum has been performed in patients with HOCM and coronary artery disease. The growing interest in this new modality is explained by the apparant ease with which this technique is performed [12].

Compared to surgery, there is far less discomfort, shorter hospital stay, less expense, and avoidance of cardiopulmonary bypass [12–22]. Both reduce LV outflow tract obstruction and symptoms. Comparisons with previous surgical studies have indicated similar results between surgical myectomy and alcohol ablation [16]. However, comparisons of current literature data [23] suggest that surgical myectomy is less subject to the risk of complete atrioventricular (AV) block requiring pacemaker implantation. Cardiovascular death was higher in the alcohol ablation group, but many of the surgical studies did not specify mortality. The two cohorts have similar mortality, ranging between 0% and 5%.

Technique of Alcohol Ablation of the Septum

Outflow tract gradients of more than 30 mm Hg at rest and more than 60 mm Hg after provocation (post-extrasystolic, Valsalva, or amylnitrite inhalation) are considered to qualify for septal ablation [9].

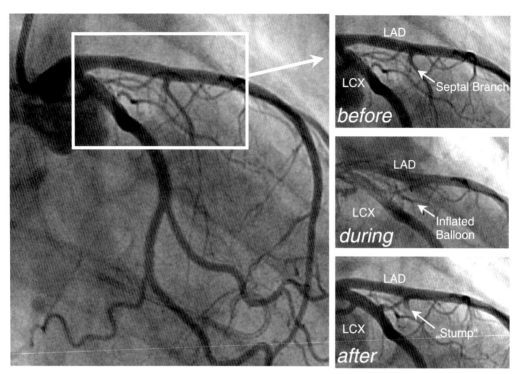

Figure 9.2 Coronary angiogram of the left coronary artery at high magnification. The left anterior descending (LAD) and the left circumflex (LCX) coronary artery can be clearly seen (*top right*) as well as the septal branch. The over-the-wire balloon catheter is introduced into the first septal branch and inflated (*middle panel*). Then 1 to 3 mL alcohol are infused over 5 minutes. The last angiogram (*bottom right*) shows that the septal branch has disappeared after alcohol injection except for a residual stump (*arrow*).

Before alcohol ablation a temporary pacemaker is placed in the right ventricle. After diagnostic coronary angiography and left ventriculography, a 6F guiding catheter is placed in the ostium of the left main coronary artery in addition to a 4F pigtail catheter (second puncture) in the apex of the left ventricle for simultaneous pressure gradient measurements. Then, a standard coronary guidewire with a floppy tip is introduced into the first, second or third septal branch. An over-the-wire balloon (1.5–2.0 mm diameter) is advanced into the septal branch and inflated with 4 to 6 bar to block the septal artery. Then, contrast material is injected to localize the ablation area under fluoroscopy. Following this procedure, echo-contrast 1 to 2 mL is injected under transthoracic echocardiography for proper localization of the ablation site (Fig. 9.2). Then, 1 to 3 mL of pure (96%) alcohol are slowly injected over 3 to 5 minutes, while the pressure gradient and the ECG are continuously recorded. At the end of the injection, there is a 4- to 5-minute wait until the balloon is deflated, to prevent alcohol backflow into the LAD. After the intervention, patients are monitored for 12 to 24 hours. The temporary pacemaker is removed after 8 to 12 hours of observation. Cardiac enzymes (creatine kinase, troponin I) are determined after 6 hours and the next morning.

Alcohol injection leads to a myocardial infarction with a creatine kinase rise to 400 to 1600 U/L. Immediately after alcohol injection, there is alcohol-induced septal hypokinesia, which leads to a reduction in outflow tract gradient. In approximately one-third of all patients the pressure gradient disappears completely and in two-thirds it decreases (Fig. 9.3). However, it takes several weeks

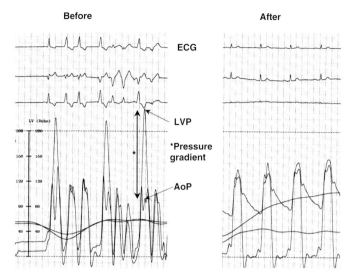

Figure 9.3 Pressure recordings in a patient with hypertrophic cardiomyopathy before and after alcohol ablation of the septum. Before the intervention there is a large pressure gradient mainly after extrasystole (150 mm Hg). The systolic pressure gradient disappears in this case completely after alcohol ablation. (AoP, aortic pressure; LVP, left ventricular pressure.)

or months (Fig. 9.4) for septal remodeling. Ventricular remodeling with a decrease in muscle mass and septal/posterior thickness takes 3 to 4 months.

Complications of Alcohol Ablation

Not all patients show a complete loss of outflow tract obstruction. Those who fail can be treated a second time. Complications include transient or permanent AV block III (Fig. 9.5, Table 9.2). Therefore, the procedure should not be done without temporary pacemaker backup. About 15% of all patients require permanent pacemaker implantation [23–29] (Table 9.2). Pre-interventional left bundle branch block or AV block I are independent predictors of AV block III after alcohol ablation. [24,30]

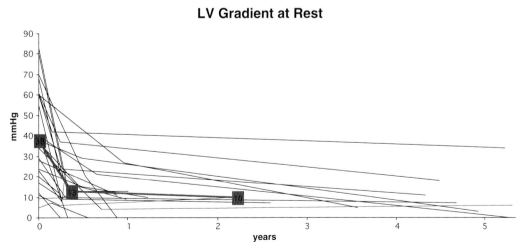

Figure 9.4 LV outflow tract gradient in patients before and after alcohol ablation (mean follow-up, 2.2 years). Data are given at rest. Pressure gradients are measured echocardiographically. Median gradients (*bold line*) decreased from 38 to 13, respectively, to 10 mm Hg during late follow-up ($p < 0.001$).

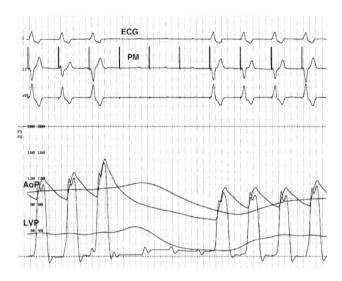

Figure 9.5 Simultaneous electrocardiogram (ECG) and pressure recordings in a patient during alcohol ablation. Electric peaks indicate pacemaker (PM) activation in the upper curve. In the case of pacing failure, aortic pressure drops significantly but atrial contractions persist. Third-degree atrioventricular (AV) block is present and continuous pacing is needed. (AoP, aortic pressure; LVP, left ventricular pressure.)

Perspectives

Alcohol ablation of the septum has become the new treatment modality in hypertrophic obstructive cardiomyopathy with a high success rate and a relatively low complication rate [15,17,31]. The most feared complication is the development of AV block, requiring prolonged rhythm control after the intervention and pacemaker implantation. In a literature overview (Table 9.2), a permanent pacemaker was required in 14% of patients after alcohol ablation [23,24,25–29]. The hypothesis that septal ablation may lead to scarring at the ablation site favoring recurrent tachyarrhythmia and NSVT[5] has not been corroborated. In contrast, previous studies have suggested that arrhythmias may even decrease due to the reduction in LV hypertrophy with a diminution of subendocardial ischemia.

Most of the studies showed a significant reduction in systolic outflow tract obstruction after alcohol ablation. The reduction in outflow tract obstruction significantly and promptly improves exercise capacity [32]. Later, LV wall thickness decreases in both septum and posterior wall. This indicates that not only the septum but also the rest of the left ventricle shows LV remodeling due to the unloading with a decrease in LV pressure gradient. This reduction in LV hypertrophy is accompanied by an improvement in diastolic function, with a reduction in LV filling pressure and an increase in diastolic filling. In a previous study [33] with septal myectomy (n = 7), a reduction in LV volume and LV filling pressure was shown during re-angiography for clinical purpose (Fig. 9.6). This figure documents very nicely the improvement in diastolic function after reduction of LV

Table 9.2 Outcome After Alcohol Ablation in a Total of 853 Patients

Author	Year	No. Patients	AV-Block III (%)	PM (%)	Death (%)
Chang et al. [24]	2003	224	14	—	—
Osterne et al. [27]	2003	18	11	11	5.5
Gietzen et al. [28]	2004	157	11	25	2.5
Talreja et al. [29]	2004	58	12	12	—
Faber et al. [30]	2005	242	10	10	1.2
Fernandes et al. [31]	2005	130	13	13	1.5
Streit et al. [23]	2007	24	13	13	0
Mean		853	12	14	2

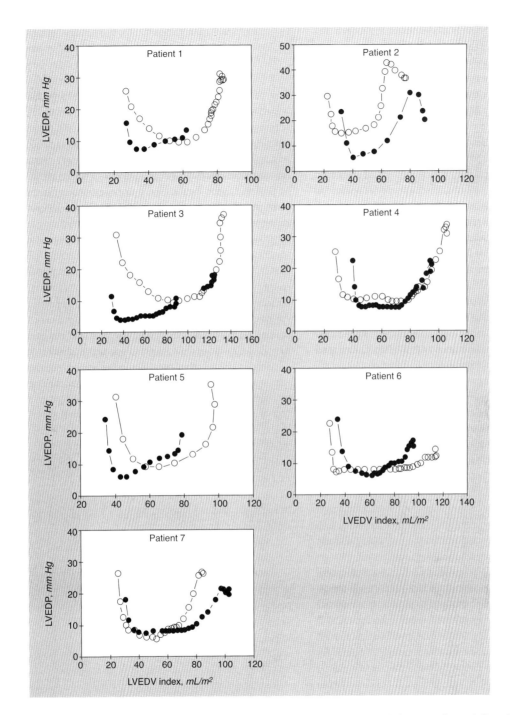

Figure 9.6 Diastolic pressure–volume relationship in 7 patients with hypertrophic cardiomyopathy before (*open circles*) and after (*solid circles*) successful myectomy. Left ventricular end-diastolic pressure (LVEDP) decreased in all patients and left ventricular end-diastolic volume (LVEDV) index decreased in 5 of the 7 subjects and increased in 2 [2,10]. An improvement in early diastolic filling was observed in 3 patients [1,4,9].

hypertrophy. However, there is much more research to do in this field, such as randomized multicenter studies to answer the question of which outcomes can be expected at a late follow-up of more
than 5 years, in particular when comparing myectomy and alcohol ablation of the septum.

References

1. Chien KR. Genomic circuits and the integrative biology of cardiac diseases. *Nature*. 2000;407:227–232.

2. Maron MS, Olivotto I, Zenovich AG, *et al.* Hypertrophic cardiomyopathy is predominantly a disease of
left ventricular outflow tract obstruction. *Circulation*.
2006;114:2232–2239.

3. Hess OM. Risk stratification in hypertrophic cardiomyopathy: fact or fiction? *J Am Coll Cardiol*.
2003;42:880–881.

4. Wigle ED, Rakowski H, Kimball BP, Williams WG.
Hypertrophic cardiomyopathy. Clinical spectrum and
treatment. *Circulation*. 1995;92:1680–1692.

5. Monserrat L, Elliott PM, Gimeno JR, Sharma S,
Penas-Lado M, McKenna WJ. Non-sustained ventricular tachycardia in hypertrophic cardiomyopathy: an
independent marker of sudden death risk in young
patients. *J Am Coll Cardiol*. 2003;42:873–879.

6. Elliott PM, Gimeno JR, Tome MT, *et al.* Left ventricular outflow tract obstruction and sudden death risk in
patients with hypertrophic cardiomyopathy. *Eur Heart
J*. 2006;27:1933–1941.

7. Maron BJ, Gardin JM, Flack JM, Gidding SS, Kurosaki
TT, Bild DE. Prevalence of hypertrophic cardiomyopa-
thy in a general population of young adults. Echocar-
diographic analysis of 4111 subjects in the CARDIA
Study. Coronary Artery Risk Development in (Young)
Adults. *Circulation*. 1995;92:785–789.

8. Spirito P, Bellone P, Harris KM, Bernabo P, Bruzzi P,
Maron BJ. Magnitude of left ventricular hypertrophy
and risk of sudden death in hypertrophic cardiomyopathy. *N Engl J Med*. 2000;342:1778–1785.

9. Sigwart U. Non-surgical myocardial reduction for
hypertrophic obstructive cardiomyopathy. *Lancet*.
1995;346:211–214.

10. Dillon A. Non-surgical reduction of the myocardial
septum. Recommendations for the National Institute for Clincal Excellence (NICE), 2004. Available at
www.nice.org.uk.

11. Maron BJ, Dearani JA, Ommen SR, *et al.* The case for
surgery in obstructive hypertrophic cardiomyopathy.
J Am Coll Cardiol. 2004;44:2044–2053.

12. Faber L, Meissner A, Ziemssen P, Seggewiss H. Percutaneous transluminal septal myocardial ablation for
hypertrophic obstructive cardiomyopathy: long term
follow up of the first series of 25 patients. *Heart*.
2000;83:326–331.

13. Boekstegers P, Steinbigler P, Molnar A, *et al.* Pressure-
guided nonsurgical myocardial reduction induced
by small septal infarctions in hypertrophic obstructive cardiomyopathy. *J Am Coll Cardiol*. 2001;38:
846–853.

14. Gietzen FH, Leuner CJ, Raute-Kreinsen U, *et al.* Acute
and long-term results after transcoronary ablation of
septal hypertrophy (TASH). Catheter interventional
treatment for hypertrophic obstructive cardiomyopathy. *Eur Heart J*. 1999;20:1342–1354.

15. Gietzen FH, Leuner CJ, Obergassel L, Strunk-Mueller
C, Kuhn H. Role of transcoronary ablation of septal
hypertrophy in patients with hypertrophic cardiomyopathy, New York Heart Association functional class
III or IV, and outflow obstruction only under provo-
cable conditions. *Circulation*. 2002;106:454–459.

16. Nagueh SF, Ommen SR, Lakkis NM, *et al.* Comparison of ethanol septal reduction therapy with
surgical myectomy for the treatment of hypertrophic obstructive cardiomyopathy. *J Am Coll Cardiol*.
2001;38:1701–1706.

17. Qin JX, Shiota T, Lever HM, *et al.* Outcome of patients with hypertrophic obstructive cardiomyopathy
after percutaneous transluminal septal myocardial ablation and septal myectomy surgery. *J Am Coll Cardiol*.
2001;38:1994–2000.

18. Knight C, Kurbaan AS, Seggewiss H, *et al.* Nonsurgical septal reduction for hypertrophic obstructive cardiomyopathy: outcome in the first series of patients.
Circulation. 1997;95:2075–2081.

19. Lakkis NM, Nagueh SF, Dunn JK, Killip D, Spencer
WH III. Nonsurgical septal reduction therapy for
hypertrophic obstructive cardiomyopathy: one-year
follow-up. *J Am Coll Cardiol*. 2000;36:852–855.

20. Kimmelstiel CD, Maron BJ. Role of percutaneous septal ablation in hypertrophic obstructive cardiomyopathy. *Circulation*. 2004;109:452–456.

21. Seggewiss H, Gleichmann U, Faber L, Fassbender
D, Schmidt HK, Strick S. Percutaneous transluminal septal myocardial ablation in hypertrophic obstructive cardiomyopathy: acute results and 3-month
follow-up in 25 patients. *J Am Coll Cardiol*. 1998;31:
252–258.

22. Wigle ED, Schwartz L, Woo A, Rakowski H. To ab-
late or operate? that is the question! *J Am Coll Cardiol*.
2001;38:1707–1710.

23. Streit S, Walpoth N, Windecker S, Meier B, Hess O. Is alcohol ablation of the septum associated with recurrent tachyarrhythmias? *Swiss Med Wkly*. 2007;137:660–668.

24. Chang SM, Nagueh SF, Spencer WH III, Lakkis NM. Complete heart block: determinants and clinical impact in patients with hypertrophic obstructive cardiomyopathy undergoing nonsurgical septal reduction therapy. *J Am Coll Cardiol*. 2003;42:296–300.

25. Osterne EC, Seixas TN, Paulo Filho W, Osterne EM, Gomes OM. Percutaneous transluminal septal alcoholization for the treatment of refractory hypertrophic obstructive cardiomyopathy: initial experience in the Federal District. *Arq Bras Cardiol*. 2003;80:359–378.

26. Gietzen FH, Leuner CJ, Obergassel L, Strunk-Mueller C, Kuhn H. Transcoronary ablation of septal hypertrophy for hypertrophic obstructive cardiomyopathy: feasibility, clinical benefit, and short term results in elderly patients. *Heart*. 2004;90:638–644.

27. Talreja DR, Nishimura RA, Edwards WD, *et al.* Alcohol septal ablation versus surgical septal myectomy: comparison of effects on atrioventricular conduction tissue. *J Am Coll Cardiol*. 2004;44: 2329–2332.

28. Faber L, Seggewiss H, Gietzen FH, *et al.* Catheter-based septal ablation for symptomatic hypertrophic obstructive cardiomyopathy: follow-up results of the TASH-registry of the German Cardiac Society. *Z Kardiol*. 2005;94:516–523.

29. Fernandes VL, Nagueh SF, Wang W, Roberts R, Spencer WH III. A prospective follow-up of alcohol septal ablation for symptomatic hypertrophic obstructive cardiomyopathy—the Baylor experience (1996–2002). *Clin Cardiol*. 2005;28:124–130.

30. Faber L, Welge D, Fassbender D, Schmidt HK, Horstkotte D, Seggewiss H. Percutaneous septal ablation for symptomatic hypertrophic obstructive cardiomyopathy: managing the risk of procedure-related AV conduction disturbances. *Int J Cardiol*. 2007;119:163–167.

31. Seggewiss H. Current status of alcohol septal ablation for patients with hypertrophic cardiomyopathy. *Curr Cardiol Rep*. 2001;3:160–166.

32. Mahboob A, Haroon TS, Iqbal Z, Iqbal F, Saleemi MA, Munir A. Fixed drug eruption: topical provocation and subsequent phenomena. *J Coll Physicians Surg Pak*. 2006;16:747–750.

33. Hess OM, Krayenbuehl HP. Management of hypertrophic cardiomyopathy. *Curr Opin Cardiol*. 1993;8:434–440.

PART III

Treatment of Left Ventricular Failure

CHAPTER 10
Biventricular Pacing

Haran Burri[1] *and Etienne Delacrétaz*[2]
[1]Cardiology Service, University Hospital of Geneva, Geneva, Switzerland
[2]Cardiology, Swiss Cardiovascular Center Bern, University Hospital Bern, Bern, Switzerland

---

Chapter Overview

- Cardiac resynchronization therapy (CRT) improves symptoms, increases functional capacity, reduces hospital admission, and prolongs life.
- Current indications apply to patients with all the following features: drug-refractory New York Heart Association (NYHA) III/IV heart failure, QRS >120 ms, left ventricular ejection fraction (LVEF) ≤ 35%.
- About 70% of patients respond favorably to biventricular pacing.
- Strategies to improve response to CRT may be implemented before implantation (by optimizing patient selection), during implantation (by optimizing lead position), and after implantation (by optimizing device programming).

Cardiac resynchronization therapy (CRT, also called biventricular pacing) has emerged as a highly effective treatment option in an important subset of heart failure patients with marked intraventricular dyssynchrony. Large multicenter trials have shown that biventricular pacing improves symptoms and functional capacity, reduces admissions for heart failure, and prolongs survival.

Overview of Cardiac Resynchronization Therapy

Heart Failure and Dyssynchrony

It is important to differentiate electrical dyssynchrony (referring to a long PR interval or a wide QRS complex) from mechanical dyssynchrony. Although these two entities may be interrelated, they are not synonymous.

Current Best Practice in Interventional Cardiology. Edited by B Meier. © 2010 Blackwell Publishing.

Atrioventricular Dyssynchrony

Patients with heart failure may have transmitral E- and A-wave fusion when examined by Doppler echocardiography. This may result from a long PR interval, from sinus tachycardia, or also from delayed left ventricular relaxation brought about by prolonged left ventricular systole. The EA fusion may result in a shortened ventricular filling time and also in diastolic mitral regurgitation (which is usually mild).

Interventricular Dyssynchrony

In the setting of left bundle branch block (LBBB) there may be a delay in ejection of the left ventricle with respect to the right ventricle. The hemodynamic consequence of interventricular dyssynchrony has not been well defined.

Intraventricular Dyssynchrony

LBBB may result in early contraction of the interventricular septum, which stretches the lateral wall of the left ventricle, and is then in turn stretched by delayed contraction of the lateral wall [1]. Dyssynchrony of the anterolateral papillary muscle may also result in reduced tethering of the mitral valve with mitral regurgitation.

Overview of Clinical Trials on CRT

In 1990, Mower and associates from Baltimore reported biventricular pacing for the first time in a canine experiment [2]. In 1991, Mower worked with Bakker from the Netherlands and their associates on a series of 12 class III/IV patients with a biventricular pacemaker, but failed to publish their work until a decade later [3]. The first publication of CRT was a case report from a group in Paris in 1994, of a patient with severe congestive heart failure and LBBB who was remarkably improved by pacing both ventricles simultaneously using a standard dual-chamber pacemaker and Y-adapters [4]. Since then, CRT has been studied in over 4000 patients included in randomized controlled trials. An overview of the major trials is presented in Table 10.1

It should be noted that all trials (apart from MUSTIC-AF) excluded patients in chronic atrial fibrillation. These trials have shown that CRT improves subjective parameters (quality of life, NYHA functional class) as well as objective parameters (6-minute walking distance, MVO_2, echographic parameters such as ventricular remodelling and reduction in mitral regurgitation). End points such as admission for heart failure and death are also improved by CRT. Both the MIRACLE [8] CARE-HF [14] trials have shown a reduction of about 50% for rate of admission for heart failure. The extended phase of the CARE-HF study [15] showed that CRT reduced total mortality, with an impressive 13% absolute risk reduction after a mean follow-up of 36 months.

Mechanisms of Effect of CRT

The mechanisms of action of CRT are mutifactorial. Some of the effects may be observed almost immediately (such as an improvements in mitral regurgitation, dP/dT, and LVEF, which continue to improve over time), and others may take weeks to months to take effect (such as left ventricular remodeling) [16]. The relative contributions of the different effects probably vary from patient to patient. It was seen in the MIRACLE and MIRACLE-

ICD trials that about 80% of patients who show a favorable response to CRT (with an improvement of $\geq$ 1 NYHA class) do so within 1 month [17].

Improvement in left ventricular contractility and LVEF may result from better synchronicity of ventricular contraction [1]. Mitral regurgitation may be acutely reduced by resynchronization of contraction of the anterolateral papillary muscle, and also by an increase of the closing force of the left ventricle [18]. Ventricular remodeling has been shown over long-term follow-up of the CARE-HF study, with a reduction in LVEDV over a 29-month follow-up [19].

As CRT has been shown to improve LVEF and ventricular contractility [16], increase in myocardial oxygen demand resulting in ischemia could be a concern in patients with coronary artery disease. However, it has been shown that CRT does not increase myocardial metabolic requirements [20–22]. This may be explained by an increase in contraction efficiency and by more homogenous myocardial glucose metabolism [23].

Device Implantation

The procedure is usually performed under local anesthesia. The coronary sinus (CS) is accessed using a specialized guiding sheath, of which several shapes are available to suit different anatomies. An occlusive venogram is then performed with a balloon catheter to choose a target vein for left ventricular lead placement (Figs. 10.1 to 10.3). Most operators chose to implant the lead in a (postero)-lateral vein if this is feasible. Valves within the CS, tortuous veins, small-caliber branches, and phrenic nerve stimulation may hinder lead placement. The leads are wedged in the vein and are stabilized by the predefined lead shape. The procedure may be technically challenging. Nevertheless, with the tools currently available, procedural success is about 95% in experienced hands and most often lasts under 2 hours. An epicardial lead may be an option in case of inability to place the left ventricular lead transvenously.

Complications include coronary sinus dissection that may be seen in about 4% of cases [8] due to traumatic manipulation of the guiding catheter when entering the CS or when inflating the balloon

Table 10.1 Overview of Published Randomized Controlled Trials of CRT

Study	Year	No. Patients	NYHA	QRS (ms)	Sinus	CRTP/CRTD	Follow-up (mo)	Primary End Point
PATH CHF [5]	1999	41	III, IV	≥120	Normal	CRTP	6	Peak VO$_2$, anaerobic VO$_2$, 6-MWT
MUSTIC SR [6]	2001	58	III	>150	Normal	CRTP	3	6-MWT
MUSTIC AF [7]	2002	43	III	>200[a]	AF	CRTP	3	6-MWT
MIRACLE [8]	2002	453	III, IV	≥130	Normal	CRTP	6	NYHA, QoL, 6-MWT
CONTAK CD [9]	2003	490	II–IV	≥120	Normal	CRTD	6	Composite (mortality + HF hosp. + VT)
MIRACLE ICD [10]	2003	369	III, IV	≥130	Normal	CRTD	6	NYHA, QoL, 6-MWT
PATH CHF II [11]	2003	89	II–IV	≥120	Normal	Both	3	Peak VO$_2$, anaerobic VO$_2$, 6-MWT
COMPANION [12]	2004	1520	III, IV	≥120	Normal	Both	12	All-cause mortality + all-cause hosp.
MIRACLE ICDII [13]	2004	186	II	≥130	Normal	CRTD	6	Peak VO$_2$
CARE HF [14]	2005	813	III, IV	≥120	Normal	CRTP	29	All-cause mortality + CV hosp.

LVEF had to be ≤ 35% for all trials; hosp., hospitalization.
[a]Paced QRS duration.

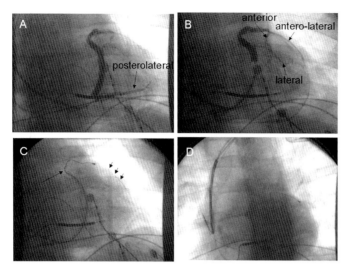

Figure 10.1 A. Balloon occlusive coronary sinus venography in the left anterior oblique projection with a posterolateral and an anterolateral branch. **B.** More distal balloon occlusion better delineates anterolateral and anterior branches. **C.** After canulation of the small anterolateral branch with a wire (*arrows*), a unipolar electrode is introduced over the wire. To allow sufficient backup, the long sheath was introduced deep into the coronary sinus (*arrow*) **D.** Final position of the leads after removal of the guiding system.

catheter, and may exceptionally result in tamponnade. Phrenic nerve stimulation by the LV lead may cause discomfort to the patient. If reprogramming the pacemaker does not solve the problem, the lead may have to be repositioned. Lead displacements, occurring in 6% of patients in the CARE-HF trial [14], also require reintervention. A rare but dreaded complication is infection, which occurs in about 1% of patients [8] (which is comparable to standard pacemaker/ICD procedures) and requires explantation of the device.

Current Indications for CRT

The European guidelines for cardiac pacing and CRT were updated in 2007 [24], and are similar to recommendations of the ACC/AHA guidelines for management of chronic heart failure dating from 2005 [25]. CRT is a class I indication (level of evidence A for CRT pacemakers and B for CRT defibrillators) in patients with all of the following:

- LVEF $\leq$ 35%
- NYHA III or IV despite optimal medical therapy

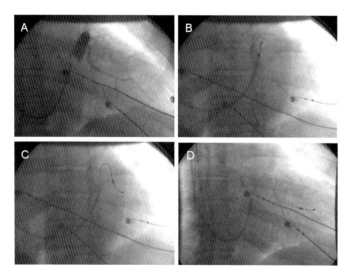

Figure 10.2 A. Balloon occlusive coronary sinus venography showing the target lateral branch in the anteroposterior view. **B.** Canulation of the branch with a wire. **C.** Positioning of the electrode. Because of instability of the electrode at that target site, it has to be advanced in a more distal position (**D**).

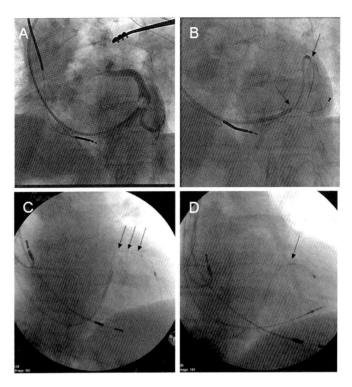

Figure 10.3 A. Balloon occlusive coronary sinus venography in the left anterior oblique projection showing a siphon-shaped ostium of the posterolateral branch. **B.** A curved telescopic sheath (*arrows*) was used to canulate the branch and allow introduction of an electrode into the branch. **C, D.** Large-size branches sometimes call for the implantation of an electrode with active fixation. After guidewire placement and delivery of the lead, the lead's lobes are deployed up to 24F diameter, firmly fixing the electrode in place and reducing the potential for dislodgment during catheter withdrawal **(D).**

- QRS $\geq$ 120 ms
- LV dilatation (LVEDD > 55 mm or > 30 mm/m^2 or > 30 mm/m height)
- Sinus rhythm (chronic AF: class IIa, level of evidence C)

Patient indications for CRT are likely to evolve over time, and may in the future include patients in NYHA class I or II heart failure (based upon results of the ongoing REVERSE and MADIT-CRT studies) and selected patients with a narrow (< 120 ms) QRS complex.

There has been much debate on selecting patients for CRT based on evidence of mechanical dyssynchrony (eg, using echocardiography) rather than electrical dyssynchrony (using the surface ECG and QRS duration). Even though QRS duration has been used as an inclusion criterion in all major trials, it has been shown that electrical dyssynchrony is not automatically associated with mechanical dyssynchrony, and vice-versa. In patients with impaired left ventricular function, mechanical dyssynchrony of the left ventricle may

be absent in about 30% of patients with congestive heart failure and intraventricular conduction delay [26,27], and present in about 40% to 50% of patients with a QRS duration $\leq$ 120 ms [26–28]. A variety of imaging techniques exist for diagnosing dyssynchrony, including echocardiography, MRI, and nuclear angiography, although it has to be borne in mind that there is no gold standard. As a means of increasing the response rate, many authors have advocated the use of echocardiography for screening candidates to CRT [29]. However, many issues still exist concerning the use of echocardiography, such as the method of choice, poor reproducibility in the clinical setting, and lack of solid evidence, as most of the data come from single-center observational studies with < 100 patients. The Predictors of Response to CRT (PROSPECT) trial is the largest report to date that prospectively evaluated 12 different echographic parameters in 426 patients, and found limited feasibility, reproducibility, and predictive value of all studied parameters [30]. As stated in the latest guidelines [24], the role of echocardiography for patient selection remains to be determined in randomized trials. Therefore one should not deny CRT to a patient who otherwise fulfils the criteria of the current guidelines, based only on the fact that mechanical dyssynchrony does not seem to be present on echocardiography.

Defining Response to CRT

It has often been stated that about 70% to 80% of patients respond to CRT (and therefore that 20% to 30% of patients are "nonresponders"). The percentage of "responders" in different studies varies between about 50% [31] to almost 90% [32], depending on the criteria used for defining response. The response rate is usually higher for studies using "soft" clinical end points such as improvement in NYHA functional class, and lower for studies using objective echographic parameters of LV function or remodeling.

Subjective parameters such as quality-of-life questionnaires and assessment of NYHA functional class are prone to a placebo effect, and therefore use of more objective parameters such as the 6-MWT or VO_2max may be useful. The 6-MWT is most often used, as it is easy to implement and does not require special equipment. This simple test has, however, never been standardized. Although never formally tested, shorter corridor lengths (eg, 15 m instead of > 30 m) may have an impact on 6-MWT performance due to the increased impact of turning. Accompaniment and verbal encouragement may influence the distance walked. Other factors, such as footwear (hospital slippers), orthopedic, respiratory, or neurologic condition (eg, Parkinson disease), may also limit the distance walked.

Echocardiographic evaluation of LV function and remodeling (assessed by changes in LV volumes) have also been used as objective parameters. Reverse remodeling with a reduction in LVESV ≥ 10% and improvement in LVEF have been shown to predict long-term survival in CRT patients, whereas clinical parameters such as improvement in quality of life, NYHA class, and 6-MWT did not [33].

A further issue is that a lack of improvement over follow-up may not necessarily mean absence of response to therapy, as CRT may in fact prevent progression of heart failure. This issue is currently being addressed in patients with NYHA class I and II heart failure in the REVERSE and the MADIT-CRT trials.

Optimization of Patient Selection

General Considerations
It must be remembered that CRT is currently indicated only in *drug-refractory* NYHA class III-IV patients. Medication still is first-line therapy, and should be prescribed in all newly diagnosed patients with heart failure, with response evaluated after at least 6 months. Reversible causes contributing to heart failure should be corrected, such as myocardial ischemia and valve disease (eg, severe aortic stenosis), as they may play a preponderant role in the patient's clinical presentation. In patients with significant lung disease, it may not be easy to evaluate the contribution of heart failure to symptoms. BNP levels may be useful in these patients during episodes of decompensation.

Etiology of Heart Failure
There has been much debate whether patients with ischemic heart disease benefit as much from CRT as patients with non-ischemic cardiomyopathy. The difference in substrate in these two populations may influence the ability of CRT to improve cardiac function.

In the MIRACLE [8,34], COMPANION [12], and CARE-HF [14] trials, about 40% to 60% of patients had ischemic cardiomyopathy, with no differences in the primary end point in these patients compared to patients with non-ischemic cardiomyopathy. CRT may have an added benefit in some patients with severe coronary artery disease by reducing drug-refractory angina [35]. In terms of reverse remodelling, however, data from the MIRACLE [34] and CARE-HF [19] trials have shown that patients with non-ischemic cardiomyopathy clearly show a greater improvement.

Selection of patients with ischemic cardiomyopathy may be improved by testing of myocardial viability. Ypenburg and associates [36] have shown using ^{18}F-FDG SPECT imaging that the extent of viability and total scar score were highly predictive for response to CRT. In another study, extent of myocardial scar studied using MRI was predictive of response to CRT [37]. Viability and myocardial contractile reserve have also been shown to be predictive of response to CRT using dobutamine stress echocardiography [38].

Cardiac Arrhythmias

Atrial Fibrillation

The MUSTIC-AF [7] trial was a small crossover study that randomized biventricular pacing to right univentricular pacing in patients with chronic AF who had undergone ablation of the AV node. Patients had an improvement in clinical parameters at 3 months follow-up [7] and at 1 year [39]. However, this study compared CRT with right ventricular apical pacing, which may by itself have detrimental effects, and therefore does not answer the question of whether CRT is superior to no pacing.

An important study [40] involved 162 patients with chronic AF who were implanted with CRT and underwent AV nodal ablation if the percentage of ventricular sensing was > 85% at the 2-month follow-up. Clinical and echographic parameters were compared over a 4-year follow-up with patients in sinus rhythm who received CRT. Patients with AF and AV nodal ablation showed similar benefits to those in sinus rhythm in terms of improvement in LVEF, functional capacity score, and reduction in LV volumes. However, patients without AV nodal ablation did not seem to derive any benefit of therapy. The study shows the importance of performing AV nodal ablation in patients with chronic AF who require CRT, unless the baseline ventricular rate is very slow and the counters show almost permanent pacing (> 90% ventricular pacing).

The PAVE trial [41] randomized right univentricular pacing to biventricular pacing in 184 patients with AF who required AV nodal ablation and had otherwise large enrollment criteria (6-MWT

< 450 ms and NYHA class I-III, with no limit on baseline LVEF or QRS duration). At 6 months, the LVEF in patients with RV pacing showed a slight but significant reduction, whereas no changes were noted in patients in the CRT arm. The 6-MWT also improved significantly in the CRT arm (and remained unchanged in the RV pacing arm), but the benefit was only seen in patients with a baseline LVEF < 0.45.

Ventricular Premature Beats

Frequent ventricular premature beats will interfere with therapy delivery, and this should be taken into consideration when considering CRT indication. Antiarrhythmic drug therapy may be initiated to suppress ventricular ectopy, and if this is ineffective, radiofrequency ablation may be required. Ablation of frequent monomorphic ventricular premature beats may by itself also have a favorable effect on left ventricular function.

Intraventricular Conduction Pattern (RBBB vs. LBBB)

As most patients with congestive heart failure with intraventricular conduction delay have a left bundle branch block (LBBB), or indeterminate pattern, patients with right bundle branch block (RBBB) are under-represented in CRT trials. In the COMPANION study, only about 10% of the total population had RBBB [42]. Although it has been shown that the majority of these patients have evidence of left ventricular mechanical dyssynchrony [28], it is unknown whether the functional consequences are similar to those with LBBB. A pooled analysis of 61 patients with RBBB randomized in the MIRACLE and CONTAK-CD trials has been reported [43]. The results indicate that NYHA functional class was improved in these patients, but there were no differences in quality of life and exercise capacity at 6 months. Therefore, there is less evidence that CRT is effective in patients with RBBB as compared to patients with LBBB.

QRS Duration

Although it has been established that dyssynchrony may be present in about 40% to 50% of patients with a QRS duration $\leq$ 120 ms [26–28], there is currently very little data on the utility of CRT in these subjects. Three nonrandomized studies have evaluated CRT in patients with a normal QRS, and have found favorable results [44–46]. The only randomized trial to date exploring CRT in patients with a "narrow" QRS is the RethinQ trial [47]. A total of 172 heart failure patients with QRS < 130 ms and echographic evidence of dyssynchrony were randomized to a standard ICD versus CRT-D. At the 6 month follow-up, there were no differences between the groups in terms of the primary end point (change in peak oxygen consumption), although patients in the CRT arm had a significantly better improvement in NYHA class.

In conclusion, even though nonrandomized trials suggest that CRT may be beneficial for selected patients with a narrow QRS complex, we have to wait for more data from randomized trials before extending indications to these patients.

CRT for Right Ventricular Pacing-Induced Dyssynchrony

In patients with right ventricular pacing, the left ventricular activation sequence is severly altered, with adverse effects on ventricular function [48]. The issue of device upgrades was not addressed in the large clinical trials; however, smaller studies have shown that these patients seem to benefit from CRT therapy [49,50]. Therefore, the upgrade of an existing pacemaker or defibrillator to a CRT device is frequently performed, and is a class IIa recommendation according to the current European guidelines [24]. Furthermore, implantation of a CRT device should be considered in patients with impaired left ventricular function needing a pacemaker because of AV conduction abnormalities if they are likely to require frequent ventricular stimulation.

Optimizing Lead Position

Right Atrial Lead Position

In most cases, the atrial lead is simply used for sensing atrial activity to trigger biventricular pacing. However, some patients may have chronotropic insufficiency and require atrial pacing. A subset of patients who have interatrial conduction delay (indi-

cated by a wide and notched P wave) may benefit from interatrial septal pacing. The delayed left atrial contraction in these patients will require programming a long AV interval in order to avoid truncating the mitral A wave. However, a long AV interval may compromise biventricular capture. Pacing the interatrial septum may shorten the interatrial conduction time, and thereby reduce left AV dyssynchrony.

Right Ventricular Lead Position

The right ventricular lead has traditionally been placed at the apex, but there is consistent evidence to suggest that this may have adverse hemodynamic effects. Alternative pacing sites, such as the interventricular septum or right ventricular outflow tract (RVOT), have been proposed, but it is still not well established whether these sites offer any benefit over the apex for standard pacing. Optimal right ventricular lead position for CRT is even less well defined. The great majority of patients included in the major trials had their lead placed at the apex, but many implanters today opt for positioning the lead on the interventricular septum or RVOT due to the hypothesis that this may improve resynchronization.

There are no randomized studies to date evaluating right ventricular lead position for CRT. However, acute hemodynamic studies suggest that there does not seem to be any overall benefit with septal pacing in this context [51,52], and that pacing of the right ventricular apex may in fact yield greater dP/dT than high septal pacing when the left ventricular lead is in an anterolateral or lateral vein [52]. Van Campen and associates [53] studied the acute effects of different combinations of right and left ventricular lead position using echocardiography to measure cardiac output. They conclude that optimal lead positions are patient-dependent and should be individually optimized.

Left Ventricular Lead Position

The rationale of CRT is to coordinate ventricular contraction, thereby leading to improved cardiac function. It therefore seems logical that the LV lead should ideally be placed at a site with delayed contraction. It has been shown that pacing the LV at the site of maximal mechanical delay evaluated by TDI in intrinsic rhythm is associated with increased reverse remodelling [54] and short-term exercise capacity [55].

Accurate evaluation of mechanical delay by TDI may, however, be difficult in the clinical setting due to the complexity of data interpretation. As a surrogate to *mechanical* delay, *electrical* delay may be used to guide LV lead positioning. Electrical delay may be measured peroperatively on the epicardial surface by the LV lead itself. Measurement of electrical delay has been used for guiding LV lead placement during the early days of CRT, until it was shown that a (postero-)lateral position yielded greater acute hemodynamic benefit compared to an anterior position [56]. As a consequence, most physicians currently aim to place the LV lead in a lateral or posterolateral branch of the coronary sinus whenever possible. However, it has been shown that the region of maximal mechanical delay varies between patients and may involve sites remote from these branches [55]. Furthermore, data showing no major difference in clinical outcome between patients implanted with a lead in an anterior versus a posterolateral position [57] raise some doubt as to the rationale for routinely targeting (postero-)lateral veins for LV lead placement.

Singh and associates [58] studied 71 patients with a standard indication for CRT by measuring the delay between the onset of the surface QRS complex to the sensed EGM on the LV lead at implantation. The authors have shown that delayed LV lead sensing (occurring during the second half of the QRS complex) is associated with better clinical outcome at 12 months.

It is probably best to avoid placing the LV lead over regions of transmural scar, as this has been shown to result in a reduced acute hemodynamic benefit [59] and absence of clinical response at follow-up [60].

Currently, options for placing the LV lead in a particular position are limited by individual variations of coronary sinus anatomy, branch takeoff angle and tortuosity, and vein diameter, as well as presence of phrenic nerve stimulation. With the advent of new tools, these limitations are being progressively overcome.

Optimizing Device Programming

Proper device programming will ensure that the patient derives maximal possible benefit from CRT. Rate response should be activated in patients with chronotropic incompetence. The upper tracking rate should be set to higher values than the default 120 bpm (eg, to 140 bpm), in order to ensure biventricular pacing during rapid heart rates during exercise. As almost 90% of patients requiring CRT have a history of atrial arrhythmia [61], automatic mode switching should be enabled in all patients. In patients with paroxysmal atrial fibrillation, antiarrhythmic therapy should be aimed at maintaining sinus rhythm.

AV Interval Optimization

Hemodynamic response to pacing may be affected by timing of the AV interval, affecting synchronicity of atrial and ventricular contraction. Some form of AV interval optimization was used in most of the major clinical trials on CRT. The optimal AV interval may be highly variable between subjects, and should therefore be individually optimized. AV optimization may be particularly useful in patients who have interatrial conduction delay and who may require particularly long AV intervals (see "Right Atrial Lead Position" earlier in the chapter).

In addition, the hemodynamic effect of CRT may also vary with the degree of fusion with intrinsic conduction, which will in turn depend on the programmed AV interval. A number of different techniques have been used for AV optimization, and are detailed below.

Echocardiography

Patients with heart failure may have E-A fusion assessed by pulsed-wave Doppler at the mitral valve leaflet tips. Shortening the AV interval by pacing the ventricle and shortening of the QRS will result in anticipation of the E wave of the following cycle, leading to separation of the E and A waves and prolongation of diastolic filling time. However, the AV interval should not be too short, as A-wave truncation will result, compromising ventricular filling.

Several techniques have been described for optimizing the AV interval:

Ritter Method

The Ritter method was initially described in patients with atrioventricular block implanted with standard pacemakers [62–64], and has been used in the Insync III trial [65]. AV intervals are programmed to a short and to a sufficiently long value that does not truncate the A wave (eg, 50 ms and 150 ms), and the delay between QRS onset and the end of the A-wave (QA interval) measured at each setting. The following formula is then used to calculate the optimal delay:

$$AV_{opt} = AV_{short} + [(AV_{long} + Q_{Along})$$
$$- (AV_{short} + QA_{short})]$$

This may be simplified to:

$$AV_{opt} = AV_{long} - (QA_{short} - QA_{long})$$

The technique only requires about 5 minutes for calculating the optimal setting (Fig. 10.4).

Iterative Method

The iterative method was used in the CARE-HF trial [14]. A long AV interval (eg, 75% of the intrinsic AV interval) is programmed and the AV interval decremented in 20-ms steps, until A-wave truncation is observed. The AV interval may then be incremented in 10-ms steps to obtain the optimal setting.

Aortic Velocity–Time Integral Method

Measurement of aortic velocity–time integral (VTI) is a surrogate of stroke volume, and may be done at different programmed AV intervals. This method was evaluated in a study of 40 patients implanted with a biventricular pacemaker randomized to either an empiric AV interval of 120 ms or to individually optimized AV intervals [66]. Patients with optimized settings had greater improvement in NYHA class and quality of life at 3 months, although there was no difference in 6-MWT distance.

Mitral Inflow VTI Method

Jansen and colleagues [67] used invasive measurement of left ventricular dP/dT$_{max}$ for compar-

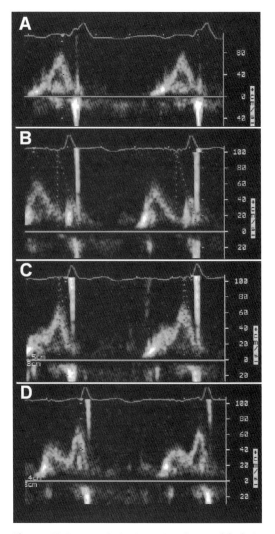

Figure 10.4 AV optimization using the simplified Ritter method. **A.** Intrinsic rhythm with EA fusion. **B.** Biventricular pacing with short AV interval (50 ms). (QA = 120 ms [*dotted line*]; note the truncated A wave.) **C.** Long AV interval. (QA = 80 ms [*dotted line*]). **D.** Optimal AV interval = 150 − (120 − 80) = 110 ms.

ing four different Doppler methods for optimizing AV intervals in patients with CRT. These were the pulsed-wave transmitral VTI (maximal VTI of E and A waves), diastolic filling time (maximal EA duration), the aortic VTI, and the Ritter formula. Measurement of the maximal VTI of mitral inflow was the most accurate method, yielding identical results to LV dP/dt$_{max}$ in 29 of 30 patients. Shortcomings of methods using VTI measurements are that they are relatively time-consuming and may have limited reproducibility in the clinical setting.

Finometer

Whinnet and coworkers optimized AV intervals using a Finometer (Finapres, Amsterdam, Holland) for measuring beat-to-beat changes in blood pressure. The technique was highly reproducible, and indicated that changes in AV intervals had a more pronounced effect on systolic blood pressure at higher-paced atrial rates than at resting heart rates, with a parabolic relationship between AV intervals and systolic blood pressure [68].

Device-Based Algorithms

Drawbacks with the different techniques mentioned so far are that they may be time-consuming, have limited reproducibility, or may require specialized material. Ideally, the device should be able to evaluate the optimal setting automatically. Several device-based algorithms exist:

1 The Boston Scientific Expert Ease for Heart Failure algorithm (derived from data of the PATH-CHF I and II studies) calculates an optimal sensed and paced AV delay based on the patient's QRS width and intrinsic AV interval [69]. In a recent trial, the algorithm performed better than the Ritter or aortic VTI methods [70].

2 The St-Jude QuickOpt algorithm analyzes the left atrial far-field electrogram on the right atrial lead to optimize AV intervals. The clinical impact of this algorithm is being evaluated.

3 Peak endocardial acceleration may be measured by a right ventricular lead equipped with a microaccelerometer located on its distal end (Sorin group, Milano, Italy). Using a specially developed algorithm and automatic AV delay scanning, the optimal AV delay measured by this method was found to closely correlate to that using echocardiography in patients with CRT [62]. The clinical impact of this feature is currently being assessed in a trial.

Limitations with these methods are that the AV intervals are optimized in a supine resting patient at a given heart rate and at specific loading conditions. These circumstances obviously do not reflect hemodynamics in a patient who is active. Scharf

and associates reported that the optimal AV interval is actually longer during exercise than at rest [71]. As no current pacemaker algorithm allows AV prolongation at increased heart rates (which may also result in ventricular pseudofusion), it may be advisable to program a fixed (nonadaptive) AV interval.

There is no general consensus as to what value the default offset between sensed and paced AV intervals should be, as these parameters will depend on intra- and inter-atrial conduction delay as well as right atrial lead position. In patients who are expected to require atrial pacing, it is therefore important to also optimize the paced AV interval, as the offset is patient-specific and may differ considerably from nominal values.

Due to growth in numbers of CRT implantations, many centers may find it difficult to perform optimization in all patients. Also, the evidence that AV optimization has an incremental benefit on clinical outcome is scant. It would nevertheless be advisable to at least evaluate transmitral flow by echocardiography after implantation to ensure absence of EA fusion or A-wave truncation, and optimize AV intervals if necessary. Furthermore, it has been shown that the optimal AV interval may vary considerably over follow-up [66], which raises the question of how often optimization should be repeated.

VV Interval Optimization

Programming of a VV interval (otherwise known as sequential biventricular pacing) may affect inter- as well as intra-ventricular synchrony, as the interventricular septum is usually activated by the right ventricular lead and the lateral left ventricular wall by the coronary sinus lead.

Different techniques have been used for optimizing VV intervals. Echocardiography may be used for measuring aortic outflow VTI at different programmed VV delays. The sample volume should be placed at exactly the same point in the aortic outflow tract at each setting. It is therefore important that a second person assists the examinator by manipulating the pacemaker programmer for changing device settings. Recordings should be taken at each delay and VTI measured offline. Impact of different settings will usually be of small magnitude, and measurement error may play a significant part in observed differences. Whinnet and associates optimized VV intervals using a Finometer and found that the effect on systolic blood pressure was less pronounced than with AV optimization [72,73]. The St-Jude QuickOpt algorithm measures the electrical delay between the right and left ventricular leads, and thereby calculates the VV delay that would lead to the best fusion of the resulting wavefronts.

Few studies have evaluated the clinical impact of VV optimization. A nonrandomized study with 34 patients showed no difference in NYHA class and 6-MWT distance after 3 months of optimized sequential pacing, as compared to patients with simultaneous pacing [74]. Results of the RHYTHM-ICD VV Optimization Phase Study have been presented [75]. Compared to 72 patients receiving simultaneous biventricular pacing, 48 patients with echocardiographically optimized VV intervals showed a nonsignificant trend in better functional outcome at 6 months. In the Insync III study [61], clinical outcome in 359 patients with optimized sequential biventricular pacing was compared with outcome in patients receiving simultaneous pacing in the MIRACLE trial. Although no changes in quality of life and NYHA functional class were noted between groups, patients with optimized sequential pacing showed a greater increase in 6-MWT distance. The DECREASE-HF trial [76] is the first randomized, double-blind study comparing simultaneous and sequential CRT (as well as left univentricular pacing) in 306 patients. There was no advantage of sequential pacing over simultaneous pacing as concerns improvement in ventricular volumes and systolic function.

Whether individually optimized sequential biventricular pacing improves outcome in patients with CRT remains to be proven. Due to the time-consuming process of VV optimization, it may be best to leave the default setting of simultaneous pacing after implantation, and optimize VV intervals in nonresponders at follow-up.

Additional Features of CRT Devices

Patient symptoms and clinical status may be correlated with device diagnostics, such as evolution of average heart rates, heart rate variability, and daily activity. Repeated measurement of intrathoracic impedance (a feature known as Optivol available in Medtronic biventricular ICDs) has been shown to identify fluid overload before onset of symptoms, and predicts admission for heart failure with 77% sensitivity, with early warning of about 2 weeks before admission [77]. As soon as the fluid index threshold is crossed, an audible alarm may alert the patient of impending decompensation, and allows the physician to titrate medication in order to avoid clinical deterioration. However, false-positive events (alerts without deterioration in clinical status or admission for heart failure) are possible, and an option would be to initially program this feature in a monitor-only mode to test the accuracy of the algorithm in a given patient. Finally, the advent of telemedicine offers novel opportunities for patient surveillance with automatic transmission of cardiac or technical events by the device.

Conclusions

Cardiac resynchronization therapy is an efficient therapy that improves symptoms, increases functional capacity, reduces hospital admission, and prolongs life in patients with symptomatic heart failure. Advances in equipment and techniques have improved the delivery of this therapy. However, CRT does not result in significant clinical improvement in 20% to 30% of patients. One of the main challenges is to reduce the number of nonresponders, by improving patient selection, optimizing lead positioning, and fine-tuning device programming.

References

1. Breithardt OA, Stellbrink C, Herbots L, *et al.* Cardiac resynchronization therapy can reverse abnormal myocardial strain distribution in patients with heart failure and left bundle branch block. *J Am Coll Cardiol.* 2003;42:486–494.
2. Lattuca J, Cohen T, Mower M. Bi-ventricular pacing to improve cardiac hemodynamics. *Clin Res.* 1990;38:882A.

3. Bakker PF, Meijburg HW, de Vries JW, *et al.* Biventricular pacing in end-stage heart failure improves functional capacity and left ventricular function. *J Interv Card Electrophysiol.* 2000;4:395–404.

4. Cazeau S, Ritter P, Bakdach S, *et al.* Four chamber pacing in dilated cardiomyopathy. *Pacing Clin Electrophysiol.* 1994;17:1974–1979.

5. Auricchio A, Stellbrink C, Block M, *et al.* Effect of pacing chamber and atrioventricular delay on acute systolic function of paced patients with congestive heart failure. The Pacing Therapies for Congestive Heart Failure Study Group. The Guidant Congestive Heart Failure Research Group. *Circulation.* 1999;99:2993–3001.

6. Cazeau S, Leclercq C, Lavergne T, *et al.* Effects of multisite biventricular pacing in patients with heart failure and intraventricular conduction delay. *N Engl J Med.* 2001;344:873–880.

7. Leclercq C, Walker S, Linde C, *et al.* Comparative effects of permanent biventricular and right-univentricular pacing in heart failure patients with chronic atrial fibrillation. *Eur Heart J.* 2002;23:1780–1787.

8. Abraham WT, Fisher WG, Smith AL, *et al.* Cardiac resynchronization in chronic heart failure. *N Engl J Med.* 2002;346:1845–1853.

9. Higgins SL, Hummel JD, Niazi IK, *et al.* Cardiac resynchronization therapy for the treatment of heart failure in patients with intraventricular conduction delay and malignant ventricular tachyarrhythmias. *J Am Coll Cardiol.* 2003;42:1454–1459.

10. Young JB, Abraham WT, Smith AL, *et al.* Combined cardiac resynchronization and implantable cardioversion defibrillation in advanced chronic heart failure: the MIRACLE ICD Trial. *JAMA.* 2003;289:2685–2694.

11. Auricchio A, Stellbrink C, Butter C, *et al.* Clinical efficacy of cardiac resynchronization therapy using left ventricular pacing in heart failure patients stratified by severity of ventricular conduction delay. *J Am Coll Cardiol.* 2003;42:2109–2116.

12. Bristow MR, Saxon LA, Boehmer J, *et al.* Cardiac-resynchronization therapy with or without an implantable defibrillator in advanced chronic heart failure. *N Engl J Med.* 2004;350:2140–2150.

13. Abraham WT, Young JB, Leon AR, *et al.* Effects of cardiac resynchronization on disease progression in patients with left ventricular systolic dysfunction, an indication for an implantable cardioverter-defibrillator, and mildly symptomatic chronic heart failure. *Circulation.* 2004;110:2864–2868.

14. Cleland JG, Daubert JC, Erdmann E, *et al.* The effect of cardiac resynchronization on morbidity and mortality in heart failure. *N Engl J Med.* 2005;352:1539–1549.

15. Cleland JG, Daubert JC, Erdmann E, *et al.* Longer-term effects of cardiac resynchronization therapy on mortality in heart failure [the CArdiac REsynchronization-Heart Failure (CARE-HF) trial extension phase. *Eur Heart J.* 2006;27:1928–1932.

16. Yu CM, Chau E, Sanderson JE, *et al.* Tissue Doppler echocardiographic evidence of reverse remodeling and improved synchronicity by simultaneously delaying regional contraction after biventricular pacing therapy in heart failure. *Circulation.* 2002;105:438–445.

17. Pires LA, Abraham WT, Young JB, Johnson KM. Clinical predictors and timing of New York Heart Association class improvement with cardiac resynchronization therapy in patients with advanced chronic heart failure: results from the Multicenter InSync Randomized Clinical Evaluation (MIRACLE) and Multicenter InSync ICD Randomized Clinical Evaluation (MIRACLE-ICD) trials. *Am Heart J.* 2006;151:837–843.

18. Breithardt OA, Sinha AM, Schwammenthal E, *et al.* Acute effects of cardiac resynchronization therapy on functional mitral regurgitation in advanced systolic heart failure. *J Am Coll Cardiol.* 2003;41:765–770.

19. Cleland JGF. CARE-HF extension results. European Society of Cardiology annual meeting. 2005. *Eur J Heart Fail.* 2005;7:1070–1075.

20. Ukkonen H, Beanlands RSB, Burwash IG, *et al.* Effect of cardiac resynchronization on myocardial efficiency and regional oxidative metabolism. *Circulation.* 2003;107:28–31.

21. Nelson GS, Berger RD, Fetics BJ, *et al.* Left ventricular or biventricular pacing improves cardiac function at diminished energy cost in patients with dilated cardiomyopathy and left bundle-branch block. *Circulation.* 2000;102:3053–3059.

22. Sundell J, Engblom E, Koistinen J, *et al.* The effects of cardiac resynchronization therapy on left ventricular function, myocardial energetics, and metabolic reserve in patients with dilated cardiomyopathy and heart failure. *J Am Coll Cardiol.* 2004;43:1027–1033.

23. Nowak B, Sinha AM, Schaefer WM, *et al.* Cardiac resynchronization therapy homogenizes myocardial glucose metabolism and perfusion in dilated cardiomyopathy and left bundle branch block. *J Am Coll Cardiol.* 2003;41:1523–1528.

24. Vardas PE, Auricchio A, Blanc JJ, *et al.* Guidelines for cardiac pacing and cardiac resynchronization therapy: the task force for cardiac pacing and cardiac resynchronization therapy of the European Society of Cardiology. Developed in collaboration with the European Heart Rhythm Association. *Eur Heart J.* 2007;28:2256–2295.

25. Hunt SA, Abraham WT, Chin MH, *et al.* ACC/AHA 2005 Guideline update for the diagnosis and management of chronic heart failure in the adult: a report of the American College of Cardiology/American Heart Association Task Force on Practice Guidelines. *Circulation.* 2005;112:1825–1852.

26. Fauchier L, Marie O, Casset-Senon D, Babuty D, Cosnay P, Fauchier JP. Reliability of QRS duration and morphology on surface electrocardiogram to identify ventricular dyssynchrony in patients with idiopathic dilated cardiomyopathy. *Am J Cardiol.* 2003;92:341–344.

27. Yu CM, Lin H, Zhang Q, Sanderson JE. High prevalence of left ventricular systolic and diastolic asynchrony in patients with congestive heart failure and normal QRS duration. *Heart.* 2003;89:54–60.

28. Bader H, Garrigue S, Lafitte S, *et al.* Intra-left ventricular electromechanical asynchrony. A new independent predictor of severe cardiac events in heart failure patients. *J Am Coll Cardiol.* 2004;43:248–256.

29. Bax JJ, Ansalone G, Breithardt OA, *et al.* Echocardiographic evaluation of cardiac resynchronization therapy: ready for routine clinical use? A critical appraisal. *J Am Coll Cardiol.* 2004;44:1–9.

30. Chung ES, Leon AR, Tavazzi L, *et al.* Results of the Predictors of Response to CRT (PROSPECT) trial. *Circulation.* 2008;117:2608–2616.

31. Penicka M, Bartunek J, De Bruyne B, *et al.* Improvement of left ventricular function after cardiac resynchronization therapy is predicted by tissue Doppler imaging echocardiography. *Circulation.* 2004;109:978–983.

32. Reuter S, Garrigue S, Barold SS, *et al.* Comparison of characteristics in responders versus nonresponders with biventricular pacing for drug-resistant congestive heart failure. *Am J Cardiol.* 2002;89:346–350.

33. Yu CM, Bleeker GB, Fung JW, *et al.* Left ventricular reverse remodeling but not clinical improvement predicts long-term survival after cardiac resynchronization therapy. *Circulation.* 2005;112:1580–1586.

34. St John Sutton MG, Plappert T, Hilpisch KE, Abraham WT, Hayes DL, Chinchoy E. Sustained reverse left ventricular structural remodeling with cardiac resynchronization at one year is a func-

tion of etiology: Quantitative Doppler echocardiographic evidence from the multicenter inSync randomized clinical evaluation (MIRACLE). *Circulation.* 2006;113:266–272.

35. Gasparini M, Mantica M, Galimberti P, *et al.* Relief of drug refractory angina by biventricular pacing in heart failure. *Pacing Clin Electrophysiol.* 2003;26:181–184.

36. Ypenburg C, Schalij MJ, Bleeker GB, *et al.* Extent of viability to predict response to cardiac resynchronization therapy in ischemic heart failure patients. *J Nucl Med.* 2006;47:1565–1570.

37. White JA, Yee R, Yuan X, *et al.* Delayed enhancement magnetic resonance imaging predicts response to cardiac resynchronization therapy in patients with intraventricular dyssynchrony. *J Am Coll Cardiol.* 2006;48:1953–1960.

38. Da Costa A, Thevenin J, Roche F, *et al.* Prospective validation of stress echocardiography as an identifier of cardiac resynchronization therapy responders. *Heart Rhythm.* 2006;3:406–413.

39. Linde C, Leclercq C, Rex S, *et al.* Long-term benefits of biventricular pacing in congestive heart failure: results from the MUltisite STimulation in cardiomyopathy (MUSTIC) study. *J Am Coll Cardiol.* 2002;40:111–118.

40. Gasparini M, Auricchio A, Regoli F, *et al.* Four-year efficacy of cardiac resynchronization therapy on exercise tolerance and disease progression: The importance of performing atrioventricular junction ablation in patients with atrial fibrillation. *J Am Coll Cardiol.* 2006;48:734–743.

41. Doshi RN, Daoud EG, Fellows C, *et al.* Left ventricular-based cardiac stimulation post AV nodal ablation evaluation (the PAVE study). *J Cardiovasc Electrophysiol.* 2005;16:1160–1165.

42. Bristow MR, Feldman AM, Saxon LA. Heart failure management using implantable devices for ventricular resynchronization: Comparison of Medical Therapy, Pacing, and Defibrillation in Chronic Heart Failure (COMPANION) trial. COMPANION Steering Committee and COMPANION Clinical Investigators. *J Card Fail.* 2000;6:276–285.

43. Egoavil CA, Ho RT, Greenspon AJ, Pavri BB. Cardiac resynchronization therapy in patients with right bundle branch block: Analysis of pooled data from the MIRACLE and Contak CD trials. *Heart Rhythm.* 2005;2:611–615.

44. Bleeker GB, Holman ER, Steendijk P, *et al.* Cardiac resynchronization therapy in patients with a narrow QRS Complex. *J Am Coll Cardiol.* 2006;48:2243–2250.

45. Yu CM, Chan YS, Zhang Q, *et al.* Benefits of Cardiac Resynchronization Therapy for Heart Failure Patients With Narrow QRS Complexes and Coexisting Systolic Asynchrony by Echocardiography. *J Am Coll Cardiol.* 2006;48:2251–2257.

46. Gasparini M, Regoli F, Galimberti P, *et al.* Three years of cardiac resynchronization therapy: Could superior benefits be obtained in patients with heart failure and narrow QRS? *Pacing Clin Electrophysiol.* 2007;30(suppl 1):S34–S39.

47. Beshai JF, Grimm RA, Nagueh SF, *et al.* Cardiac-Resynchronization Therapy in Heart Failure with Narrow QRS Complexes. *N Engl J Med.* 2007;357:2461–2471.

48. Sweeney MO, Prinzen FW. A new paradigm for physiologic ventricular pacing. *J Am Coll Cardiol.* 2006;47:282–288.

49. Eldadah ZA, Rosen B, Hay I, *et al.* The benefit of up-grading chronically right ventricle-paced heart failure patients to resynchronization therapy demonstrated by strain rate imaging. *Heart Rhythm.* 2006;3:435–442.

50. Horwich T, Foster E, De Marco T, Tseng Z, Saxon L. Effects of resynchronization therapy on cardiac function in pacemaker patients "upgraded" to biventricular devices. *J Cardiovasc Electrophysiol.* 2004;15:1284–1289.

51. Hay I, Melenovsky V, Fetics BJ, *et al.* Short-term effects of right-left heart sequential cardiac resynchronization in patients with heart failure, chronic atrial fibrillation, and atrioventricular nodal block. *Circulation.* 2004;110:3404–3410.

52. Shimano M, Inden Y, Yoshida Y, *et al.* Does RV lead positioning provide additional benefit to cardiac resynchronization therapy in patients with advanced heart failure? *Pacing Clin Electrophysiol.* 2006;29:1069–1074.

53. van Campen LCM, Visser FC, de Cock CC, Vos DHS, Kamp O, Visser CA. Comparison of the hemodynamics of different pacing sites in patients undergoing resynchronization therapy: need for individualization and optimal lead localization. *Heart.* 2006;92:1795–1800.

54. Murphy RT, Sigurdsson G, Mulamalla S, *et al.* Tissue synchronization imaging and optimal left ventricular pacing site in cardiac resynchronization therapy. *Am J Cardiol.* 2006;97:1615–1621.

55. Ansalone G, Giannantoni P, Ricci R, Trambaiolo P, Fedele F, Santini M. Doppler myocardial imaging to evaluate the effectiveness of pacing sites in patients receiving biventricular pacing. *J Am Coll Cardiol.* 2002;39:489–499.

56. Butter C, Auricchio A, Stellbrink C, *et al.* Effect of resynchronization therapy stimulation site on the systolic function of heart failure patients. *Circulation.* 2001;104:3026–3029.

57. Gasparini M, Mantica M, Galimberti P, *et al.* Is the left ventricular lateral wall the best lead implantation site for cardiac resynchronization therapy? *Pacing Clin Electrophysiol.* 2003;26:162–168.

58. . Singh JP, Fan D, Heist EK, *et al.* Left ventricular lead electrical delay predicts response to cardiac resynchronization therapy. *Heart Rhythm.* 2006;3:1285–1292.

59. Van Gelder BM, Janssen A, Bracke F, *et al.* Electrophysiological and hemodynamic consequences of myocardial scar tissue in cardiac resynchronization therapy (abstract). *Heart Rhythm.* 2006;3:S24.

60. Bleeker GB, Kaandorp TAM, Lamb HJ, *et al.* Effect of posterolateral scar tissue on clinical and echocardiographic improvement after cardiac resynchronization therapy. *Circulation.* 2006;113:969–976.

61. Leon AR, Abraham WT, Brozena S, *et al.* Cardiac resynchronization with sequential biventricular pacing for the treatment of moderate-to-severe heart failure. *J Am Coll Cardiol.* 2005;46:2298–2304.

62. Ritter P, Padeletti L, Dellnoy PP, Garrigue S, Silvestre J. AV Delay optimisation by peak endocardial acceleration in cardiac resynchronisation therapy: comparison with standard echocardiographic procedure. *Europace.* 2004;6(suppl):209.

63. Kindermann M, Frohlig G, Doerr T, Schieffer H. Optimizing the AV delay in DDD pacemaker patients with high degree AV block: mitral valve Doppler versus impedance cardiography. *Pacing Clin Electrophysiol.* 1997;20:2453–2462.

64. Dupuis JM, Kobeissi A, Vitali L, *et al.* Programming optimal atrioventricular delay in dual chamber pacing using peak endocardial acceleration: comparison with a standard echocardiographic procedure. *Pacing Clin Electrophysiol.* 2003;26:210–213.

65. Leon AR, Abraham WT, Curtis AB, *et al.* Safety of Transvenous cardiac resynchronization system implantation in patients with chronic heart failure: Combined results of over 2,000 patients from a multicenter study program. *J Am Coll Cardiol.* 2005;46:2348–2356.

66. Sawhney N, Waggoner A, Garhwal S, Chawla M, Faddis M. Randomized prospective trial of atrioventricular delay programming for cardiac resynchronization therapy. *Heart Rhythm.* 2004;1:526–567.

67. Jansen AH, Bracke FA, van Dantzig JM, *et al.* Correlation of echo-Doppler optimization of atrioventricular

delay in cardiac resynchronization therapy with invasive hemodynamics in patients with heart failure secondary to ischemic or idiopathic dilated cardiomyopathy. *Am J Cardiol.* 2006;97:552–557.

68. Whinnett Z, Davies D, Willson K, *et al.* Determination of optimal atrioventricular delay for cardiac resynchronization therapy using acute non-invasive blood pressure. *Europace.* 2006;8:358–366.

69. Gold MR, Niazi I, Giudici M, *et al.* A new automated algorithm for optimizing AV delay to improve global LV contractile function with cardiac resynchronization therapy. *Heart Rhythm.* 2005;2:S287.

70. Giudici M, Gold MR, Niazi I, *et al.* A new AV delay optimization algorithm increases LV global contractile function in CRT patients compared with echo-derived methods of AV delay programming. *Heart Rhythm.* 2005;2:S248.

71. Scharf C, Li P, Muntwyler J, *et al.* Rate-dependent AV delay optimization in cardiac resynchronization therapy. *Pacing Clin Electrophysiol.* 2005;28:279–284.

72. Whinnett ZI, Davies JER, Willson K, *et al.* Haemodynamic effects of changes in atrioventricular and interventricular delay in cardiac resynchronisation therapy show a consistent pattern: analysis of shape, magnitude and relative importance of atrioventricular and interventricular delay. *Heart.* 2006;92:1628–1634.

73. Whinnett Z, Davies J, Willson K, *et al.* The haemodynamic response to changes in atrioventricular and interventricular delay of cardiac resynchronization therapy closely fits a parabola, which may allow more efficient optimization. *J Am Coll Cardiol.* 2006;47:22A.

74. Mortensen PT, Sogaard P, Mansour H, *et al.* Sequential biventricular pacing: evaluation of safety and efficacy. *Pacing Clin Electrophysiol.* 2004;27:339–345.

75. Baker JH, Turk K, Peres LA, Kowal RC, Pacifico A, Mc Kenzie JP. Optimization of interventricular timing delay in biventricular pacing: Results from the RHYTHM ICD V-V optimization phase study. *Heart Rhythm.* 2005;2:S205–S206.

76. Rao RK, Kumar UN, Schafer J, Viloria E, De Lurgio D, Foster E. Reduced ventricular volumes and improved systolic function with cardiac resynchronization therapy: A randomized trial comparing simultaneous biventricular pacing, sequential biventricular pacing, and left ventricular pacing. *Circulation.* 2007;115:2136–2144.

77. Yu CM, Wang L, Chau E, *et al.* Intrathoracic impedance monitoring in patients with heart failure: correlation with fluid status and feasibility of early warning preceding hospitalization. *Circulation.* 2005;112:841–848.

CHAPTER 11

Percutaneous Left Ventricular Assist Devices

Georgios Sianos[1] *and Pim J. de Feyter*[2]

[1]1st Department of Cardiology, AHEPA University Hospital, Thessaloniki, Greece
[2]Department of Cardiology, Erasmus University, Rotterdam, The Netherlands

---

Chapter Overview

- The use of percutaneous left ventricular devices (pLVADs) requires adequately trained personnel and experienced interventionists.
- pLVADs more effectively improve LV hemodynamics than the intra-aortic balloon pump.
- pLVADs improve cardiac hemodynamics in patients with cardiogenic shock but do not reduce mortality.
- pLVADs facilitate a complicated PCI procedure in very high risk patients, but cannot be recommended as a routine procedure.
- The role of pLVADs in routine clinical practice has not yet been established.

The intra-aortic balloon pump (IABP) has always been used as the first-choice device to provide hemodynamic support in case of a failing heart pump. However, the IABP relies on the existence of a certain level of remaining left ventricular function and requires accurate synchronization with the cardiac cycles, which precludes its use in persistent tachyarrhythmias or ventricular fibrillation. In many instances with severe depression of the left ventricular function, the use of an IABP falls short in reversing the unstable hemodynamic situation.

Two effective devices have been developed and clinically tested to provide hemodynamic support in the catheterization laboratory: the Tandem Heart and the Impella Recover LP2.5. These devices can be used in various clinical situations:

1 To hemodynamically support patients with an acute myocardial infarction complicated with cardiogenic shock.

2 In patients with abrupt closure of a large vessel during percutaneous coronary intervention and severe hemodynamic instability.

3 To support and facilitate percutaneous coronary intervention of very high risk patients/lesions to prevent significant deterioration of the hemodynamic situation during intracoronary instrumentation and manipulation.

The Tandem Heart Percutaneous Left Ventricular Assist Device

The Tandem Heart percutaneous left ventricular assist device (pLVAD) is a low-speed centrifugal continuous-flow pump with a low blood surface contrast area design to minimize the likelihood of hemolysis and formation of thromboemboli. The Tandem Heart pLVAD consists of four major components (Fig. 11.1):

- A 21F left atrial drainage cannula
- An extracorporeal centrifugal pump rotating at 7500 rpm (maximum)

Current Best Practice in Interventional Cardiology. Edited by B Meier. © 2010 Blackwell Publishing,

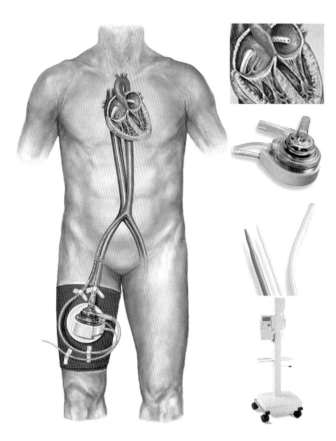

Figure 11.1 The Tandem Heart LVAD system includes a left atrial transseptal inflow cannula, arterial return cannula, a centrifugal blood pump, and a system controller.

• A femoral artery cannula (15–17 F) that extends into the iliac artery

• A microprocessor-based pump controller

The pump is powered by an electromagnetic motor that drives the plastic impeller at a speed of 3000 to 7500 rpm, provides a blood-flow rate up to 4 L/min and as such can completely substitute the left heart if necessary. The pump incorporates an infusion line to provide local anticoagulation. The device operates on AC current or batteries.

The Tandem Heart pump is percutaneously implanted. After transseptal puncture according to the Brockenbrough procedure and pre-dilatation of the fossa ovalis with a plastic dilater, the left atrial cannula is positioned under fluoroscopic control into the left atrial atrium. Aortic iliac and femoral angiography is recommended before insertion of the arterial cannula to ensure adequate vessel size. After careful air removal, the cannulae are connected to the extracorporeal centrifugal

pump. Oxygenated blood is withdrawn from the left atrium and pumped into the femoral artery. Bilateral femoral artery access can also be used with 12F to 14F arterial cannulae. An activated clotting time of 180 to 200 seconds is recommended during pump support. The Tandem Heart is (relatively) contraindicated in patients with predominant right ventricular failure (unless a right heart Tandem support is used) or severe aortic insufficiency. The iatrogenic atrial septal defect from transseptal cannulation seems to resolve after 4 to 6 weeks.

Impella Recover LP PLVAD

The Impella Recover LP pLVAD comes in two sizes. The Impella Recover LP5 is a microaxial pump delivering a continuous flow of maximally 5 L/min. With a cannula size of 21F it has to be surgically implanted and is rarely used through the femoral

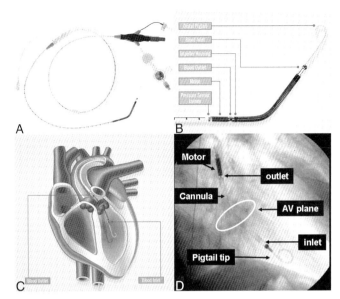

Figure 11.2 A. an overall view of the Impella p-LVAD system with catheter and connections. **B.** The distal part of the Impella system with distal pigtail, blood inlet, Impella housing, blood outlet, motor, pressure sensor. **C.** Impella p-LVAD in the left ventricle. **D.** The p-LVAD in a patient with blood inlet in the left ventricle and blood outlet in the aorta.

artery but typically with thoracotomy. The Impella Recover LP 2.5 is capable of delivering a continuous flow of up to 2.5 L/min. The cannula size is 12F, allowing percutaneous implantation. The pump incorporates an impeller driven by an electrical motor with a maximum of 50,000 revolutions per minute. The device is equipped with a pigtail catheter at the tip to ensure stable position in the left ventricle and to prevent perforation or adherence to the myocardium. The pump is placed through the aortic valve and aspirates blood from the left ventricular cavity and expels it in the aorta. Because of the positioning of the pump through the aorta, the pump cannot be used in the presence of a mechanical aortic valve or aortic stenosis, and the pump may be rather inefficient in severe aortic regurgitation. An overview of the Impella LP 2.5 is depicted in Figure 11.2

An overview of the technical characteristics of these LVADs is presented in Table 11.1.

Left Ventricular Assist Devices for Postmyocardial Infarction Complicated with Cardiogenic Shock

The incidence of cardiogenic shock complicating acute myocardial infarction is on average about 7.1%. Patients who develop cardiogenic shock have a significantly higher risk of dying during hospitalization compared to those without cardiogenic shock (71.7% vs. 12% respectively, $p < 0.001$) [1].

The use of pLVADs providing active left ventricular function support may be beneficial in patients with post-MI cardiogenic shock. These devices are

Table 11.1 Technical Characteristics of pLVADs

	Tandem Heart	Impella Recover LP 2.5	Impella Recover LP 5.0
Atrial catheter size	12–15F	12	21
Venous cannula size	21		
Flow (L/min)	4.0 (max)	2.5 (max)	5.0 (max)
Pump rpm	7500 (max)	50,000 (max)	50,000 (max)
Anticoagulation	+	+	+

mainly used as a bridge to recovery. Thiele and associates [2] reported on the safety and efficacy of the Tandem Heart LVAD in 18 consecutive patients with cardiogenic shock after myocardial infarction. The mean LVAD flow was 3.2 ± 0.6 L/min. The mean duration of cardiac assistance was 4 ± 3 days. The cardiac index significantly improved from 1.7 ± 0.3 L/min/m^2 to 2.4 ± 0.6 L/min/m^2 after LVAD implantation. The mean blood pressure increased from 63 ± 8 mm Hg to 80 ± 9 mm Hg. The pulmonary capillary wedge pressure, central venous pressure, and pulmonary arterial pressure decreased from 21 ± 4, 13 ± 4, and 31 ± 8 mm Hg to 14 ± 4, 9 ± 3, and 23 ± 6 mm Hg, respectively. The overall mortality rate at 30 days was 44%.

A randomized multicenter clinical study evaluated the safety and efficacy of the Tandem Heart LVAD compared to conventional treatment with IABP for treatment of cardiogenic shock [3]. Fourteen patients were randomized to IABP and 19 to Tandem Heart treatment. There were no differences in the baseline characteristics between the two groups, and the mean duration of support was approximately 2.5 days. The Tandem Heart LVAD achieved significantly greater increases in cardiac index and mean arterial blood pressure, and decrease in pulmonary capillary wedge pressure (Fig. 11.3). The 30-day survival free of occurrence of severe adverse events was not different, 53% in the Tandem Heart group versus 64% in the IABP group. Hemolysis was present in 1 patient in the

Tandem Heart group and 1 patient in the IABP group.

Thiele and coworkers [4] reported the outcome of a randomized comparison of IABP versus the Tandem Heart LVAD in patients with acute myocardial infarction complicated by cardiogenic shock. Twenty patients were randomized to IABP and 21 patients to Tandem Heart LVAD support. The majority of patients (95%) underwent percutaneous coronary intervention. The patient characteristics were similar in both groups. The primary end point, the cardiac power index, defined as the CI × mean arterial pressure × 0.0022, improved more effectively by LVAD support than by IABP support, as was also the case for other hemodynamic and metabolic variables (Table 11.2). The 30-day mortality was similar for the IABP group 45% versus the LVAD group 43%. Complications including severe bleeding or limb ischemia occurred much more frequently in the LVAD group (19 vs. 8, $p = 0.002$; and 7 vs. 0, $p = 0.009$). The axial flow pump Impella LVAD LP5 was investigated in an animal experiment to demonstrate that myocardial infarction size could be reduced in a sheep model with myocardial infarction induced by occlusion of the left anterior descending coronary artery [5]. The animals were allocated to four groups: (1) no support, (2) full support during ischemia and reperfusion, (3) full support during reperfusion, and (4) partial support during reperfusion. The infarct size was significantly reduced in the pump-supported animals.

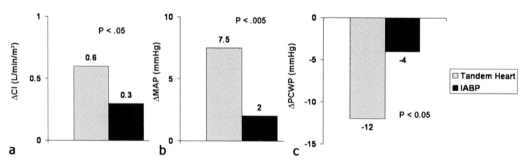

Figure 11.3 The functional efficiency of the Tandem Heart-compared to IABP on cardiac index (a), mean arterial pressure (b), and pulmonary wedge pressure (c). (CI, cardiac index; MAP, mean arterial pressure; PCWP, pulmonary capillary wedge pressure.)

Table 11.2 Hemodynamic and Metabolic Variables Before and After IABP and LVAD Implantation

	Before Implantation			After Implantation		
	IABP	LAVD	p-value	IABP	LAVD	p-value
CPI (W/m^2)	0.22	0.22	0.72	0.28	0.37	0.004
CI (L/min/m^2)	1.5	1.7	0.35	1.7	2.3	0.005
Mean blood pressure (mm Hg)	64	63	0.50	67	74	0.38
PCWP (mm Hg)	27	20	0.02	22	16	0.003
CVP (mm Hg)	13	11	0.29	12	10	0.06
PAP mean (mm Hg)	33	28	0.45	29	25	0.007
Serum lactate (mmol/L)	3.8	4.5	0.53	3.3	2.8	0.03

Percutaneous Left Ventricular Assist Devices to Support High-Risk Percutaneous Coronary Interventions

Periprocedural LV support during high-risk percutaneous coronary intervention may facilitate the procedure, and in case of flow impairment during instrumentation or in case of abrupt vessel closure may effectively support an abruptly failing left ventricle and may prevent acute periprocedural mortality.

Only a few studies with small numbers of patients have been reported. Lemos and colleagues reported on 7 patients at high risk who received the Tandem Heart LVAD support before, during, and after the procedure [6]. Patients were considered high risk in case of severely depressed left ventricular function (5 patients) or in overt cardiogenic shock (2 patients). A total of 13 lesions were successfully treated. The baseline characteristics and hemodynamic variables are presented in Table 11.3.

The mean systemic arterial pressure was 87 ± 24 mm Hg before and 103 ± 20 mm Hg after LVAD implantation. The pulmonary wedge pressure was 19 ± 9 mm Hg before and 14 ± 5 mm Hg during pump support. In-hospital death occurred in 1 patient who was in cardiogenic shock. The 30-day follow-up of the remaining 6 patients was uneventful. An example of a high-risk PCI supported by the Tandem Heart LVAD is presented in Figure 11.4.

Aragon and coworkers reported about use of Tandem Heart LVAD in 8 patients considered to be at high risk because of severely compromised left ventricular function who were scheduled for percutaneous coronary intervention of complex coronary lesions [7]. The mean ejection fraction was $30\% \pm 9\%$. There was 100% success, and on average 3 ± 1 drug-eluting stents were implanted. During the procedure the Tandem Heart LVAD provided a stable hemodynamic condition. The device

Table 11.3 Baseline Characteristics and Hemodynamics Before and After LVAD Implantation

Patients	Vessels Diseased	EF %	Duration of Support (hr)	Mean SBP Pre (mm Hg)	Mean SBP Post (mm Hg)	PCWP Pre	PCWP Post	Access Site Bleeding
1	3	20	22	76	111	11	—	
2	3	38	269	71	102	18	16	+
3	3	20	4	97	105	32	7	+
4	1	18	6	75	70	28	20	
5	2	19	7	79	85	14	10	
6	3	30	50	137	133	13	15	+
7	3	19	27	71	114	—	—	+

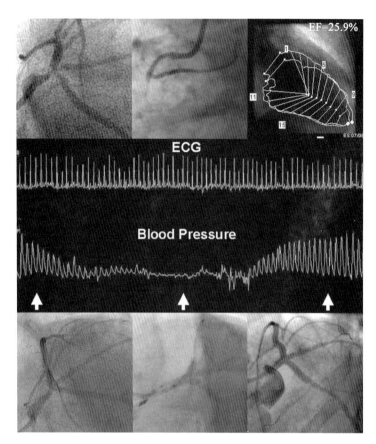

Figure 11.4 High-risk PCI in a patient with occluded right coronary artery, severe left main trifurcation disease, and ejection fraction (EF) 26% (*top frames*) supported by the Tandem Heart LVAD. During intervention of the LM with triple kissing balloon postdilatation following stent implantation of all branches, there is full circulatory support by the LVAD with complete depulsation of the heart with quick reverses after deflation of the balloons.

was removed immediately after the procedure and there were no access site problems. One patient died 10 days post PCI and another patient required hemodialysis for acute renal failure. Six patients were event free and symptom free at about 6-months follow-up.

Henriques and associates reported about the safety and feasibility of elective high-risk percutaneous coronary intervention procedures with Impella Recover LP 2.5 left ventricular support in 19 patients who were poor candidates for bypass surgery [8]. The patients were elderly (84% > 60 years of age), 74% had had previous myocardial infarction, and 63% had LVEF ≤ 25%. The device was used only during the procedure. All patients remained stable during the procedure. No limb pain was reported. There were no procedural deaths,

and two device-unrelated in-hospital late deaths. In 12 patients aortic regurgitation was monitored by echocardiography. There was no important increase or new onset of aortic regurgitation. The authors concluded that the use of the Impella 2.5 LP device is safe and appears to adequately support the hemodynamic situation of severe dysfunctional left ventricles.

Valgimigli and colleagues [9] reported the clinical, hemodynamic, and biochemical profile the safety and efficacy of the Impella Recover LP 2.5 LVAD during elective high-risk percutaneous coronary interventions in 12 patients. Using PV loop analysis and measurement of free hemoglobin (fHb), B-type natriuretic peptide, catecholamines, aldosterone, angiotensin II, and endothelin were assessed before, every 40 minutes as average during the procedure, and at 3, 12, 24 and 48 hours after intervention. The Impella catheter was used for 144 ± 88 min and was removed immediately after the procedure in all but 1 patient. In 6, 3, and 2 patients, fHb levels increased above 1, 5, and 10 times the upper limit of normal, respectively. No significant effect was found on the tested biomarkers in Impella-supported procedures. The PV analysis showed the occurrence of an acute volume increase in the majority of patients immediately after Impella insertion that tended to persist even at maximal pump speed. The study, although limited by the sample size, does not encourage the routine use of Impella Recover LP 2.5 in high-risk percutaneous interventions.

Conclusion

The Tandem Heart pLVAD and the Impella Recover LVAD provide active circulatory support by unloading the left ventricle, which results in improvement of hemodynamic and metabolic parameters in patients with postmyocardial infarction cardiogenic shock. It has been shown in relatively small studies that these devices are more effective than IABP, but improvement in mortality was not demonstrated. The use of the devices requires intensive monitoring of hemodynamic and metabolic parameters in a high-tech facility by highly skilled nurses and physicians. The use of these devices is associated with intrinsic complications due to the highly invasive procedure and the extracorporeal support. The use of the LVAD to facilitate high-risk PCI and to support or prevent an abrupt failing left ventricle is safe and feasible but it remains difficult to provide recommendations in which patients these devices should be used, and whether this procedure is actually lifesaving and cost-effective. The use of pLVAD is in its infancy, and more studies are needed to establish its role in clinical practice, also considering the option of biventricular support if required.

References

1. Goldberg RJ, Samad NA, Yarzebski J, Gurwitz J, Bigelow C, Gore JM. Temporal trends in cardiogenic shock complicating acute myocardial infarction. *N Engl J Med*. 1999;340:1162–1168.
2. Thiele H, Lauer B, Hambrecht R, Boudriot E, Cohen HA, Schuler G. Reversal of cardiogenic shock by percutaneous left atrial-to-femoral arterial bypass assistance. *Circulation*. 2001;104:2917–2922.
3. Burkhoff D, Cohen H, Brunckhorst C, O'Neill WW; TandemHeart Investigators Group. A randomized multicenter clinical study to evaluate the safety and efficacy of the TandemHeart percutaneous ventricular assist device versus conventional therapy with intraaortic balloon pumping for treatment of cardiogenic shock. *Am Heart J*. 2006;152:e1–e8.
4. Thiele H, Sick P, Boudriot E, *et al.* Randomized comparison of intra-aortic balloon support with a percutaneous left ventricular assist device in patients with revascularized acute myocardial infarction complicated by cardiogenic shock. *Eur Heart J*. 2005;26: 1276–1283.
5. Meyns B, Stolinski J, Leunens V, Verbeken E, Flameng W. Left ventricular support by catheter-mounted axial flow pump reduces infarct size. *J Am Coll Cardiol*. 2003;41:1087–1095.
6. Lemos PA, Cummins P, Lee CH, *et al.* Usefulness of percutaneous left ventricular assistance to support high-risk percutaneous coronary interventions. *Am J Cardiol*. 2003;91:479–481.
7. Aragon J, Lee M, Kar S, Makkar R. Percutaneous left ventricular assist device: "TandemHeart" for high-risk coronary intervention. *Cath Cardiovasc Interv*. 2005;65:346–352.
8. Henriques JP, Remmelink M, Baan J Jr., *et al.* Safety and feasibility of elective high-risk percutaneous coronary intervention procedures with left ventricular support of the Impella Recover LP 2.5. *Am J Cardiol*. 2006;97:990–992.
9. Valgimigli M, Steendijk P, Serruys PW, *et al.* Use of Impella Recover LP 2.5 left ventricular assist device during high-risk percutaneous coronary interventions; clinical, hemodynamic and biochemical findings. *EuroIntervention*. 2006;2:91–100.

CHAPTER 12

Treatment of Left Ventricular Failure

Roger Hullin

Départment de Médecine Interne, Centre Hospitalier Universitaire Vaudois, Lausanne, Switzerland

---

Chapter Overview

- Biventricular pacing reverses LV remodeling and increases cardiac output by optimal timing of atrial systole with ventricular diastolic filling.
- Cardiac resynchronization lowers morbidity and mortality in patients with interventricular conduction delay who remain in functional class III or IV heart failure despite optimal medical therapy.
- Chronic heart failure patients with cardiac resynchronization should receive medical treatment that is in accordance with the appropriate guidelines.
- In acute heart failure patients on percutaneous circulatory mechanical (PVAD) support, oxygen saturation should be maintained within the normal range (95–98%).
- In general, anticoagulation in patients on PVAD support should be established in accordance with the recommendations of the manufacturer.
- Improvement of hemodynamics is the goal of treatment of acute heart failure, and inotropic agents may be useful and lifesaving even in patients on PVAD support.

Drug Therapy with Cardiac Resynchronization Therapy

Rationale of Resynchronization

The rationale of cardiac resynchronization therapy (CRT) is the observation that atrioventricular, interventricular, and intraventricular conduction delay may aggravate LV dysfunction in patients with CHF. Atrioventricular dyssynchrony, as indicated by a prolonged PR interval on the surface ECG, is present in up to 35% of patients with severe CHF. Interventricular conduction delay with a QRS duration ≥ 120 ms has a prevalence of 25% to 50%, and left bundle branch block is found in 15% to 27% in this patient population [1]. Functionally, a left ventricular bundle branch block causes wall seg-

Current Best Practice in Interventional Cardiology. Edited by B Meier. © 2010 Blackwell Publishing,

ments to contract asynchronously, and this altered sequence of LV contraction favors mitral valve insufficiency.

CRT and Cardiac Remodeling

Biventricular pacing with optimal timing of atrial systole with ventricular diastolic filling immediately increases left ventricular filling, and thus cardiac output. In addition, synchronization of papillary muscle activity decreases pre-systolic mitral regurgitation. Noncontrolled studies indicate that sustained resynchronization reverses LV remodeling, decreases left ventricular end-systolic and end-diastolic volumes, and increases left ventricular ejection fraction. These benefits are attributed to CRT, since discontinuation of pacing results in loss of improvement in cardiac function [2]. Thus, cardiac remodeling is the important target of biventricular pacing in CHF, suggesting that CRT treats myocardial particularities associated with interventricular conduction delay such as redistribution of regional blood flow, alteration in the regional metabolism, or disturbance of local calcium handling [3–7] in the background of optimal medical therapy.

Effect of CRT on Outcome

The CARE-HF trial demonstrated that the beneficial effect of continued CRT is sustained during a mean follow-up of 29 months [8], with a mean decrease of 0.5 to 0.8 points in the functional NYHA class [9,10]. Of importance, the CARE-HF trial demonstrated in the CRT group a 36% risk reduction in mortality, and a 37% risk reduction for the composite end point of death and hospitalization for major cardiovascular events ($p < 0.001$). Mortality had decreased in initial CARE-HF trial mainly due to a marked reduction in CHF-related deaths; however, the extension study of the CARE-HF trial with a follow-up of 37 months showed an additional 46% reduction in the risk of sudden death occurring late [11]. In summary, CRT in heart failure lowers morbidity and mortality in patients with interventricular conduction delay who remain in functional class III or IV heart failure despite optimal medical therapy.

CRT and Heart Failure Therapy

Optimal medical therapy in heart failure patients with functional NYHA class III or IV follows the guidelines issued by the European Society of Cardiology [12] and the American Heart Association Task Force [13]. The usual criteria for patient enrollment in CRT studies were (1) CHF in functional NYHA class III and IV despite optimal medical therapy, (2) a left ventricular ejection fraction < 35%, (3) a left ventricular end-diastolic diameter > 55 mm, and (4) a QRS duration > 120 or 150 ms [14]. The usual treatment of CHF patients in functional NYHA class III and IV consists of angiotensin-converting enzyme inhibitors (ACE-Is) and/or angiotensin II type 1 receptor blockers (ARBs), beta-adrenergic blockers, aldosterone receptor antagonists, diuretics, digoxin, and antithrombotics. These drugs will be discussed next.

ACE-Is are recommended as first-line therapy in all heart failure patients with a left ventricular ejection fraction < 40% to 45%, irrespective of clinical

symptoms. Administration of ACE-Is in these patients improves survival, symptoms, and functional capacity, and reduces the number of hospitalizations (class of recommendation I, level of evidence A). Of note, titration of ACE-Is should not be based on symptomatic improvement alone (class of recommendation I, level of evidence C). Instead, ACE-Is should be up-titrated slowly and, if possible, to the dosages shown to be effective in the large, controlled heart failure trials (class of recommendation I, level of evidence A) [12].

The beneficial effect of ACE-Is is apparent over the full range of left ventricular function. A meta-analysis in 12,763 patients with left ventricular dysfunction or heart failure [15] demonstrated that ACE-Is reduce mortality, admissions for heart failure, as well as re-infarction. These effects are independent of age, sex, and baseline use of diuretics, acetylsalicylic acid, and beta-blockade, and are reciprocal to the severity of heart failure [16].

Various randomized controlled trials demonstrated the beneficial effect of CRT against the background of optimal medical therapy. Despite the fact that CRT may improve heart failure symptoms in the individual patient, up-titration of drug dosages to levels shown to be effective is recommended. In cases with ACE-I treatment at the highest dosage level, maintenance is reasonable when contraindications are absent [54].

Important adverse effects associated with ACE-Is are cough, hypotension, renal insufficiency, hyperkalemia, angioedema, and syncope. Severe cough may lead to discontinuation of ACE-I therapy. Though some patients may tolerate reinstitution after a drug-free period, the substitute will be an ARB most often. Changes in systolic and diastolic blood pressure are usually small in normotensive patients. Low systolic blood pressure (< 90 mm Hg) during ACE-I treatment is acceptable if patients remain asymptomatic. Usually, creatinine levels will remain stable or decrease towards pre-treatment values during continued treatment with ACE-Is in patients with mild or moderate heart failure. In patients with severe heart failure, serum creatinine may increase by 10% to 15% irrespective of baseline serum creatinine [17]. It is well accepted that moderate renal insufficiency (< 250 μmol/L creatinine) and systolic blood pressure ≤ 90 mm Hg are relative contraindications to ACE-I treatment. Mild hyperkalemia is not a contraindication to ACE-I treatment, whereas serum potassium levels > 5.5 mmol/L are. Bilateral renal artery stenosis and angioedema during previous ACE-I therapy are contraindications to ACE-I treatment.

Diuretics

Diuretics are essential for treatment of fluid overload, especially in patients with pulmonary congestion or peripheral edema. Usually, diuretics improve dyspnea and increase exercise tolerance (class of recommendation I, level of evidence A) [18].

No larger controlled, randomized trials have assessed the effects of diuretics on symptoms or survival; however, a meta-analysis of smaller trials support a trend towards reduced mortality [19]. In general, diuretics should always be administered in combination with beta-blockers or ACE-Is (class of recommendation I, level of evidence C).

Often treatment of severe heart failure requires increasing doses of furosemide because of decreasing diuresis. In such cases, torasemide should replace furosemide, because the bioavailability of torasemide is not reduced in patients in severe heart failure [12,20]. While single thiazide diuretic treatment is less effective when the glomerular filtration rate falls below 30 mL/min, a synergistic effect with loop diuretics remains even when renal function is decreased in the context of severe heart failure [12,21].

After implementation of CRT, frequent clinical control of volemia should guide dosing of diuretics in order to avoid hypovolemia due to over-diuresis.

Beta-Adrenoceptor Antagonists

Beta-adrenergic blockers are recommended for the treatment of all heart failure patients in functional NYHA class II-IV who present with reduced left ventricular ejection fraction due to ischemic or non-ischemic cardiomyopathies. In these patients, beta-blockers should complete the standard treatment with ACE-Is and diuretics, unless there is a contraindication (class of recommendation I, level of evidence A).

Beta-adrenergic blocker treatment reduces the number of all hospitalizations (all, cardiovascular, and heart failure). In addition, beta-lockers improve functional class and reduce worsening of heart failure symptoms irrespective of age, gender, functional class, left ventricular ejection fraction, and the etiology of heart failure (class of recommendation I, level of evidence B).

Because of pharmacologic differences among the various beta-blockers in heart failure [22,23], only bisoprolol, carvedilol, metoprolol succinate, and nebivolol are recommended (class of recommendation I, level of evidence A).

Most often, initiation of beta-blocker treatment is associated with a biphasic response of initial worsening followed by long-term improvement. Therefore, careful monitoring is mandatory when beta-blocker treatment is initiated, and increments in dosing should be small with up-titration adapted to the individual responses. Analysis of the dose–response curves in the CIBIS II and the MERIT-HF trials indicate a significant reduction in the risk of mortality even in the study groups with lower beta-blocker dosage [24,25]. Because of the linearity of this relationship, up-titration of beta-blocker doses should attempt the highest dosage tolerated, even after successful CRT. Of note, beta-blockers may prolong atrioventricular conduction, and in these cases the atrioventricular delay of the pacemaker should be adjusted. Furthermore, up-titration of the beta-blocker can induce sinus bradycardia, necessitating atrial pacing. In such patients, adjustments of the atrioventricular delay of the pacemaker are necessary.

Aldosterone Receptor Antagonists

Aldosterone antagonists are recommended in addition to ACE-I, beta-blockers, and diuretics when patients are in heart failure with functional NYHA class III-IV (class of recommendation I, level of evidence B).

Spironolactone was developed as a diuretic agent. Today it plays an additional important therapeutic role in the treatment of more severe heart failure, but at a lower dosage level. Physiologic action of aldosterone promotes myocardial and vascular fibrosis, potassium and magnesium depletion, sympathetic activation and parasympathetic inhibition, as well as baroreceptor dysfunction. Synthesis of aldosterone is suppressed insufficiently by ACE-Is alone; therefore the aldosterone receptor antagonists spironolactone [26] or eplerenone [27] decrease mortality and morbidity when added to ACE-Is, beta-blockers, and diuretics. It remains unclear whether symptomatic improvement after CRT should motivate discontinuation of aldosterone receptor antagonist treatment, especially when the functional NYHA class improves to ≤ II. In fact, favorable pharmacologic effects on the turnover of the extracellular matrix turnover may persist, especially when the extracellular matrix turnover is high [28].

ARBs

ARBs may be used in symptomatic heart failure patients who do not tolerate ACE-Is. In these patients ARBs improve morbidity and mortality (class of recommendation I, level of evidence B).

ARBs and ACE-Is seem to have a similar efficacy in chronic heart failure on morbidity and mortality (class of recommendation IIa, level of evidence B). However, the study results suggest that high target doses of ARBs are required [29].

ARBs may be considered in combination with ACE-Is when patients remain symptomatic with signs of heart failure despite standard therapy. Addition of ARBs reduces mortality in these patients (class of recommendation IIa, level of evidence B) and heart failure-related hospitalizations (class of recommendation I, level of evidence A). However, careful monitoring and individual tailoring of these drugs is mandatory because of the higher rate of discontinuation due to hypotension/dizziness, renal impairment, or hyperkalemia. Both ARBs and aldosterone antagonists reduce morbidity and mortality in NYHA class III patients who remain symptomatic despite standard therapy [26,30,31]. At the moment, it remains unclear whether the addition of an ARB or an aldosterone antagonist is more beneficial in these patients.

Anticoagulation

Patients with CHF have a high risk of thromboembolic events. Factors predisposing to thromboembolism are low cardiac output with relative stasis of blood in dilated cardiac chambers, poor contractility, regional wall abnormalities, and atrial fibrillation [32]. The reported annual risk for stroke is 1% to 2% in controlled heart failure studies (V-HeFT, SAVE trial), while < 0.5% in the general population aged 50 to 75 years. The risk of stroke increases when patients are older or ejection fraction is lower [33,34]. However, there is little evidence in the literature that antithrombotic therapy reduces the risk of death or vascular events. The consensus is that CHF patients with underlying coronary artery disease should receive anti-platelet therapy for the prevention of myocardial infarction and death (class of recommendation IIa, level of evidence B) [35]. Furthermore, patients with previous myocardial infarction and a left ventricular mural thrombus should receive oral anticoagulation (class of recommendation IIa, level of evidence C). Nevertheless, acetylsalicylic acid therapy should be avoided in patients with recurrent hospitalizations for heart failure (class of recommendation IIb, level of evidence B).

Antithrombotic therapy in the immediate post CRT implantation period should follow the recommendations of the implanting physician; however, oral anticoagulation is recommended when the left ventricular lead was placed transseptally, and mandatory when atrial fibrillation is documented.

Problems of Drug Therapy with Resynchronization

Supraventricular tachycardia, such as atrial fibrillation or atrial flutter, may reveal the need for additional antiarrhythmic drug therapy in order to preserve the beneficial effects of resynchronization. Often, these drugs entail negative chronotropic effects, which necessitate adjustments of the atrioventricular delay of the pacemaker when sinus bradycardia occurs. In addition, negative inotropic effects may decrease the clinical efficacy of resynchronization therapy. Furthermore, proarrhythmic effects with increased extrasystoly may result in a loss of resynchronization. If amiodarone or its derivatives will be used in such cases, it is necessary to control the lead thresholds, which may change.

Some patients may present with fast atrioventricular conduction, which can reduce the benefits resulting from electrical coordination of atrioventricular action. These patients demand antiarrhythmic agents that slow atrioventricular conduction such as beta-blockers, verapamil, digitalis, or any combination of these drugs. In rare cases, ablation of the atrioventricular node may be necessary.

Cardiac Rehabilitation

In patients with stable CHF, cardiac rehabilitation and aerobic exercise training have emerged as a valuable strategy to maintain functional capacity and alleviate heart failure symptoms [55]. Supervision in a monitored environment is ideal, but third-party reimbursement may be limiting. Therefore, general recommendations are minimum walking at home, or encouragement for daily physical activity for 30 to 40 minutes starting with 5 minutes of continuous walking and increments of 2 to 4 minutes every few days. However, trials investigating the effect of cardiac rehabilitation after resynchronization have not been published.

Drug Therapy with Percutaneous Assist Devices

Percutaneous circulatory mechanical assistance may be indicated in patients with acute heart failure when the response to conventional therapy is inadequate. The general consensus is to consider these devices only in case of the potential for myocardial recovery, or as a bridge to surgical interventions or heart transplantation (class of recommendation IIb, level of evidence B).

The main principle of left ventricular assistance is the partial replacement of the mechanical work of the left ventricle in order to decrease myocardial work. In parallel, left ventricular assist devices should increase peripheral and end-organ flow [36], and thus prevent the development of end-organ failure. This may bridge these patients to surgical LVAD implantation [37] or heart trans-

plantation. However, percutaneous assist devices (PVADs) may also assist as temporary circulatory support during percutaneous high-risk coronary interventions such as mainstem percutaneous angioplasty. Those patients who need prolonged PVAD support most often require supplementary medical treatment with oxygen or ventilatory assistance, and medical treatment with vasodilators, inotropics, diuretics, anticoagulation, and morphine or its analogues. The manner of medical support needed will be discussed in the following sections.

Oxygen and Ventilatory Assistance

The main priority in the treatment of acute heart failure patients is the achievement of adequate oxygenation levels at the cellular level. Adequate oxygenation should prevent end-organ dysfunction and the onset of multiple organ failure. In general, the maintenance of an oxygen saturation within the normal range (95–98%) is recommended to maximize tissue oxygenation (class of recommendation I, level of evidence C).

There is strong consensus that noninvasive ventilation such as CPAP or NIPPV should be applied prior to endotracheal intubation [38,39] (class of recommendation IIa, level of evidence A) in order to reduce breathing work and thus the overall metabolic demand. However, endotracheal intubation is always indicated when noninvasive methods fail to improve tissue oxygenation (class of recommendation IIa, level of evidence C).

Morphine and Its Analogues

Morphine and its analogues are usually indicated in patients with acute heart failure, especially when patients present with restlessness and dyspnea (class of recommendation II, level of evidence B). These drugs will relieve breathlessness and thus partially reduce breathing work. In addition, cardiovascular effects such as venous and mild arterial dilatation, as well as the reduction of heart rate, may play a role [40]. However, in cases with reduced renal function, morphine analogues without secondary accumulation due to renal insufficiency should be administered.

Anticoagulation

Antithrombotic treatment is well established for the acute coronary syndrome, as well as for atrial fibrillation with or without heart failure. In the setting of a PVAD, however, specific recommendations of the manufacturer for the guidance of anticoagulation should be taken into account. Most important, careful monitoring of the coagulation system is mandatory, as there is often concomitant liver dysfunction in acute heart failure, which may decrease the hepatic synthesis of various coagulation factors.

Vasodilators

Vasodilation is always indicated when acute heart failure is associated with peripheral hypoperfusion and low diuresis, especially when systemic blood pressure is adequate.

Intravenous nitrate is a potent vasodilating agent that relieves pulmonary congestion, particularly in patients with acute coronary syndrome, but without compromising the stroke volume or increasing myocardial oxygen demand (class of recommendation I, level of evidence B). In addition, the combination of low-dose furosemide with intravenous nitrates at the highest dosage tolerated treats severe pulmonary congestion more effectively than treatment with furosemide alone [41]. However, intravenous nitrate treatment is limited by the development of tolerance, which occurs within 16 to 24 hours, especially when doses are high.

Intravenous sodium nitroprusside is indicated in patients with severe heart failure due to increased afterload or severe mitral regurgitation (class of recommendation I, level of evidence C). However, controlled trials documenting its efficacy in acute heart failure are lacking. Likewise, administration of nitroprusside has yielded inconsistent results in patients with acute myocardial infarction [42]. Pathophysiologic studies suggest a "coronary steal syndrome" caused by sodium nitroprusside [43], which may explain the clinical findings in patients with coronary artery disease. Therefore, nitrates should be favored in patients with acute heart failure due to coronary artery disease.

Diuretics

Diuretics are indicated in patients with acute heart failure when symptoms of fluid retention are present (class of recommendation I, level of evidence B). So far, the obvious symptomatic benefit has precluded a formal evaluation of diuretics in large–scale, randomized clinical trials. Therefore, safety and efficacy profiles are not established, as well as the impact of diuretics on outcome.

Inotropic Agents

Inotropic agents are indicated in acute heart failure whenever peripheral hypoperfusion is present, or when pulmonary edema persists despite optimal diuretic or vasodilator treatment (class of recommendation II, level of evidence C).

The clinical course and the prognosis of acute heart failure depend critically on hemodynamics. Thus, improvement of hemodynamics is the goal of treatment of acute heart failure, and inotropic agents may be useful and lifesaving. However, the beneficial effects of improved hemodynamics may be partially counteracted by the increased risk of arrhythmias and myocardial ischemia as oxygen demand increases [44]. Left ventricular unloading by PVAD may decrease the need for inotropic support and thus decrease the risk for severe arrythmias; however, only rare cases may get along without positive inotropic therapy.

Dobutamine is a positive inotropic agent that stimulates both the β_1-adrenergic and the β_2-adrenergic receptors in a 3:1 ratio [45]. Its pharmacologic action is a dose-dependent positive inotropic and chronotropic effect [46]. Clinically, dobutamine at low doses will induce mild vasodilation, while higher doses induce vasoconstriction [47]. The magnitude of benefits may vary in the individual patient, especially when patients received prior beta-blocker treatment. In this setting, pharmacologic specificities play an important role, with metoprolol demanding high doses of dobutamine for an inotropic effect [48] while patients on carvedilol treatment respond with increased pulmonary vascular resistance to dobutamine treatment [49]. On the other hand, the inotropic effect of dobutamine in combination with a phosphodiesterase inhibitor is greater than each drug alone because of their synergistic pharmacologic action [50].

Levosimendan treatment results in a dose-dependent increase in stroke volume, a decrease in pulmonary wedge pressure and pulmonary vascular resistance, a decrease in systemic vascular resistance and blood pressure, and a slight heart rate increase [51]. The effect of levosimendan on mortality remains debated [51,52]; however, symptoms of fatigue and dyspnea improve, and the BNP level drops. Pharmacologically, different mechanisms of action have been identified for levosimendan: (1) Ca^{2+} sensitization of the contractile proteins, which is responsible for inotropic action at the low-dose level; and (2) phosphodiesterase inhibition mediating positive inotropic and lusitropic effects at the high-dose level. In addition, levosimendan induces opening of the smooth-muscle K^+ channel, which results in dose-dependent vasodilation. Because of these pharmacologic properties, the actual recommendation is to use levosimendan primarily in patients with symptomatic low output but without severe hypotension (class of recommendation IIa, level of evidence B). Of note, the hemodynamic response of levosimendan maintained, or even increased, in patients with concomitant beta-blocker therapy [51]. Furthermore, the metabolites of levosimendan have a half-life of $\sim$80 hours, which probably explains the clinical effect lasting beyond the usual 24-hour infusion [53].

Vasopressor Agents

In general, vasopressor therapy with epinephrine or norepinephrine is indicated when the combination of fluid challenge and inotropic agents fails to restore circulatory stability and organ perfusion despite improvement of cardiac output. Since cardiogenic shock is usually associated with high systemic peripheral resistance, any vasopressor may increase the afterload of the failing heart and decrease cardiac output. Therefore, vasopressors should be used with caution, as they may further decrease end-organ blood supply. In this setting, PVAD support should decrease the need of vasopressor agents, favor reverse remodeling of the left ventricle by mechanical unloading, and favor end-organ supply with oxygen.

References

1. Hawkins NM, Petrie MC, MacDonald MR, Hogg KJ, McMurray JJ. Selecting patients for cardiac resynchronization therapy: electrical or mechanical dyssynchrony? *Eur Heart J*. 2006;27:1270–1281.
2. Duncan A, Wait D, Gibson D, *et al.* Left ventricular remodeling and hemodynamic effects of multisite pacing in patients with left ventricular dysfunction and activation disturbances in sinus rhythm: sub-study of the MUSTIC trial. *Eur Heart J*. 2003;24:430–441.
3. Vernooy K, Verbeek XAAM, Peschar M, *et al.* Left bundle branch block induces left ventricular remodelling and functional septal hypoperfusion. *Eur Heart J*. 2005;26:91–98.
4. Spragg DD, Leclerq C, Loghmani M, *et al.* Regional alterations in protein expression in dyssynchronous failing heart. *Circulation*. 2003;108:929–932.
5. Nowak B, Sinha A, Schaefer W, *et al.* Cardiac resynchronization therapy homogenizes myocardial glucose metabolism and perfusion in dilated cardiomyopathy and left bundle brunch block. *J Am Coll Cardiol*. 2003;41:1523–1528.
6. Ukkonen H, Beanlands R, Burwash I, *et al.* Effect of cardiac resynchronization on myocardial efficiency and regional oxidative metabolism. *Circulation*. 2003;107:28–31.
7. Sundell J, Egblom E, Koistinen J, *et al.* The effect of cardiac resynchronization therapy on left ventricular function, myocardial energetics and metabolic reserve in patients with dilated cardiomyopathy and heart failure. *J Am Coll Cardiol*. 2004;43:1027–1033.
8. Cleland JGF, Daubert LC, Erdmann E, *et al.* The effect of cardiac resynchronization therapy on morbidity and mortality in heart failure (the Cardiac Resynchronization-Heart Failure [CARE-HF] Trial). *N Engl J Med*. 2005;352:1539–1549.
9. Aurricchio A, Stellbrink C, Sack S, *et al.* Pacing therapies in congestive heart failure (PATH-CHF) Study Group. Long-term effect of hemodynamically optimized cardiac resynchronization therapy in patients with heart failure and ventricular conduction delay. *J Am Coll Cardiol*. 2002;39:2026–2033.
10. Higgins S, Hummel J, Niazi I, *et al.* Cardiac resynchronization therapy for the treatment of heart failure in patients with intraventricular conduction delay and malignant ventricular tacharrythmias. *J Am Coll Cardiol*. 2003;42:1454–1459.
11. Cleland JGF, Daubert JC, Erdmann E, *et al.* Longer-term effects of cardiac resynchronization therapy on mortality in heart failure (the Cardiac

Resynchronization-Heart Failure [CARE-HF] trial extension phase). *Eur Heart J*. 2006;27:1928–1932.

12. Swedberg K, Cleland JG, Dargie H, *et al.* Guideline for the diagnosis and treatment of chronic heart failure: full text (update 2005). *Eur Heart J*. 2005;26:1115–1140.

13. Hunt SA, Abraham WT, Chin MH, *et al.* ACC/AHA guideline update for the diagnosis and management of chronic heart failure in the adult: a report of the American College of Cardiology/Amaerican Heart Association Task Force in Practice Guidelines (Writing Committee to update the 2001 guidelines for the evaluation and management of heart failure): developed in a collaboration with the American College of Chest Physicians and the International Society of Heart and Lung Transplantation: endorsed by the Heart Rhythm Society. *Circulation*. 2005, e154–e235.

14. Vardas PE, Aurrichio A, Blanc JJ, *et al.* Guidelines for cardiac pacing and cardiac resynchronization therapy. The Task Force for Cardiac Pacing and Cardiac Resynchronization Therapy of the European Society of Cardiology. Developed in collaboration with the European Heart Rhythm Society. *Eur Heart J*. 2007;28:2256–2295.

15. Flather M, Yusuf S, Kober L, *et al.* Long-term ACE inhibitor therapy in patients with heart failure or left-ventricular dysfunction. A systematic overview of data from individual patients. *Lancet*. 2000;355:1575–1581.

16. The Consensus Trial Study Group. Effects of enalapril on mortality in severe congestive heart failure. Results of the Cooperative North Scandinavian Enalapril Survival Study (CONSENSUS). *N Engl J Med*. 1987;316:1429–1435.

17. Ljungman S, Kjekshus J, Swedberg K. Renal function in severe congestive heart failure during treatment with enalapril. The Cooperative North Scandinavian Enalapril Survival Study (CONSENSUS). *Am J Cardiol*. 1992;70:479–487.

18. Kaddoura S, Patel D, Parameshwar J, *et al.* Objective assessment of the response to the treatment of severe heart failure using a 9-minute walk test on a patient-powered treadmill. *J Card Fail*. 1996;2: 133–139.

19. Paris R, Flather M, Purcell H, *et al.* Current evidence supporting the role of diuretics in heart failure: a meta analysis of randomized controlled trials. *Int J Cardiol*. 2002;82:140–158.

20. Vargo DL, Kramer WG, Black PK, *et al.* Bioavailability, pharmacokinetics, and pharmacodynamics of torasemide and furosemide in patients

with congestive heart failure. *Clin Pharmacol Ther*. 1995;57:601–609.

21. Channer KS, McLean KA, Lawson-Matthew P, *et al.* Combination diuretic treatment in severe heart failure: a randomized controlled trial. *Br Heart J*. 1994;71:146–150.

22. The Beta Blocker Evaluation of Survival Trial Investigators. A trial of the beta-blocker bucindolol in patients with advanced heart failure. *N Engl J Med*. 2001;344:1659–1667.

23. Poole-Wilson PA, Swedberg K, Cleland JG, *et al.* Comparison of cardvedilol and metoprolol on clinical outcomes in patients with CHF in the Cardvedilol Or Metoprolol Eurpoean Trial (COMET): randomized controlled trial. *Lancet*. 2003;362:7–13.

24. Simon T, Mary-Krause M, Funck-Bentano C, *et al.* Bisoprolol dose-response relationship in patients with congestive heart failure: a subgroup analysis in the cardiac insufficiency bisoprolol study (CIBIS II). *Eur Heart J*. 2003;24:552–559.

25. Wikstrand J, Hjalmarson A, Waagstein F, *et al.* Dose of metoprolol CR/XL and clinical outcomes in patients with heart failure: analysis of the experience in metoprolol CR/XL randomized intervention trial in CHF (MERIT-HF). *J Am Coll Cardiol*. 2002;40:491–498.

26. Pitt B, Zannad F, Remme WJ, *et al.* The effect of spironolactone on morbidity and mortality in patients with severe heart failure. Randomized Aldosterone Evaluation Study Investigators. *N Engl J Med*. 1999;341:709–717.

27. Pitt B, Remme W, Zannad F, *et al.* Eplerenone, a selective aldosterone blockerin patients with left ventricular dysfunction after myocardial infarction. *N Engl J Med*. 2003;348:1309–1321.

28. Zannad F, Alla F, Dousset B, Perez A, Pitt B. Limitation of excessive extracellular matrix turnover may contribute to survival benefit of spironolactone thaerapy in patients with congestive heart failure therapy: insights from the randomized aldosterone evaluation study (RALES). Rales Investigators. *Circulation*. 2000;102:2700–2706.

29. Young JB, Dunlap ME, Pfeffer MA, *et al.* Mortality and morbidity reduction with candesartan in patients with CHF and left ventricular systolic dysfunction. Results of the CHARM-Low Left Ejection Fraction Trials. *Circulation*. 2004;110:2618–2625.

30. Cohn JN, Tognoni G. A randomized trial of the angiotensin-receptor blocker valsartan. *N Engl J Med*. 2001;345:1667–1675.

31. McMurray JJ, Ostergren J, Swedberg K, *et al.* Effects of candesartan in patients with CHF and reduced

left-ventricular systolic function taking angiotensin-converting enzyme inhibitors: the CHARM Added trial. *Lancet*. 2003;362:767–771.

32. Jafri SM. Hypercoagulatbility in heart failure. *Semin Thromb Hemost*. 1997;53:543–545.

33. Cohn JN, Johnson H, Ziesche S, *et al.* A comparison of enalapril with hydralazine-isosorbide dinitrate in the treatment of congestive heart failure. *N Engl J Med*. 1991;325:303–310.

34. Pfeffer MA, Braunwald E, Moye LA, *et al.* Effect of captopril on mortality and morbidity in patients with left ventricular dysfunction after myocardial infarction. Results of the survival and ventricular enlargement trial. The SAVE investigators. *N Engl J Med*. 1992;327:669–677.

35. Collaborative meta-analysis of randomized trials of antiplatelet therapy for prevention of death, myocardial infarction, and stroke in high risk patients. *BMJ*. 2002;324:71–86.

36. Delgado DH, Rao V, Ross HJ, Verma S, Smedira NG. Mechanical circulatory assistance: state of the art. *Circulation*. 2002;106:1046–1050.

37. Idelchik GM, Simpson L, Civitello AB, *et al.* Use of the percutaneous left ventricular assist device in patients with severe cardiogenic shock as a bridge to long-term left ventricular assist device implantation. *J Heart Lung Transplant*. 2008;27:106–111.

38. Pang D, Keenan SP, Cook DJ, Sibbald WJ. The effect of positive airway pressure support on mortality and the need for intubation in cardiogenic shock pulmonary edema: a systematic review. *Chest*. 1998;114:1185–1192.

39. Masip J, Betbese AJ, Paez J, *et al.* Non-invasive positive pressure support ventilationversus conventional oxygen therapy in acute cardiogenic pulmonary edema: a randomized trial. *Lancet*. 2000;356:2126–2132.

40. Lee G, DeMaria AN, Amsterdam EA, *et al.* Comparative effects of morphine, meperidine, and pentazocine on cardiocirculatory dynamics in patients with acute myocardial infarction. *Am J Med*. 1976;60:949-955.

41. Cotter G, Metzkor E, Kaluski E, *et al.* Randomized trial of high-dose isosorbide dinitrate plus low-dose furosemide versus high-dose furosemide plus low-dose isosorbide dinitrate in severe pulmonary edema. *Lancet*. 1998;351:389–393.

42. Cohn JN, Franciosa JA. Vasodilator therapy in heart failure *N Engl J Med*. 1977;297:254–258.

43. Reves JG, Erdmann W, Mardis M, Karp RB, King M, Lell WA. Evidence for the existence of intramyocardial steal. *Adv Exp Med Biol*. 1977;94:755–760.

44. Katz AM. Potential deleterious effects of inotropic agents in the therapy of chronic heart failure. *Circulation*. 1986;73:III184–III190.

45. Leier CV, Binkley PF. Parenteral inotropic support for advanced congestive heart failure. *Prog Cardiovasc Dis*. 1998;41:207–224.

46. Fowler MB, Laser JA, Hopkins GL, Minobe W, Bristow MR. Assessment of the beta-adrenergic receptor pathway in the intact failing heart: progressive receptor-downregulation and subsensitivity to agonist response. *Circulation*. 1986;74: 1290–1302.

47. Jain P, Massie BM, Gattis WA, Klein L, Gheorghiade M. Current medical treatment for the exacerbation of chronic heart failure resulting in hospitalization. *Am Heart J*. 2003;145:S13–S17.

48. Lowes BD, Tsvetkova T, Eichhorn EJ, Gilbert EM, Bristow MR. Milrinone versus dobutamine in heart failure subjects treated chronically with carvedilol. *Int J Cardiol*. 2001;81:141–149.

49. Metra M, Nodari S, D'Aloia A, *et al.* Beta-blocker therapy influences the hemodynamic response to inotropic agents in patients with heart failure: a randomized comparison of dobutamine and enoximone before and after chronic treatment with metoprolol or carvedilol. *J Am Coll Cardiol*. 2002;40: 1248–1258.

50. Gilbert EM, Hershberger RE, Wiechmann RJ, Movesian MA, Birstow MR. Pharmacologic and hemodynamic effects of combined beta-agonist stimulation and phosphodiesterase inhibition in the failing heart. *Chest*. 1995;108: 1524–1532.

51. Follath F, Cleland JG, Just H, *et al.* Efficacy and safety of intravenous levosimendan compared with dobutamine in severe low output heart failure (the LIDO study). *Lancet*. 2002;360:196–202.

52. Mebazaa A, Nieminen MS, Packer M, *et al.* Levosimendan vs. dobutamine for patients with acute decompensated heart failure: the SURVIVE randomized trial. *JAMA*. 2007;297:1883–1891.

53. Kivikko M, Lehtonen L, Colucci WS. Sustained hemodynamic effects of intravenous levosimendan. *Circulation*. 2003;107:81–86.

54. Abraham WT, Yancy CW. Cardiac resynchronization therapy: a practical guide for patient management after device implantation. *Congest Heart Fail*. 2006;12:219–222.

55. Smart N, Fang ZY, Marwich TH. A practical guide to exercise training for heart failure patients. *J Card Fail*. 2003;9:49–58.

PART IV
Cardiovascular Imaging

CHAPTER 13

Computed Tomography for Screening and Follow-Up

Stephan Achenbach
Department of Cardiology, University of Erlangen, Erlangen, Germany

---

Chapter Overview

- Computed tomography allows imaging of the heart and coronary arteries with increasing robustness.
- Sufficient image quality provided, coronary artery stenoses can be detected with a high sensitivity and negative predictive value.
- Specificity and positive predictive values are lower.
- The main application of coronary CT angiograophy is to rule out coronary artery stenoses in selected patients.
- Imaging of stents is more difficult and currently not recommended.
- Coronary CT angiography can also detect nonobstructive plaque, but it is not yet a clinical application for risk stratification of asymptomatic individuals.

Cardiac computed tomography (CT), and in particular CT imaging of the coronary arteries, has been receiving rapidly growing interest during the recent years. In fact, it is has been incorporated in the clinical workup of selected patients with known or suspected coronary artery disease in more and more practice settings. Improvements in CT technology and a growing number of scientific studies that have demonstrated high accuracy of CT imaging for the detection of coronary artery stenoses have been the reasons behind this very visible development.

The interventional community has been following this development with mixed feelings of interest and reluctance—there is justified concern that the technique is still of inferior diagnostic accuracy as compared to the invasive angiogram, and that

it may be used inadequately and in patients who do not need this kind of test; while on the other hand it may be a potentially useful tool for the invasive and interventional cardiologist that could take some of the purely diagnostic load off of the catheterization suite, identify patients with acute coronary syndromes earlier than the current clinical workup, or even provide useful information in the context of complex coronary interventions.

Catheter-based coronary angiography has been and remains the gold standard for visualizing the coronary artery lumen. Noninvasive visualization of the coronary vessels is a challenging task. In spite of the impressive image quality that "coronary CT angiography" often provides (Fig. 13.1), CT is not yet ready to generally replace the invasive angiogram as the standard test for the diagnosis of coronary artery stenoses. The small dimensions and the rapid motion of the coronary arteries pose tremendous challenges for noninvasive imaging, and only the recent substantial improvements in scanner technology have made it

Current Best Practice in Interventional Cardiology. Edited by B Meier. © 2010 Blackwell Publishing.

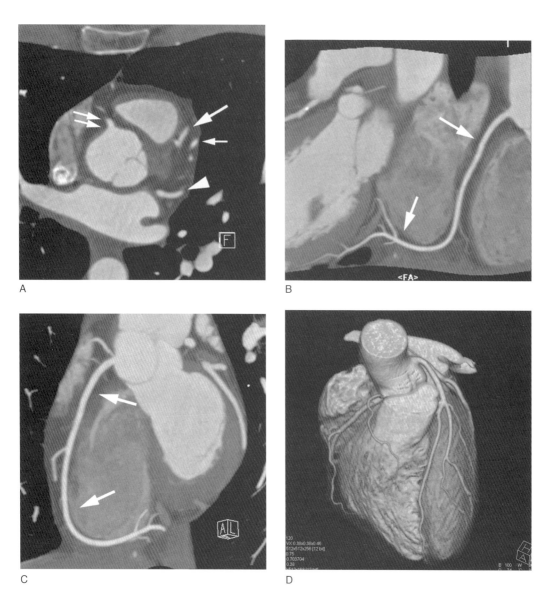

A

B

C

D

Figure 13.1 Typical data set of coronary CT angiography. After intravenous injection of contrast agent, the blood lumen is brightly enhanced. **A.** Thin transaxial image shows a section of the left anterior descending coronary artery (*large arrow*) and a diagonal branch (*small arrow*) as well as the left circumflex coronary artery (*arrowhead*) and the origin of the right coronary artery from the aortic root (*double arrows*).

B. Curved multiplanar reformat image shows the entire course of the right coronary artery (*arrows*). **C.** Maximum-intensity projection image, here with 5.0-mm thickness, depicts the right coronary artery (*arrows*) in a fashion similar to invasive coronary angiography. **D.** Three-dimensional reconstruction that shows the heart and coronary arteries.

possible to perform "coronary CT angiography" (often called coronary CTA) outside highly specialized centers and extremely selected patients. All the same, through the ability to noninvasively and

quickly detect or rule out coronary artery stenoses, coronary CTA has the potential to substantially impact on the management of many patients with suspected or—to some extent—with known coronary artery disease. However, the somewhat limited spatial and temporal resolution of CT (which most likely will not continue to improve at a similarly rapid rate as in the past) causes limitations, and it is important to understand them in order to avoid unreasonable applications or misinterpretation of scan results. Many very valuable scientific studies have become available during the past year and have contributed to clarifying the role that coronary CTA can play as a diagnostic tool.

CT Technology

Coronary artery imaging requires high spatial and temporal resolution. Clinical applications crucially depend on the technology that is used. Sixty-four-slice CT with gantry rotation times between 330 and 420 ms constitutes the widely accepted minimum requirement for coronary CT angiography [1–3]. With half-scan reconstruction (which means that data sampled during one-half rotation are used to reconstruct each transaxial image), the temporal resolution of 64-slice CT is approximately 165 to 210 ms. So-called multisegment reconstruction algorithms can be used to improve temporal resolution by combining data samples during several consecutive heartbeats [2]. However, the limited temporal resolution of CT is one of its main limitations. It has been convincingly shown that low heart rates improve image quality in 64-slice CT [3–7], and it is currently recommended to lower the patient's heart rate to below 65/min or, optimally, 60/min in order to achieve optimal image quality when coronary CTA is performed with 64-slice CT equipment [1,2]. This is sometimes perceived as a major limitation of CT angiography, but experienced users of coronary CT angiography uniformly agree that the clinical value of coronary CT angiography when performed with 64-slice equipment critically depends on lowering heart rate because of the substantial effects on image quality and diagnostic accuracy. Oral or intravenous short-acting beta blockade are most often used to lower heart rate in preparation for coronary CT angiography.

Beyond 64-slice CT, manufacturers have chosen different approaches to further develop cardiac CT technology. Continuing along the line of 4-, 16-, and 64-slice CT, two manufacturers have chosen to further increase the number of simultaneously acquired slices by creating 256-slice and 320-slice systems. This is meant to allow coverage of the entire volume of the heart in one single rotation [8,9], requiring only one single heartbeat for data acquisition while spatial resolution and temporal resolution of each individual cross-sectional image remain unchanged. This approach makes cardiac CT imaging less susceptible to arrhythmias, requires less contrast, and will potentially reduce radiation dose [9].

Another manufacturer has introduced the Dual Source CT (DSCT) system, which combines two x-ray tubes and detectors in a single gantry, arranged at an angle of 90 degrees. This provides a twofold increase in temporal resolution as compared to 64-slice CT: only one-quarter rotation is necessary to collect the x-ray data necessary for reconstruction of an axial image, and with a rotation time of 0.28 ms, the system thus provides a temporal resolution of 75 ms. Initial publications demonstrate that this noticeably reduces problems caused by motion artefacts [10–13]. First investigations that compared coronary imaging by DSCT to invasive coronary angiography have demonstrated high diagnostic accuracy for detection of coronary stenoses even without systematic pre-treatment to lower heart rate [13–18].

Coronary CT Angiography for the Detection of Stenoses

Accuracy

Clinical applications of coronary CT angiography will critically depend on its accuracy for detection of significant coronary artery stenoses (Fig. 13.2). Numerous recent studies have assessed the accuracy of coronary CT angiography for stenosis detection in comparison to invasive, catheter-based coronary angiography. Using 40-slice CT [19–22], 64-slice CT [23–32], or dual source CT [14–18],

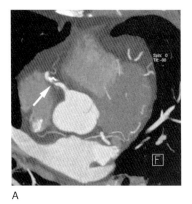
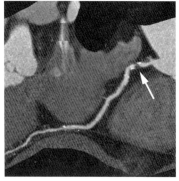
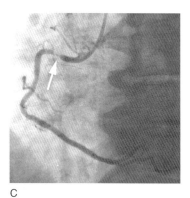

A   B   C

Figure 13.2 High-grade stenosis of the proximal right coronary artery depicted by contrast enhanced coronary CT angiography. **A.** Transaxial image. The atherosclerotic plaque that leads to a stenosis of the right coronary artery is partly calcified, partly noncalcified (*arrow*).

B. Curved multiplanar reconstruction, which also shows the stenosis of the right coronary artery (*arrow*). **C.** Corresponding invasive coronary angiogram (*arrow* = stenosis).

the sensitivity for the detection of coronary artery stenoses has ranged from 86% to 100% and specificity was reported to be between 91% and 98 %. Accuracy values are not uniform across all patients. Several trials have demonstrated that high heart rates and extensive calcification negatively influence accuracy [3,33,34]. Usually, a degraded image will lead to false-positive rather than false-negative findings [33], and specificity and positive predictive value will therefore be affected worst.

Recently, a thorough meta-analysis has become available that carefully analyzed the accuracy data that are available for coronary CT angiography with various generations of CT technology [3].

The authors were able to demonstrate a significant increase in the sensitivity and specificity for stenosis detection as scanner technology evolved from 4- slice to 16-slice and 64-slice equipment (Table 13.1). For 64-slice CT, the authors report a pooled sensitivity of 93% and specificity of 96% based on a per-segment analysis, as well as a sensitivity of 99% and specificity of 93% based on a per-patient analysis (in a total of 363 patients). While these pooled results confirm the high accuracy values that had been found in the previously published smaller studies, it has to be taken into account that all available results were obtained in highly specialized centers. In addition,

Table 13.1 Sensitivity and Specificity of Coronary CT Angiography Versus Invasive Coronary Angiography for Detection of Coronary Artery Stenoses (meta-analysis of pooled data)

Scanner Type	No. Studies	Per-Segment Analysis		Per-Patient Analysis	
		Sensitivity (%)	Specificity (%)	Sensitivity (%)	Specificity (%)
4-slice CT	22	84	93	91	83
16-slice CT	26	83	96	97	81
64-slice CT	6	93	96	99	93

From Vanhoenacker PK, Heijenbrok-Kal MH, Van Heste R, et al. Diagnostic performance of multidetector CT angiography for assessment of coronary artery disease: meta-analysis. *Radiology*. 2007;244:419–428.

patients in all of the trials were somewhat selected: all had a stable sinus rhythm and usually a low heart rate, ability to cooperate and perform at least a 10-second breathhold, as well as absence of renal failure, previously implanted coronary stents, or previous bypass surgery. Most likely, results will be somewhat inferior in less experienced centers and less selected patient populations.

The uniformly high negative predictive value that was found in all published trials (ranging from 95% to 100%) indicates that coronary CTA will be able to reliably rule out coronary artery stenoses, at least in patients comparable to those that were included in these published trials. Based on considerations of pre-test likelihood, the predictive power would be altered in patient groups with higher prevalence of disease. In a recent publication by Meijboom and associates, the diagnostic accuracy of coronary CT angiography was put in relation to the clinical presentation and pre-test likelihood of coronary artery disease [35]. It was clearly shown that the diagnostic value of CT angiography was highest in patients with a relatively low pre-test likelihood of disease and lowest in those patients in whom the clinical presentation suggested a high likelihood that coronary stenoses would be present. Therefore, the clinical use of CT angiography will be most beneficial whenever the clinical situation implies a relatively low pre-test likelihood of coronary disease, but still requires further workup to rule out significant coronary stenoses. In high-risk patients with a high likelihood of coronary artery stenoses, coronary CT angiography will be less useful (Table 13.2).

Potential Clinical Applications

In spite of the impressive image quality—which continues to improve—coronary CT angiography will not constitute a general replacement for invasive, catheter-based diagnostic coronary angiography in the foreseeable future. Spatial resolution and temporal resolution are substantially lower than in invasive angiography. In addition, arrhythmias—most prominently atrial fibrillation—high heart rates, and inability to perform a 10-second breathhold may preclude CT angiography in a significant number of patients who require a workup for coronary artery disease. Similarly, in patients with diffuse, severe disease, with substantial coronary calcification or with small coronary arteries (as often encountered, for example, in patients with diabetes), the spatial resolution of CT may not be sufficiently high to allow reliable interpretation of the coronary system. For challenging cases like these, invasive angiography will remain the best diagnostic option.

On the other hand, CT angiography does make it possible to reliably exclude the presence of coronary artery stenoses if image quality is good, and in many patients the clinical situation may mandate ruling out coronary artery disease even though the pre-test likelihood is not very high. Often CT image quality can be expected to be high in these patients, and CT angiography will be clinically useful. Based on clinical considerations, CT angiography is not as likely to be useful in patients with a high pre-test likelihood of disease. First of all, patients with a high pre-test likelihood of disease or with previously known coronary disease often have reduced

Table 13.2 Diagnostic Performance of 64-Slice CT Depending on Clinical Pre-test Likelihood of Coronary Artery Disease in 254 Patients

Pre-test Probability[a]	No. Patients	Sensitivity (%)	Specificity (%)	Pos. Pred. Value (%)	Neg. Pred. Value (%)
High	105	98	74	93	89
Intermediate	83	100	84	80	100
Low	66	100	93	75	100

[a]Estimated with the Duke Clinical Risk Score.
From Meijboom WB, van Mieghem CA, Mollet NR, et al. 64-slice computed tomography coronary angiography in patients with high, intermediate, or low pretest probability of significant coronary artery disease. *J Am Coll Cardiol.* 2007;50:1469–1475.

image quality due to the above-named reasons, such as substantial calcification and small coronary diameters, so that the accuracy of CT angiography will likely be reduced. Second, coronary CTA—as opposed to invasive angiography—does not offer an option for immediate intervention, and referring patients with a high likelihood of stenoses to the catheterization suite makes more sense than subjecting them to a CT angiogram first. Similarly, imaging of entirely asymptomatic patients cannot be recommended, since "screening" for coronary artery stenoses is not likely to improve prognosis.

In the past year, several studies were published that have specifically addressed the accuracy of coronary CTA in some clinical situations that are typically associated with a low to intermediate likelihood of disease, but in which invasive angiography is currently frequently performed in order to rule out stenoses. For example, Andreini and coworkers studied 61 patients with heart failure of unknown etiology and reported a sensitivity of 99% and specificity of 96% to identify patients with coronary artery stenoses using a 16-slice CT scanner [36]. In a similar, small study, Manghat and colleagues found 100% accuracy for the identification of patients with coronary stenoses among 18 patients presenting with cardiomyopathy [37]. Gosthine and associates evaluated the accuracy of 64-slice coronary CT angiography in 66 patients with left bundle-branch block and reported a sensitivity of 97%, specificity of 95%, as well as a negative predictive value of 97% for the detection of patients who had significant coronary artery stenoses [34].

Two studies addressed the utility of coronary CT angiography to rule out coronary stenoses in patients who require noncoronary cardiac surgery. Meijboom and associates used 64-slice CT to study 145 consecutive patients with aortic valve stenosis who required surgery; 48 patients could not be scanned by CT because of atrial fibrillation, renal failure, or other reasons. In the remaining 70 patients, the authors found a sensitivity of 100% (18 of 18 stenoses detected) and specificity of 92% for the detection of coronary artery stenoses [38]. In 50 patients requiring aortic valve replacement for severe regurgitation, Scheffel and colleagues reported 100% sensitivity and 95% specificity for the iden-

tification of subjects who had significant coronary stenoses [39].

Another situation in which the use of a noninvasive imaging technology to rapidly and reliably rule out coronary stenoses could be of tremendous clinical value is the setting of acute chest pain. Especially if the ECG is normal and myocardial enzymes are not elevated, the likelihood of coronary disease is low, but the possibility of myocardial infarction requires a rapid and definite diagnosis. In initial trials, CT angiography has been shown to be both accurate and safe to stratify patients with acute chest pain and absence of ECG changes as well as myocardial enzyme elevation [28,40–43] (Fig. 13.3). One study demonstrated a cost advantage of incorporating CT angiography in the workup of low-likelihood acute chest pain patients as compared to the standard of care [42].

Some recently published official documents offer recommendations as to the clinical use of coronary CTA. A Scientific Statement of the American Heart Association on the assessment of coronary artery disease by cardiac computed tomography states the following:

> Especially in the context of ruling out stenosis in patients with low to intermediate pretest likelihood of disease, CT coronary angiography may develop into a clinically useful tool. CT coronary angiography is reasonable for the assessment of obstructive disease in symptomatic patients (Class IIa, Level of Evidence: B) [44].

A group of U.S.-based professional societies (both cardiology and radiology) have jointly issued a statement of appropriateness criteria for cardiac CT and MR imaging, which lists several situations in which coronary CT angiography is considered to be of clinical value [48]. They include the use of CT coronary angiography to rule out coronary artery stenoses in patients who are symptomatic, but who have an uninterpretable or equivocal stress test, who are unable to exercise, or who have an uninterpretable ECG. Furthermore, the document considers the use of coronary CT angiography appropriate for patients with new-onset heart failure and for patients who present with acute chest pain and an intermediate pre-test likelihood of coronary artery disease, but who have a normal ECG and absence of enzyme elevation (Table 13.3) [45]. In

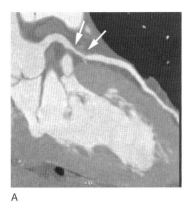
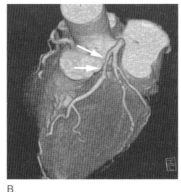
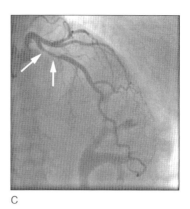

A B C

Figure 13.3 69-year-old patient with an episode of chest pain at rest, but normal ECG and normal myocardial enzymes upon arrival at the emergency room. **A.** Curved multiplanar reconstruction of the left main and left anterior descending coronary artery shows a long, noncalcified stenosis of the very proximal LAD (*arrows*). **B.** 3-dimensional reconstruction that also demonstrates the stenosis (*arrows*). **C.** Corresponding invasive coronary angiogram (*arrows* = stenosis).

addition, the use of CT angiography is considered "appropriate" to evaluate patients with anomalous coronary arteries [45].

Imaging of Patients with Bypass Grafts and Stents

Coronary CT angiography has substantial limitations in patients with previous coronary revascularization. In patients after bypass surgery, assess-

ing the native coronary arteries can be extremely difficult because of their often small diameters and severe calcifications. For detecting occlusion or stenoses in bypass grafts themselves, the reported accuracies are high [46–51]. However, accuracy for detecting and ruling out stenoses in nongrafted and runoff vessels is substantially lower [47,49]. A recent study performed by 64-slice CT found a sensitivity and specificity of only 86% and 76% for the

Table 13.3 "Appropriate" Indications for CT Coronary Angiography According to an Expert Consensus Document

Detection of CAD with prior test results—evaluation of chest pain syndrome
Uninterpretable or equivocal stress test result (exercise, perfusion, or stress echo)
Detection of CAD: symptomatic—evaluation of chest pain syndrome
Intermediate pre-test probability of CAD, ECG uninterpretable, or unable to exercise
Detection of CAD: symptomatic—acute chest pain
Intermediate pre-test probability of CAD, no ECG changes, and serial enzymes negative
Evaluation of coronary arteries in patients with new-onset heart failure to assess etiology
Detection of CAD: symptomatic
Evaluation of suspected coronary anomalies

From Hendel RC, Patel MR, Kramer CM, et al. ACCF/ACR/SCCT/SCMR/ASNC/NASCI/SCAI/SIR 2006 appropriateness criteria for cardiac computed tomography and cardiac magnetic resonance imaging: a report of the American College of Cardiology Foundation Quality Strategic Directions Committee Appropriateness Criteria Working Group, American College of Radiology, Society of Cardiovascular Computed Tomography, Society for Cardiovascular Magnetic Resonance, American Society of Nuclear Cardiology, North American Society for Cardiac Imaging, Society for Cardiovascular Angiography and Interventions, and Society of Interventional Radiology. *J Am Coll Cardiol*. 2006;48:1475–1497.

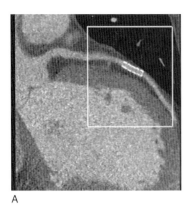
A

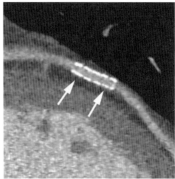
B

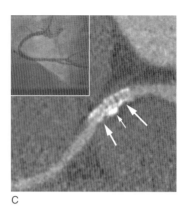
C

Figure 13.4 CT imaging of stents. **A,B.** Demonstration of absence of in stent restenosis in a data set of high quality, without artifacts (**arrows** in **B** = stent). **C.** In a different patient, visualization of a stent in the proximal right coronary artery (*large arrows*) is impaired by artefact caused by motion and a small calcification (*small arrow*). The stent lumen cannot clearly be demonstrated to be patent and free of in-stent stenosis. However, invasive angiography (*inset*) demonstrates absence of in-stent stenosis.

detection of stenoses in the native coronary arteries after patients with bypass surgery [49].

Similarly, assessment of coronary artery stents is often unreliable (Fig. 13.4). The dense metal of the stents can cause artifacts that impair evaluability. The ability to assess stents concerning in-stent restenosis depends on many factors which include stent type and diameter [52] as well as the overall quality of the data set [53–57]. Some recently published studies suggest that the analysis of large stents (eg, stents implanted in the left main coronary artery [53]) may be possible by CT. In some studies, sensitivities of up to 95% for the detection of in-stent restenosis have been reported [55–57]. However, the overall number of included stents was small and patients were heavily selected (eg, in one of the studies, the mean weight of the patient was 61 kg), so that the results cannot be generalized. Also, positive predictive values were low (54–94%). Most experts still do not encourage the use of coronary CTA to assess patients with implanted stents.

Coronary CTA and Ischemia

Coronary CTA, like invasive angiography, is a purely anatomic imaging modality and cannot demonstrate ischemia. The functional relevance of a coronary lesion is beyond the reach of coronary

CTA. Especially in the case of lesions with borderline degree of stenosis, this may be a limitation. It is not surprising that coronary CTA is a better predictor of angiographic findings than testing for ischemia [58–60]. Schuijf and associates demonstrated that among patients with intermediate risk for coronary artery disease, only 19 of 33 patients in whom stenoses were demonstrated by coronary CTA had ischemia in SPECT myocardial perfusion imaging. On the other hand, 28 of them had obstructive coronary lesions in invasive coronary angiography. However, all 25 patients in whom coronary CTA ruled out the presence of obstructive stenoses also had a "negative" coronary angiogram [58]. Similarly, Hacker and colleagues showed in 38 patients that the demonstration of coronary artery stenoses by CTA had a negative predictive value of 94%, but a positive predictive value of only 32% to predict ischemia in SPECT perfusion imaging [60].

These results underscore that a "negative" coronary CTA result is a very reliable predictor to rule out the presence of coronary artery stenoses and the need for revascularization, and that it may therefore be used as a "gatekeeper" to avoid invasive angiograms. On the other hand, coronary CTA, like invasive angiography, should not be performed in an unselected patient population and not for "screening" purposes. A positive CT scan by itself does not strongly predict the need for revascularization [61].

Imaging of Coronary Atherosclerotic Plaque

Under favorable conditions, coronary CT angiography makes it possible to visualize nonstenotic, noncalcified coronary atherosclerotic plaque (Fig. 13.5). In comparison to intravascular ultrasound (IVUS), accuracy for detecting noncalcified plaque was approximately 80% to 90% [62–64]. To a certain extent, coronary CT angiography allows plaque characterization: on average, the CT attenuation within fibrous plaques is higher than within lipid-rich plaques (mean attenuation values of 91–116 HU versus 47–71 HU) [64–68]. However, the variability of density measurements within plaque types is large [68], and density measurements are influenced heavily by the contrast attenuation of surrounding structures [69]. Therefore, accurate classification of plaque composition by coronary CTA is not currently possible. Besides measurements of plaque attenuation, other parameters that might contribute to the detection of vulnerable plaques and that can be assessed by CT in-

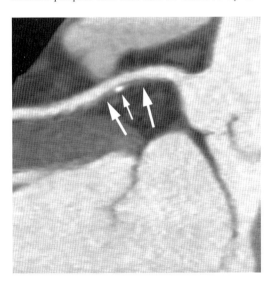

Figure 13.5 Nonstenotic coronary atherosclerotic plaque visualized in the proximal left anterior descending coronary artery (*large arrows*). The plaque is largely noncalcified and contains a small calcification (*small arrow*).

clude plaque volume and the degree of remodelling [70–72]. The clinical utility of these observations is uncertain. Several smaller studies have retrospectively analyzed CT plaque characteristics by CT in patients after acute coronary syndromes. They found a higher percentage of non-calcified plaque and more positive remodeling lesions responsible for acute cardiac events as compare to stable lesions [73,74]. A very recent analysis showed that very low CT attenuation values (less than 30 HU) are more frequently found in lesions associated with an acute coronary syndrome [74]. However, it is problematic that CT data acquisition in all of these studies was performed *after* the ischemic event, and plaque rupture with subsequent thrombus formation may have contributed to morphologic changes of the atherosclerotic lesion as seen in CT.

In 2007, a first prospective trial concerning the predictive value of atherosclerotic plaque seen in coronary CT angiography concerning future cardiovascular events became available. Pundzuite and associates followed 100 symptomatic patients who underwent CT coronary angiography for a mean period of 16 months and were able to demonstrate that patients with nonobstructive plaque detected by MDCT had a higher cardiovascular event rate than individuals without any plaque [75]. Thus while there is some rather indirect evidence that assessment of non-calcified plaque by coronary CT angiography may allow risk stratification, superiority over other methods of risk prediction has not been shown, and the available data are far too limited to justify the use of coronary CT angiography to stratify asymptomatic individuals concerning their future risk for cardiovascular disease events.

Coronary CT Angiography in the Context of Percutaneous Coronary Interventions

CT angiography may provide information that may be helpful in the context of coronary artery interventions. In addition to demonstrating the coronary lumen, CT imaging allows visualization of the amount and type of plaque, permits quantifying the amount of calcification, and can provide accurate, three-dimensional information on the angle of vessel bifurcations [76]. A recent publication described

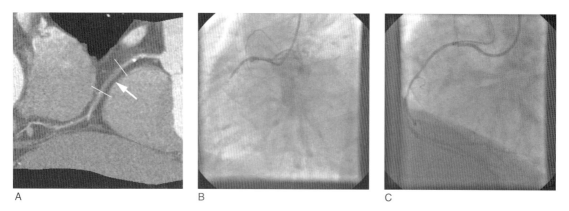

Figure 13.6 Chronic total occlusion of the right coronary artery. **A.** Coronary CT angiography (here: 16-slice CT) demonstrates that there is no calcification in the occluded vessel segment (*arrow*). **B,C.** Successful interventional recanalization.

that coronary CT angiography allows accurate classification of coronary bifurcation lesions [77]. Older work, published by Mollet and colleagues in 2005, has demonstrated that CT angiography—by quantifying lesion length and degree of calcification—is more accurate than invasive angiography to predict the success of percutaneous treatment of chronic total coronary occlusions (Fig 13.6) [78].

Radiation Exposure

There is increasing awareness of the radiation exposure associated with coronary CT angiography. The radiation dose to the patient depends on many patient-related (eg, size of scan field) and scanner-related parameters, and it will vary substantially, depending on the scan protocol that is used. Typical radiation doses range from approximately 5 to 20 mSv [79–82]. Some measures that make it possible to substantially reduce radiation dose are the use of ECG-correlated tube current modulation (which can lower radiation dose by approximately 50% [79]) and the use of 100 kV instead of 120 kV tube voltage [79]. The use of sequential ("step and shoot") scan algorithms instead of standard spiral acquisition may be a further opportunity to lower radiation exposure and has been evaluated in some initial trials [83,84]. Using these new scan algorithms, mean radiation doses have been reported to be as low as 2.1 mSv [84] (Fig. 13.7).

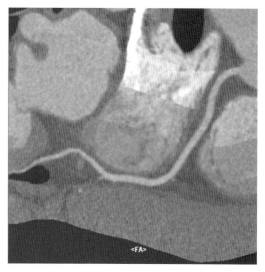

Figure 13.7 Visualization of the right coronary artery in a patient scanned with a low radiation exposure protocol. By reducing tube voltage to 100 kV and using prospective triggering (step-and-shoot acquisition), radiation dose for the entire data set was only 1.7 mSv.

Future Perspectives

CT technology has been evolving rapidly over the past several years, and it is reasonable to assume that it will continue to improve, albeit at a somewhat slower pace. Given certain prerequisites, such as a rather slow and stable heart rate and absence of pronounced coronary calcification, coronary CT angiography is already quite accurate to detect and rule out coronary artery stenoses and may be useful in selected patients and specific clinical situations to rule out coronary stenoses and avoid diagnostic invasive angiograms with a negative result. It is reasonable to assume that image quality will become more stable in the coming years, and that more trials will identify clinical situations in which performing coronary CT angiography is beneficial for the patient. Most likely, CT will assume an increasing role in the emergency room setting and evaluation of acute chest pain. Clearly, inappropriate applications in unsuited patients should currently be avoided. On the other hand, the method has tremendous potential to help in patient management and deserves great efforts to thoroughly evaluate its clinical utility, develop new applications, and further improve technology in the years to come.

References

1. Achenbach S. Cardiac CT. State of the art for the detection of coronary arterial stenosis. *J Cardiovasc CT*. 2007;1:3–20.

2. Schoepf UJ, Zwerner PL, Savino G, Herzog C, Kerl JM, Costello P. Coronary CT angiography. *Radiology*. 2007;244:48–63.

3. Vanhoenacker PK, Heijenbrok-Kal MH, Van Heste R, *et al.* Diagnostic performance of multidetector CT angiography for assessment of coronary artery disease: meta-analysis. *Radiology*. 2007;244: 419–428.

4. Leschka S, Wildermuth S, Boehm T, *et al.* Noninvasive coronary angiography with 64-section CT: effect of average heart rate and heart rate variability on image quality. *Radiology*. 2006;241:378–385.

5. Herzog C, Arning-Erb M, Zangos S, *et al.* Multidetector row CT coronary angiography: influence of reconstruction technique and heart rate on image quality. *Radiology*. 2006;238:75–86.

6. Ghostine S, Caussin C, Daoud B, *et al.* Non-invasive detection of coronary artery disease in patients with left bundle branch block using 64-slice computed tomography. *J Am Coll Cardiol*. 2006;48:1929–1934.

7. Wintersperger BJ, Nikolaou K, von Ziegler F, *et al.* Image quality, motion artifacts, and reconstruction timing of 64-slice coronary computed tomography angiography with 0.33-second rotation speed. *Invest Radiol*. 2006;41:436–342.

8. Mori S, Kondo C, Suzuki N, Hattori A, Kusakabe M, Endo M. Volumetric coronary angiography using the 256-detector row computed tomography scanner: comparison in vivo and in vitro with porcine models. *Acta Radiol*. 2006;47:186–191.

9. Kido T, Kurata A, Higashino H, *et al.* Cardiac imaging using 256-detector row four-dimensional CT: preliminary clinical report. *Radiat Med*. 2007;25:38–44.

10. Flohr TG, McCollough CH, Bruder H, *et al.* First performance evaluation of a dual-source CT (DSCT) system. *Eur Radiol*. 2006;16:256–268.

11. Achenbach S, Ropers D, Kuettner A, *et al.* Contrast-enhanced coronary artery visualization by dual-source computed tomography—initial experience. *Eur J Radiol*. 2006;57:331–335.

12. Johnson TR, Nikolaou K, Wintersperger BJ, *et al.* Dual-source CT cardiac imaging: initial experience. *Eur Radiol*. 2006;16:1409–1415.

13. Reimann AJ, Rinck D, Birinci-Aydogan A, *et al.* Dual-source computed tomography: advances of improved temporal resolution in coronary plaque imaging. *Invest Radiol*. 2007;42:196–203.

14. Scheffel H, Alkadhi H, Plass A, *et al.* Accuracy of dual-source CT coronary angiography: first experience in a high pre-test probability population without heart rate control. *Eur Radiol*. 2006;16:2739–2747.

15. Heuschmid M, Burgstahler C, Reimann A, *et al.* Usefulness of noninvasive cardiac imaging using dual-source computed tomography in an unselected population with high prevalence of coronary artery disease. *Am J Cardiol*. 2007;100:587–592.

16. Ropers U, Ropers D, Pflederer T, *et al.* Influence of heart rate on the diagnostic accuracy of dual-source tomography computed angiography. *J Am Coll Cardiol*. 2007;50:2393–2398.

17. Leber AW, Johnson T, Becker A, *et al.* Diagnostic accuracy of dual-source multi-slice CT-coronary angiography in patients with an intermediate pretest likelihood for coronary artery disease. *Eur Heart J*. 2007;28:2354–2360.

18. Weustink AC, Meijboom WB, Mollet NR, *et al.* Reliable high-speed coronary computed tomography in symptomatic patients. *J Am Coll Cardiol*. 2007;50:786–794.

19. Lim MCL, Wong TW, Yaneza LO, De Larrazabal C, Lau JK, Boey HK. Non-invasive detection of significant coronary artery disease with multi-section computed tomography angiography in patients

with suspected coronary artery disease. *Clin Radiol.* 2006;61:174–180.

20. Halon DA, Gaspar T, Adawi S, *et al.* Uses and limitations of 40 slice multi-detector row spiral computed tomography for diagnosing coronary lesions in unselected patients referred for routine invasive coronary angiography. *Cardiology.* 2007;108:200–209.

21. Watkins MW, Hesse B, Green CE, *et al.* Detection of coronary artery stenosis using 40-channel computed tomography with multisegment reconstruction. *Am J Cardiol.* 2007;99:175–181.

22. Grosse C, Globits S, Hergan K. Forty-slice spiral computed tomography of the coronary arteries: assessment of image quality and diagnostic accuracy in a non-selected patient population. *Acta Radiol.* 2007;48:36–44.

23. Ropers D, Rixe J, Anders K, *et al.* Usefulness of multidetector row computed tomography with 64 × 0.6 mm collimation and 330-ms rotation for the noninvasive detection of significant coronary artery stenoses. *Am J Cardiol.* 2006;97:343–348.

24. Fine JJ, Hopkins CB, Ruff N, Newton FC. Comparison of accuracy of 64-slice cardiovascular computed tomography with coronary angiography in patients with suspected coronary artery disease. *Am J Cadiol.* 2006;97:173–174.

25. Nikolaou K, Knez A, Rist C, *et al.* Accuracy of 64-MDCT in the diagnosis of ischemic heart disease. *AJR.* 2006;187:111–117.

26. Schlosser T, Mohrs OK, Magedanz A, *et al.* Noninvasive coronary angiography using 64-detector-row computed tomography in patients with a low to moderate pretest probability of significant coronary artery disease. *Acta Radiol.* 2007;48:300–307.

27. Mühlenbruch G, Seyfarth T, Soo CS, Pregalathan N, Mahnken AH. Diagnostic value of 64-slice multidetector row cardiac CTA in symptomatic patients. *Eur Radiol.* 2007;17:603–609.

28. Meijboom WB, Mollet NR, Van Mieghem CA, *et al.* 64-slice computed tomography coronary engiography in patients with non-ST elevation acute coronary syndrome. *Heart.* 2007;93:1386–1392.

29. Herzog C, Zwerner PL, Doll JR, *et al.* Significant coronary artery stenosis: Comparison on per-patient and per-vessel or per-segment basis at 64-section CT angiography. *Radiology.* 2007;244:112–120.

30. Ehara M, Surmely JF, Kawai M, *et al.* Diagnostic accuracy of 64-slice computed tomography for detecting angiographically significant coronary artery stenosis in an unselected consecutive patient population. *Circ J.* 2007;70:564–571.

31. Hausleiter J, Meyer T, Hadamitzky M, *et al.* Noninvasive coronary computed tomographic angiography for patients with suspected coronary artery disease: the Coronary Angiography by Computed Tomography with the Use of a Submillimeter Resolution (CACTUS) trial. *Eur Heart J.* 2007;28:3034–3041.

32. Shabestari AA, Abdi S, Akhlaghpoor S, *et al.* Diagnostic performance of 64-channel multislice computed tomography in assessment of significant coronary artery disease in symptomatic subjects. *Am J Cardiol.* 2007;99:1656–1661.

33. Hoffmann U, Moselewski F, Cury RC, *et al.* Predictive value of 16-slice multidetector spiral computed tomography to detect significant obstructive coronary artery disease in patients at high risk for coronary artery disease: patient-versus segment-based analysis. *Circulation.* 2004;110:2638–2643.

34. Gosthine S, Caussin C, Daoud B, *et al.* Non-invasive detection of coronary artery disease in patients with left bundle branch block using 64-slice computed tomography. *J Am Coll Cardiol.* 2006;48:1929–1934.

35. Meijboom WB, van Mieghem CA, Mollet NR, *et al.* 64-slice computed tomography coronary angiography in patients with high, intermediate, or low pretest probability of significant coronary artery disease. *J Am Coll Cardiol.* 2007;50:1469–1475.

36. Andreini D, Pontone G, Pepi M, *et al.* Diagnostic accuracy of multidetector computed tomography coronary angiography in patients with dilated cardiomyopathy. *J Am Coll Cardiol.* 2007;49:2044–2450.

37. Manghat NE, Morgan-Hughes GJ, Shaw SR, *et al.* Multi-detector row CT coronary angiography in patients with cardiomyopathy—initial single-centre experience. *Clin Radiol.* 2007;62:632–638.

38. Meijboom WB, Mollet NR, Van Mieghem CA, *et al.* Pre-operative computed tomography coronary angiography to detect significant coronary artery disease in patients referred for cardiac valve surgery. *J Am Coll Cardiol.* 2006;48:1658–1665.

39. Scheffel H, Leschka S, Plass A, *et al.* Accuracy of 64-slice computed tomography for the preoperative detection of coronary artery disease in patients with chronic aortic regurgitation. *Am J Cardiol.* 2007;100:701–706.

40. Hoffmann U, Nagurney JT, Moselewski F, *et al.* Coronary multidetector computed tomography in the assessment of patients with acute chest pain. *Circulation.* 2006;114:2251–2260.

41. Gallagher MJ, Ross MA, Raff GL, Goldstein JA, O'Neill WW, O'Neil B. The diagnostic accuracy of 64-slice computed tomography coronary angiography

compared with stress nuclear imaging in emergency department low-risk chest pain patients. *Ann Emerg Med.* 2007;49:125–136.

42. Goldstein JA, Gallagher MJ, O'Neill WW, Ross MA, O'Neil BJ, Raff GL. A randomized controlled trial of multi-slice coronary computed tomography for evaluation of acute chest pain. *J Am Coll Cardiol.* 2007;49:863–871.

43. Coles DR, Wilde P, Oberhoff M, Rogers CA, Karsch KR, Baumbach A. Multislice computed tomography coronary angiography in patients admitted with a suspected acute coronary syndrome. *Int J Cardiovasc Imaging*, 2007. Available online.

44. Budoff MJ, Achenbach S, Blumenthal RS, *et al.* Assessment of coronary artery disease by cardiac computed tomography: a scientific statement from the American Heart Association Committee on Cardiovascular Imaging and Intervention, Council on Cardiovascular Radiology and Intervention, and Committee on Cardiac Imaging, Council on Clinical Cardiology. *Circulation.* 2006;114:1761–1791.

45. Hendel RC, Patel MR, Kramer CM, *et al.* ACCF/ACR/SCCT/SCMR/ASNC/NASCI/SCAI/SIR 2006 appropriateness criteria for cardiac computed tomography and cardiac magnetic resonance imaging: a report of the American College of Cardiology Foundation Quality Strategic Directions Committee Appropriateness Criteria Working Group, American College of Radiology, Society of Cardiovascular Computed Tomography, Society for Cardiovascular Magnetic Resonance, American Society of Nuclear Cardiology, North American Society for Cardiac Imaging, Society for Cardiovascular Angiography and Interventions, and Society of Interventional Radiology. *J Am Coll Cardiol.* 2006;48:1475–1497.

46. Chiurlia E, Menozzi M, Ratti C, Romagnoli R, Modena MG. Follow-up of coronary artery bypass graft patency by multislice computed tomography. *Am J Cardiol.* 2005;95:1094–1097.

47. Salm LP, Bax JJ, Jukema JW, *et al.* Comprehensive assessment of patients after coronary artery bypass grafting by 16-detector-row computed tomography. *Am Heart J.* 2005;150:775–781.

48. Anders K, Baum U, Schmid M, Ropers D, *et al.* Coronary artery bypass graft (CABG) patency: assessment with high-resolution submillimeter 16-slice multidetector-row computed tomography (MDCT) versus coronary angiography. *Eur J Radiol.* 2006;57:336–344.

49. Ropers D, Pohle FK, Kuettner A, *et al.* Diagnostic accuracy of noninvasive coronary angiography in pa-

tients after bypass surgery using 64-slice spiral computed tomography with 330-ms gantry rotation. *Circulation.* 2006;114:2334–2341.

50. Meyer TS, Martinoff S, Hadamitzky M, *et al.* Improved noninvasive assessment of coronary artery bypass grafts with 64-slice computed tomographic angiography in an unselected patient population. *J Am Coll Cardiol.* 2007;49:946–950.

51. Feuchtner GM, Schachner T, Bonatti J, *et al.* Diagnostic performance of 64-slice computed tomography in evaluation of coronary artery bypass grafts. *AJR Am J Roentgenol.* 2007;189:574–580.

52. Maintz D, Seifarth H, Raupach R, *et al.* 64-slice multidetector coronary CT angiography: in vitro evaluation of 68 different stents. *Eur Radiol.* 2006;16:818–826.

53. Van Mieghem CA, Cademartiri F, Mollet NR, *et al.* Multislice spiral computed tomography for the evaluation of stent patency after left main coronary artery stenting: a comparison with conventional coronary angiography and intravascular ultrasound. *Circulation.* 2006;114:645–653.

54. Rixe J, Achenbach S, Ropers D, *et al.* Assessment of coronary artery stent restenosis by 64-slice multi-detector computed tomography. *Eur Heart J.* 2006;27:2567–2572.

55. Oncel D, Oncel G, Karaca M. Coronary stent patency and in-stent restenosis: determination with 64-section multidetector CT coronary angiography—initial experience. *Radiology.* 2007;242:403–409.

56. Ehara M, Kawai M, Surmely JF, *et al.* Diagnostic accuracy of coronary in-stent restenosis using 64-slice computed tomography. *J Am Coll Cardiol.* 2007;49:951–959.

57. Cademartiri F, Schuijf JD, Pugliese F, *et al.* Usefulness of 64-slice multislice computed tomography coronary angiography to assess in-stent restenosis. *J Am Coll Cardiol.* 2007;49:2204–2210.

58. Schuijf JD, Wijns W, Jukema JW, *et al.* Relationship between noninvasive coronary angiography with multi-slice computed tomography and myocardial perfusion imaging. *J Am Coll Cardiol.* 2006;48:2508–2514.

59. Hacker M, Jakobs T, Hack N, *et al.* Combined use of 64-slice computed tomography angiography and gated myocardial perfusion SPECT for the detection of functionally relevant coronary artery stenoses. First results in a clinical setting concerning patients with stable angina. *Nuklearmedizin.* 2007;46:29–35.

60. Hacker M, Jakobs T, Hack N, *et al.* Sixty-four slice spiral CT angiography does not predict the functional

relevance of coronary artery stenoses in patients with stable angina. *Eur J Nucl Med Mol Imaging.* 2007;34:4–10.

61. Berman DS, Hachamovitch R, Shaw LJ, *et al.* Roles of nuclear cardiology, cardiac computed tomography, and cardiac magnetic resonance: noninvasive risk stratification and a conceptual framework for the selection of noninvasive imaging tests in patients with known or suspected coronary artery disease. *J Nucl Med.* 2006;47:1107–1118.

62. Achenbach S, Moselewski F, Ropers D, *et al.* Detection of calcified and noncalcified coronary atherosclerotic plaque by contrast-enhanced, submillimeter multidetector spiral computed tomography: a segment-based comparison with intravascular ultrasound. *Circulation.* 2004;109:14–17.

63. Leber AW, Knez A, Becker A, Becker C, von Ziegler F, Nikolaou K, *et al.* Accuracy of multidetector spiral computed tomography in identifying and differentiating the composition of coronary atherosclerotic plaques: a comparative study with intracoronary ultrasound. *J Am Coll Cardiol.* 2004;43:1241–1247.

64. Leber AW, Becker A, Knez A, *et al.* Accuracy of 64-slice computed tomography to classify and quantify plaque volumes in the proximal coronary system: a comparative study using intravascular ultrasound. *J Am Coll Cardiol.* 2006;47:672–627.

65. Schroeder S, Kopp AF, Baumbach A, *et al.* Noninvasive detection and evaluation of atherosclerotic coronary plaques with multislice computed tomography. *J Am Coll Cardiol.* 2001;37:1430–1435.

66. Caussin C, Ohanessian A, Ghostine S, *et al.* Characterization of vulnerable nonstenotic plaque with 16-slice computed tomography compared with intravascular ultrasound. *Am J Cardiol.* 2004;94:99–100.

67. Carrascosa PM, Capunay CM, Garcia-Merletti P, Carrascosa J, Garcia MF. Characterization of coronary atherosclerotic plaques by multidetector computed tomography. *Am J Cardiol.* 2006;97:598–602.

68. Pohle K, Achenbach S, MacNeill B, *et al.* Characterization of non-calcified coronary atherosclerotic plaque by multi-detector row CT: comparison to IVUS. *Atherosclerosis.* 2007;190:174–180.

69. Cademartiri F, Mollet NR, Runza G, *et al.* Influence of intracoronary attenuation on coronary plaque measurements using multislice computed tomography: observations in an ex vivo model of coronary computed tomography angiography. *Eur Radiol.* 2005;15:1426–1431.

70. Achenbach S, Ropers D, Hoffmann U, *et al.* Assessment of coronary remodeling in stenotic and non-

stenotic coronary atherosclerotic lesions by multidetector spiral computed tomography. *J Am Coll Cardiol.* 2004;43:842–847.

71. Moselewski F, Ropers D, Pohle K, *et al.* Comparison of measurement of cross-sectional coronary atherosclerotic plaque and vessel areas by 16-slice multidetector computed tomography versus intravascular ultrasound. *Am J Cardiol.* 2004;94:1294–1297.

72. Bruining N, Roelandt JR, Palumbo A, *et al.* Reproducible coronary plaque quantification by multislice computed tomography. *Catheter Cardiovasc Interv.* 2007;69:857–865.

73. Hoffmann U, Moselewski F, Nieman K, *et al.* Noninvasive assessment of plaque morphology and composition in culprit and stable lesions in acute coronary syndrome and stable lesions in stable angina by multidetector computed tomography. *J Am Coll Cardiol.* 2006;47:1655–1662.

74. Motoyama S, Kondo T, Sarai M, *et al.* Multislice computed tomographic characteristics of coronary lesions in acute coronary syndromes. *J Am Coll Cardiol.* 2007;50:319–326.

75. Pundzuite G, Schuijf JD, Jukema JW, *et al.* Prognostic value of multislice computed tomography coronary angiography in patients with known or suspected coronary artery disease. *J Am Coll Cardiol.* 2007;49:62–70.

76. Pflederer T, Ludwig J, Ropers D, Daniel WG, Achenbach S. Measurement of coronary artery bifurcation angles by multidetector computed tomography. *Invest Radiol.* 2006;41:793–798.

77. Van Mieghem CA, Thury A, Meijboom WB, *et al.* Detection and characterization of coronary bifurcation lesions with 64-slice computed tomography coronary angiography. *Eur Heart J.* 2007;28:1968–1976.

78. Mollet NR, Hoye A, Lemos PA, *et al.* Value of preprocedure multislice computed tomographic coronary angiography to predict the outcome of percutaneous recanalization of chronic total occlusions. *Am J Cardiol.* 2005;95:240–243.

79. Hausleiter J, Meyer T, Hadamitzky M, *et al.* Radiation disease estimates from cardiac multislice computed tomography in daily practice. *Circulation.* 2006;113:1305–1310.

80. Einstein AJ, Henzlova MJ, Rajagopalan S. Estimating risk of cancer associated with radiation exposure from 64-slice computed tomography coronary angiography. *JAMA.* 2007;298:317–323.

81. Stolzmann P, Scheffel H, Schertler T, *et al.* Radiation

dose estimates in dual-source computed tomography coronary angiography. *Eur Radiol*. September 2007. Available online.

82. Francone M, Napoli A, Carbone I, *et al*. Noninvasive imaging of the coronary arteries using a 64-row multidetector CT scanner: initial clinical experience and radiation dose concerns. *Radiol Med (Torino)*. 2007;112:31–46.

83. Hsieh J, Londt J, Vass M, Li J, Tang X, Okerlund D.Step-and-shoot data acquisition and reconstruction for cardiac x-ray computed tomography. *Med Phys*. 2006;33:4236-4248.

84. Husmann L, Valenta I, Gaemperli O, *et al*. Feasibility of low-dose coronary CT angiography: first experience with prospective ECG-gating. *Eur Heart J*. 2008;29:191–197.

CHAPTER 14

Magnetic Resonance for Functional Testing and Interventional Guidance

Simon Koestner

Cardiology, Cardiovascular Department, University Hospital Bern, Bern, Switzerland

---

Chapter Overview

- Owing to its excellent spatial and contrast resolution and to free spatial orientation of imaging plans, cardiovascular magnetic resonance (CMR) provides high-quality anatomic and functional information.
- In the context of ischemic heart disease, delayed contrast enhancement technique allows for imaging of post-infarction scar and determination of myocardial viability.
- Dobutamine stress magnetic resonance and adenosine magnetic resonance myocardial perfusion imaging are robust techniques for ischemia detection.
- Coronary magnetic resonance angiography is helpful for the evaluation of anomalous coronary artery anatomy and coronary aneurysms.
- MR imaging of the atherosclerotic plaque is raising hope for the identification of vulnerable plaques.
- The application fields of magnetic resonance imaging (MRI) guided interventions include endovascular therapy, interventional electrophysiology procedures, and myocardial therapy.
- The broad spectrum of imaging techniques offered by CMR open perspectives for integrated imaging of the cardiovascular system.
- Given the rapid development of new applications for CMR, regular updates of clinical guidelines will be needed.

Cardiovascular magnetic resonance (CMR) imaging has undergone major improvements in the past several years and is increasingly used in clinical settings. Owing to its high spatial resolution and contrast, free spatial orientation of imaging planes, and ability for tissue characterization, CMR can provide precise anatomic and functional information. Thus it is today recognized for its value in the assessment and monitoring of a wide range of cardiac pathology. Besides precise measurements of ventricular volumes, mass, and function, the spectrum of indications for CMR comprises the evalua-

tion of congenital heart disease, intra- or extracardiac tumors, arrhythmogenic right ventricular cardiomyopathy/dysplasia (ARVC/D), pericardial disease, and thoracic and abdominal vessels. In the field of ischemic heart disease (IHD), CMR allows for localization and sizing of myocardial infarction (MI), detection of hibernating myocardium, imaging of myocardial perfusion, and stress examinations, thus giving insights into myocardial viability and ischemia detection. Coronary artery imaging and catheter guidance are new, promising applications calling for further research and developments. The purpose of this chapter is to review the technical aspects and the diagnostic accuracy of CMR applications related to IHD, and to summarize the available recommendations.

Current Best Practice in Interventional Cardiology. Edited by
B Meier. © 2010 Blackwell Publishing,

System Requirements, Personnel Qualifications, and Safety

System Requirements/ECG Gating

The systems generally used for CMR are 1.5 or 3 Tesla(T) MR scanners. Synchronization should be performed with a multichannel ECG (vector ECG) to allow for reliable triggering in the presence of strong magnetic fields, and at high heart rates (eg, in order to obtain sufficient image quality during stress examinations). In case of insufficient quality of the ECG signal, the peripheral pulse wave can be used for triggering. In order to improve the so-called signal-to-noise ratio (SNR) and to make the field of view smaller (thus reducing acquisition time and improving spatial resolution), *surface coils* are placed on the body surface to receive the signal emitted by the *body coil* (integrated into the scanner).

Personnel Qualifications

The qualifications recommended for physicians and other personnel involved in CMR can be found in the guidelines of the Society for Cardiovascular Magnetic Resonance (SCMR) [1] and in the guidelines of the American College of Radiology (ACR) [2].

Safety/Contraindications

Before starting with an MR examination, the patient has to be informed about the procedure, the use of contrast agents, and the contraindications (Table 14.1). In order to obtain good-quality images, complete instructions for the breathholding are mandatory.

MRI safety issues are constantly evolving. Up to date information can be retrieved on the website of the Institute for Magnetic Resonance Safety, Education, and Research (www.imrser.org). In patients with severely impaired kidney function, gadolinium-based contrast agents may induce nephrogenic systemic fibrosis (NSF) [3]. Because of this, contrast agents are contraindicated in patients with a glomerular filtration rate (GFR) < 30 mL/min/1.73 m^2.

Table 14.1 Contraindications to MRI

Absolute Contraindications[a]
Cardiac pacemakers, defibrillators, neurostimulators
Pumps (eg, for insulin)
Ear implants
Neurosurgical clips
Metal splinters
Swan-Ganz catheters
Pregnancy (first trimester)

Relative Contraindications
Claustrophobia
Obesity
Pregnancy (second and third trimesters)

[a]Artificial valves (including the Starr-Edwards type) are no longer contraindicated. In the first 2 months after surgical implantation of any device, only patients with nonferromagnetic implants are allowed to undergo MRI. Go to *www.imrser.org* for further information.

Ventricular Volumes and Function

Owing to its excellent spatial, contrast, and temporal resolution and to free spatial orientation of imaging plans, CMR provides high-quality anatomic information throughout the cardiac cycle, thus allowing for precise, highly reproducible, three-dimensional volumetric quantification (without bias linked to geometric assumptions) as well as for regional functional analysis. As a consequence, CMR has today become the gold standard for mass, volume, and functional measurements of both the left ventricle (LV) [4] and right ventricle (RV) [5]. This high accuracy, as well as the excellent inter-observer and interstudy reproducibility [5], make CMR useful for patient follow-up, clinical research with small sample sizes, or large drug trials.

Technical Considerations

Cine imaging relies on the use of balanced steady-state free-precession (SSFP) gradient-echo pulse sequences (bright blood imaging), for which no contrast is needed. To improve spatial resolution, triggered segmented cine imaging (with data acquired on several cardiac cycles) is generally used. Retrospective triggering, allowing for data acquisition throughout the entire cardiac cycle, is preferably used. However, since the resulting cine is a sum of several cardiac cycles, irregular heartbeat (atrial fibrillation, frequent premature atrial or ventricular beats) will lead to blurring of the images. This can be overcome by the use of different strategies like prospective gating, arrhythmia detection algorithms, or real-time imaging, the latter providing "live" images with poorer resolution.

In general, three long-axis views (4-chamber, 3-chamber, and 2-chamber views, for qualitative analysis) and a stack of short-axis views (usually around 10 slices, for qualitative and quantitative analysis) encompassing the entire ventricle are acquired.

Interpretation/Measurements

A first visual evaluation of cine imaging provides information on both global and segmental function of the ventricles. The assessment of regional wall motion abnormalities (WMAs) should be done in accordance to the standard 17-segment model of the American Heart Association (AHA) [6] and the following terms: normal, hyperkinetic, hypokinetic, akinetic, and dyskinetic. In the case of MI with significant WMAs, intracavitary thrombi can be identified using cine imaging. Further characterization of the thrombus can be made using contrast agents (perfusion and late enhancement). For research purposes, the analysis of regional wall motion and thickening can be assisted by software (centerline method).

The volumes are calculated by delineation of the endocardial contours for each short-axis slice, multiplication of the resulting area by the sum of the slice thickness and the interslice distance, and adding the resulting volumes. End-diastolic volume (EDV) and end-systolic volume (ESV), and thus stroke volume (SV), ejection fraction (EF), cardiac output (CO), and all related normalized values, can be calculated for both ventricles. The calculation of myocardial mass is made in a similar manner and requires delineation of the epicardial borders. Maceira and associates reported the normal values for both LV [7] and RV [8] using SSFP imaging. Although myocardial tagging is not used in standard clinical settings, it has been shown

to be a very useful supplemental tool to precisely analyze regional systolic and diastolic function, strain, and torsion [9,10].

Although (transesophageal) echocardiography will provide more detailed anatomic information on the valves, SSFP imaging offers the possibility of both morphologic and functional evaluation of the valves due to the excellent contrast between blood and myocardial or valvular structures. Also, turbulences caused by valvular regurgitation or stenosis generate flow voids, seen as black jets on SSFP images. Moreover, flow quantification using phase contrast velocity imaging allows for acquisition of velocity maps and calculation of cardiac output at the level of the aorta and pulmonary artery (PA). Thus, comparison of CO calculated both with volumetric ventricular analysis and flow quantification in the aorta or PA permits calculation of mitral and tricuspid regurgitation fractions. Velocity mappings at the level of the mitral valve, inferior or superior vena cava, and pulmonary veins also allow for assessment of diastolic function [10,11].

Scar Detection/Assessment of Viability

Delayed Contrast Enhancement

CMR with delayed contract enhancement (DCE) allows for high-resolution detection of myocardial edema or fibrosis using gadolinium chelates as contrast agents. This highly reproducible technique plays an important role in the evaluation of patients with ischemic heart disease as well as nonischemic conditions like dilated, hypertrophic, or infiltrative cardiomyopathies or myocarditis [12]. In the setting of MI, the location (coronary territory), transmural extent, and mass of scar tissue can be precisely assessed and has been shown to have an important prognostic value (see below). Thanks to its excellent spatial resolution, this technique is able to detect microinfarcts, for instance after PCI [13]. Moreover, the detection of RV infarction has been shown to be more frequent with DCE than with standard techniques [14].

The determination of myocardial viability after MI using DCE has been validated in animal models [15] and against positron emission tomography (PET) as standard of reference for imaging areas of decreased perfusion and metabolism as markers of MI [16]. The thickness of the residual rim of viable myocardium has actually been shown to better correlate with myocardial viability assessed by PET than the total end-diastolic wall thickness [17].

Technical Considerations

After intravenous administration (bolus 0.10 – 0.20 mmol/kg), gadolinium-based extracellular contrast agents accumulate in areas of an expanded extracellular compartment like (sub-) acute (edema, cellular disruption) or chronic (fibrous tissue replacement, fatty dysplasia) infarction scar with a time delay of 10 to 15 minutes. Thus the acquisition of the images has to be started in practice 10 to 20 minutes after the administration of the contrast. Gadolinium induces T1 shortening, resulting in increased signal on T1-weighted images, which is the reason why a segmented inversion recovery T1-weighted gradient echo pulse sequence is generally used for image acquisition. As a consequence on DCE images, bright areas will correlate with scar ("bright is dead"). To lower the risk of artifacts, image acquisition is made during diastolic standstill. To allow for sufficient coverage of all ventricular segments and making direct comparison possible, the views should be the same as for cine imaging (see ventricular volumes and function) with standard long-axis views (4-, 3-, and 2-chamber) and a complete stack of short-axis. If needed, additional views will be planned to confirm or rule out suspected areas of enhancement.

To enhance the signal of areas of contrast (white), the myocardium has to be "nulled" (ie, made as black as possible) by adjusting the inversion time (TI, time interval between an inversion pulse that prepares water protons and the start of actual image acquisition) during the acquisition of the images. Image acquisition can be made either slice by slice using multiple breathholds or using a multislice single shot sequence. The latter will lead to somewhat lower image quality, but is helpful in challenging situations (irregular heartbeat, difficulty in breath holding). The acquisition of cine

delayed-enhancement MR in order to combine information on both contractility and infarction localization has been described recently [18]. The interpretation of the images is made on the basis of the 17-segment model of the AHA [6].

Comparison with Other Techniques

Wagner and associates [19] showed that single photon emission computed tomography (SPECT) and DCE using CMR detect transmural infarcts at similar rates. However, owing to its better special resolution, DCE systematically detects *subendocardial* infarcts that are missed by SPECT [20]. This higher spatial resolution also leads to more frequent scar detection with DCE than with PET [16]. A study comparing MR to a combined SPECT/PET protocol found similar results [21]. In comparison with SPECT, the sensitivity, specificity, and accuracy of DCE in the prediction of viable myocardium were significantly higher [22]. Comparing DCE, dobutamine stress MR (DSMR, described later in the chapter), end-diastolic wall thickness, and SPECT in patients with highly impaired LV function, DCE has been shown to be the best technique for predicting viability [23]. Adding to the value of CMR, the radiation burden of SPECT and PET has to be taken in consideration.

Prognostic Value of Late Enhancement

The transmural extent of infarction as detected by DCE has been shown to correlate directly with the degree of resting regional dysfunction in chronic IHD [24] and to be a critical determinant of contractile recovery. Kim and associates [25] were able to show that segments of myocardium with less than 25% of enhancement of the wall thickness were likely to recover after percutaneous or surgical revascularization (positive and negative predictive values of 71% and 79%, respectively). In contrast, segments with more than 50% of late enhancement had < 10% probability of functional improvement. Further studies confirmed that the proportion of remaining viable myocardium predicts the global functional recovery of the LV after revascularization in chronic ischemic cardiomyopathy [26,27]. In clinical practice, the cutoff value of

50% of enhanced wall thickness is broadly used. The heterogeneity of scar tissue after myocardial infarction can also be assessed and has been shown to correlate well with the susceptibility to ventricular arrhythmias [28].

In the setting of acute MI, DCE has shown to predict functional improvement of stunned myocardium [29]. This technique is also superior to early EF in predicting recovery in patients with initially depressed EF after MI. Rubenstein and colleagues showed that patients with an early EF after MI < 35% and an infarct size > 34% do not show any significant functional improvement at 3 months follow-up [30]. However, the significance of DCE extent for sudden cardiac death is not known yet. Lund and coworkers [31] showed that an infarct size of 24% or more of the LV area constitutes an important threshold to predict remodeling. The characterization of the peri-infarct zone by DCE also seems to be a predictor of post-MI mortality [32].

Additional Value of DCE: Microvascular Obstruction (MVO)

The use of delayed contrast enhancement in the setting of AMI also allows for visualization of microvascular obstruction (MVO). Zones of MVO actually correspond to areas of microvascular injury and no reflow. Thus, since no contrast at all can reach these areas, MVO will appear on the images as subendocardial black zones surrounded by enhanced infracted tissue (Fig. 14.1). Nijveldt and associates [33] showed in 60 patients that the presence of MVO early after acute MI was a stronger predictor of both global and regional functional recovery than other angiographic (TIMI flow, myocardial blush), electrocardiographic (ST-segment resolution), or DCE (transmural extent) characteristics of microvascular injury.

Ischemia Detection

The detection of myocardial ischemia using wall motion analysis or perfusion measurements plays a growing role in clinical decision–making, since narrowing of the epicardial coronary lumen alone does not necessarily predict its hemodynamic con-

sequences to the underlying myocardium [34,35]. Stress echocardiography and SPECT have been successfully used for this purpose for many years. Today CMR is increasingly used due to its high spatial resolution and the absence of ionizing radiation.

Dobutamine Stress Magnetic Resonance

Technical Aspects

The technical developments in CMR made it possible to perform cine imaging of the heart also under stress conditions, and to keep a consistently high temporal and spatial resolution up to heart rates of 200 beats per minute. Thus, along with an appropriate sequence type (described later), dobutamine stress magnetic resonance (DSMR) permits detection of stress-induced WMAs in a similar manner as dobutamine stress echocardiography [36].

Dobutamine is a sympathomimetic drug with dose-dependent effects. Low-dose ($\leq$10 µg/kg/min) intravenous infusion of dobutamine mainly increases cardiac contractility. At higher doses (up to a maximum of .50 µg/kg/min), both heart rate and myocardial oxygen consumption increase, leading to contraction abnormalities in myocardial segments supplied by stenotic coronary arteries due to a mismatch between oxygen demand and availability. In principle, both dobutamine or adenosine can be used for stress MR. However, it has been shown that dobutamine is superior to adenosine for the detection of inducible WMAs related to coronary stenoses >50% with a diagnostic accuracy of 86% for DSMR and 58% for adenosine stress MR [37]. Stress can also be achieved using an MR-compatible cycle ergometer. However, the handling of this equipment during MR scanning is complex, which is why the technique is mainly used for research purposes.

Using dobutamine, the pharmacologic stress protocol for DSMR follows the standard high-dose dobutamine/atropine regimen as used in stress echocardiography. First, standard rest cine scans (4-, 3-, and 2-chamber views as well as 3 short-axis views) are acquired using an SSFP pulse sequence (see also "Ventricular Volumes and Function" earlier in the chapter) combined with parallel imaging (eg, SENSE) and retrospective gating. After

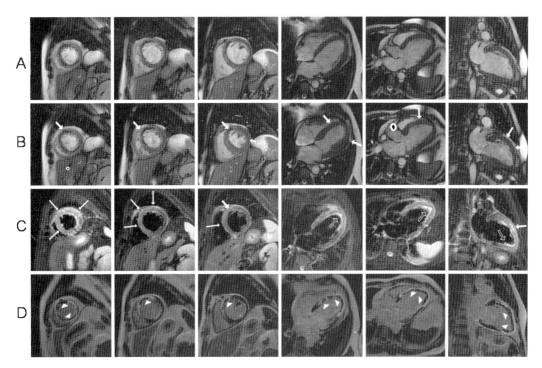

Figure 14.1 CMR of a 50-year-old patient 3 days after anterior MI. Each column shows a different view (from left to right: short axis apical, mid and basal; 4-, 3-, and 2-chamber views of the LV). **A, B.** Bright-blood cine imaging with end-diastolic **(A)** and end-systolic **(B)** phases. The *arrows* show areas of hypokinesia or akinesia. **C.** T2-wheighted images (STIR) showing areas of myocardial edema (*bright, full arrows*). The *empty arrows* show areas of slow flow caused by the presence of trabeculation. This phenomenon is normal and should not be confounded with edema. **D.** Delayed contrast enhancement (DCE) showing bright areas of myocardial necrosis and edema. The dark subendocardial rim (*arrowheads*) is typical of microvascular obstruction (MVO). MVO seen with this technique is stable between 2 and 9 days following myocardial infarction. Then, MVO will progressively disappear and be replaced by the typical pattern of chronic MI with subendocardial late enhancement and wall thinning. Please note that a dark rim is also seen on the short axis cines (A, B) because the patient received contrast between acquisition of long axis cines (made first, no dark rim) and short axis cines.

this, intravenous dobutamine is administered at 3-minute stages at doses of 10, 20, 30, and 40 mg/kg/min, followed by atropine in 0.25-mg fractions (maximal dose 2 mg) if target heart rate is not reached at maximal dobutamine dose. All standard views are repeated at each level. Termination criteria are similar to stress echocardiography. Heart rate and rhythm need to be monitored throughout the examination. Because of the effect of high magnetic fields, the ECG recorded in the scanner is not diagnostic for repolarization disturbances. However, since wall motion abnormalities occur before ST-changes in the ischemic cascade, monitoring these (using real-time cine imaging if necessary [38]) will allow for early detection of ischemia during the examination.

The analysis of the cine scans can be made on a second console during the examination. For the assessment of LV wall motion per segment, the 17-segment model of the AHA [6] serves as reference in combination with the standard 4-point scoring system (1 = normokinesis, 2 = hypokinesis, 3 = akinesis, 4 = dyskinesis). Ischemia is defined as ≥ 1 segment(s) showing WMA or a biphasic response. Using dedicated software for quantification of LV wall motion and thickening (the so-called center-line method) is feasible but time consuming and rarely used in standard clinical settings. Although the role for myocardial tagging during DSMR has been investigated by several groups [39,40], this technique is not used in daily practice at the moment.

Safety

Contraindications to DSMR include severe systemic hypertension (systolic blood pressure >220 mm Hg and/or diastolic blood pressure >120 mm Hg), unstable angina pectoris, higher-grade ventricular arrhythmia, higher-grade aortic stenosis (valve opening area <1.0 cm^2), and hemodynamically relevant obstructive hypertrophic cardiomyopathy. Myocarditis, endocarditis, and pericarditis are also contraindicated for DSMR. However, in standard clinical settings, high-dose DSMR was shown to be feasible and extremely safe. Wahl and colleagues reported only one case of sustained ventricular tachycardia with successful emergent defibrillation in 1000 consecutive patients [41].

Diagnostic Accuracy

High-dose DSMR proved to be highly accurate for the detection of inducible WMAs. In a prospective study including 172 patients and comparing high-dose DSMR with dobutamine stress echocardiography, Nagel and associates [42] demonstrated superior sensitivity and specificity of DSMR (86% and 86%) compared with dobutamine echocardiography (74% and 70%, $p < 0.05$). Comparing DSMR and dobutamine echocardiography in patients with poor acoustic windows, Hundley and coworkers [43] found similar results. For detection of ischemia in patients after revascularization, Wahl and colleagues [44] showed a sensitivity and specificity of DSMR of 89% and 84%, respectively. In a recent meta-analysis by Nandalur and associates [45] analyzing a total of 37 studies on DSMR (14 studies) or magnetic resonance myocardial perfusion imaging (MRMPI), stress-induced WMA imaging demonstrated a sensitivity of 0.83 (95% confidence interval [CI] 0.79–0.88) and specificity of 0.86 (95% CI 0.81–0.91) on a patient level (disease prevalence 70.5%).

Prognostic Value

Hundley and associates [46] showed that in patients without evidence of inducible myocardial is-chemia and an LV resting EF of more than 40%, the cardiac prognosis in the 2 years after DSMR was excellent with occurrence of MI or cardiac death in 2% of the patients over 2 years. Kuijpers and colleagues [47] showed a positive and negative predictive value of 95% and 93% respectively for development of major adverse cardiac events (clinically indicated coronary revascularization, nonfatal MI, and cardiac death). Survival rates without any cardiac event in patients with suspected myocardial ischemia and negative DSMR was 96.2% (average follow-up 24 months). At low-dose dobutamine levels, DSMR was found to be highly predictive of functional improvement of resting WMAs after coronary revascularization procedures for chronic IHD (detection of viable myocardium; see also "Scar Detection/Assessment of Viability" earlier in the chapter) [48].

Magnetic Resonance Myocardial Perfusion Imaging (MRMPI)

Technical Aspects

Adenosine MRMPI aims at the detection of ischemia in the very early phases of the ischemic cascade. This technique depicts the distribution (regionality) and the extent (transmurality) of ischemia. MRMPI presents several advantages compared to SPECT. First, this technique is more comfortable for the patient. The examination is done in one session (no separate day protocols), without ionizing radiation. It offers a higher spatial resolution than nuclear techniques and is therefore more sensitive in detecting small subendocardial perfusion defects. Moreover, it allows for simultaneous assessment of viability with the help of DCE techniques (described earlier) and offers highly precise evaluation of both LV and RV function. The pharmacologic stress is classically achieved with adenosine or dipyridamole. The latter has a longer duration of vasodilation with a half-life of approximately 30 minutes versus <10 seconds for adenosine. Despite its higher cost, the advantage of adenosine is that the side effects of the drug are self-limiting. In principle, a bicycle ergometer can also be used, as discussed earlier. Adenosine induces myocardial hyperemia by increasing myocardial

Figure 14.2 Magnetic resonance myocardial perfusion imaging (MRMPI) at apical (A), mid-ventricular (B), and basal (C) levels, in a 61-year-old patient with chest pain. First-pass perfusion shows a reversible perfusion defect (*arrows*) in the territory of the left anterior descending (LAD) artery. On the end-diastolic (ED) and end-systolic (ES) frames of bright-blood cine scans, an area of hypokinesia or akinesia is clearly visible in the same territory (*arrows*). Since no myocardial infarction (no subendocardial enhancement) can be seen on DCE images (*last column*), these findings suggest the presence of hybernating myocardium. The conventional coronary angiogram showed a significant stenosis in the proximal LAD.

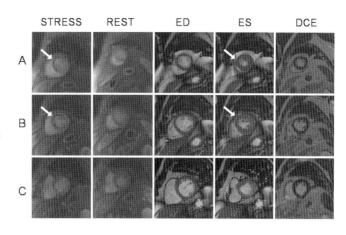

blood flow by three to four times, yielding to the so-called steal phenomenon (perfusion increases in regions supplied by nondiseased coronary arteries, and increases less or even decreases in regions supplied by hemodynamically significant stenotic coronary arteries). Adenosine induces also an increase of heart rate, without significant changes in blood pressure. The drug is administered intravenously at a rate of 140 μg/kg/min for a maximum of 6 minutes. The acquisition of contrast-enhanced first-pass images begins at least 3 minutes after adenosine has been started. The effect of adenosine is blocked by theophylline, caffeine, and xanthine-containing products. Therefore, coffee, tea, bananas, and chocolate are proscribed during the 24 hours preceding the test. Also, no beta-blockers should be taken the day of the examination.

Gadolinium-based extravascular contrast agents (described in "Scar Detection/Assment of Viability" earlier in the chapter) serve as flow tracer during their first pass through the myocardial vasculature (Fig. 14.2). Using an automatic injector, contrast is given intravenously (0.05–0.1 mmol/kg at a rate of 3–5 mL/sec) through a separate venous access. A saline chaser is given after each contrast injection. The pulse sequence used for perfusion imaging has to make possible the acquisition of a great number of images per unit of time (ideally 1 image every heartbeat at three different anatomic levels—apex, mid, and base) in order to obtain both an adequate temporal resolution during first pass of the contrast and a sufficient LV coverage. Thus, a breath-hold T1-weighted sequence is combined with parallel imaging in single-shot images (preferably 1 image <150 ms). Although rest perfusion would in principle not be mandatory, this should always be done in order to differentiate endocardial artefacts from true perfusion defects. Rest perfusion is also needed for the assessment of myocardial perfusion reserve in the case of (semi-)quantitative perfusion measurements (discussed later). Perfusion defects due to chronic infarction might be undetectable on rest perfusion images due to the previous administration of contrast for stress perfusion.

In clinical practice, functional assessment, ischemia detection, and scar imaging are combined in a time-effective way. For example, the evaluation of a patient with suspected CAD using adenosine MRMPI will usually start with standard localizers and long-axis cine sequences, immediately followed by intravenous administration of adenosine. After at least 3 minutes under adenosine, first-pass perfusion images are acquired. After withdrawal of adenosine, approximately 10 minutes are needed for recovery. During this time, standard short-axis coverage can be acquired, followed by first-pass perfusion at rest. Approximately 5 minutes after the last injection of contrast, delayed enhancement images can be obtained. The whole protocol generally lasts 50 to 60 minutes.

The analysis of myocardial perfusion can be made in three different manners, using the 17-segment model of the AHA [6]. In standard clinical settings, the usual practice is visual assessment of perfusion. This method is fast, but requires experienced physicians and has a low reproducibility. For research purposes, myocardial perfusion can be assessed in a semiquantitative manner from the upslope of signal intensity (SI) versus time curves [49]. This method has a much higher reproducibility, but the analysis is time-consuming and used in general for research purposes only. Finally, quantitative assessment of myocardial perfusion reserve (MPR) is a technique requiring the conversion of signal intensity into absolute concentrations of contrast and subsequently of perfusion in absolute values (mL/g/min). Quantitative measurements have been shown to have high degrees of agreement with both invasive fractional flow reserve (FFR) and QCA measurements and minimal operator dependency [50]. These results call for further standardization of quantitative techniques.

Safety

Adenosine and dipyridamole are contraindicated in patients with severe conduction alterations, obstructive pulmonary disease (COPD and asthma), severe carotid stenosis, and pregnancy. An asthmatic exacerbation can be stopped by the use of theophylline. However, it should be emphasized that asthmatic reactions to adenosine are extremely rare. More frequent complications include bradycardia, first- and second-degree AV-block (1 in 15 patients); third-degree AV-block (1 in 125 patients), headache, dizziness, and palpitations. The heart rate, blood pressure, and symptoms of the patient have to be repeatedly monitored before, during, and after the test. Equipment and qualified personnel for life support and resuscitation need to be available.

Diagnostic Accuracy

A review article by Gerber and colleagues [51] summarized the results of 9 studies including a total of 618 patients. Overall the sensitivity and specificity of MRMPI were 89% and 81%, respectively, for detection of >75% coronary artery stenoses on a per-patient basis. In the meta-analysis by Nandalur and associates [45], 24 studies including 1516 patients were analyzed. MRMPI demonstrated a sensitivity of 0.91 (95% CI 0.88–0.94) and a specificity

of 0.81 (95% CI 0.77–0.85) on a per-patient basis (disease prevalence 57.4%). The diagnostic performance of MRMPI was comparable, if not superior, to SPECT and stress echocardiography. The recently published MR-IMPACT trial by Schwitter and associates [52] confirms these findings. The combination of perfusion and infarction imaging (using DCE) using a defined interpretation algorithm has been demonstrated to further improve the diagnostic accuracy of CMR for the detection of CAD [53].

Prognostic Value

The predictive value of MRMPI and DSMR in patients with suspected coronary artery disease has been evaluated by Jahnke and associates [54] in 533 patients with chest pain or dyspnea. Over a median follow-up of 2.3 years, ischemia by perfusion CMR was found to be the single best predictor of cardiac death or nonfatal myocardial infarctions and was superior to ischemia on DSMR. Presence of a normal perfusion test was predictive of a 99% chance of a 3-year event-free survival. In an earlier study, Ingkanisorn and coworkers [55] reported an excellent negative predictive value of MRMPI in patients with chest pain and excluded MI.

Coronary Magnetic Resonance Angiography

The gold standard method for visualization of the coronary arteries is selective x-ray coronary angiography. This technique allows for precise assessment of the anatomy and of the lumen of the coronary arteries in any incidence. Currently, there is a rapidly growing interest in noninvasive imaging techniques like coronary magnetic resonance angiography (CMRA) or computed tomography coronary angiography (CTCA) using multidetector CT (MDCT) scanners that have 16 to 256 rows of detectors. Both techniques have strengths and limitations, which will be discussed later.

The main application fields for CMRA today are the evaluation of anomalous coronary arteries and of coronary artery aneurysms (mainly Kawasaki disease or ectatic form of atherosclerotic disease), detection of native vessel coronary stenoses, and assessment of coronary artery by-pass grafts (CABGs). However, thanks to its ability to characterize soft tissues and to differentiate between fat, fibrous tissue, calcium, and thrombus, MR is currently investigated for many promising applications for imaging the atherosclerotic plaque, raising hope for the identification of vulnerable plaques. For example, ultrasmall particles of iron oxide (USPIO) administered intravenously have been shown to be taken up by macrophages present in vulnerable plaques. USPIO and other nanoparticle agents targeting various receptors are currently under investigation [56].

Technical Aspects

A detailed description of the techniques involved in CMRA is beyond the scope of this chapter. The main challenges in CMRA are related to (1) the small size and tortuosity of coronary arteries, the reason why sufficient volumetric coverage and high spatial resolution and contrast are needed; and (2) cardiac motion and breathing, which must be compensated. For imaging coronary arteries, both black-blood (two-dimensional spin-echo CMRA) and bright-blood (two- or three-dimensional breathhold segmented gradient-echo CMRA, free-breathing three-dimensional navigator-gated whole-heart CMRA) techniques exist. For further information, the reader may refer to a recently published review article [57].

Intravenous contrast agents are not necessary, but can be used for improving the contrast between blood and surrounding tissue. However, conventional extracellular contrast agents quickly extravasate into the extracellular space, the reason why data has to be collected during first-pass with breathholding. Because of this, investigations have been made with intravascular contrast agents [58] in order to obtain a prolonged time window for data collection, thus enabling the use of real-time navigator technology and three-dimensional data collection with high spatial resolution.

Diagnostic Accuracy

For the evaluation of coronary artery anomalies, both two-dimensional breathhold segmented gradient-echo [59] and three-dimensional CMRA

[60] were reported to have a better diagnostic accuracy than conventional x-ray angiography. These properties make CMRA particularly useful for evaluation of young patients with suspected anomalous coronary arteries.

In a multicenter single-vendor trial, Kim and associates [61] reported a sensitivity, specificity, and positive and negative predictive values of 93%, 42%, 70%, and 81%, respectively, for detection of native vessel coronary stenoses. Both sensitivity and negative predictive value were 100% for detection of left-main or 3-vessel disease. Several single-center trials using free-breathing navigator-gated whole-heart CMRA reported sensitivities of 80% to 90% and specificities >90%.

Although numerous trials showed the ability of different CMRA techniques (free-breathing ECG-gated two-dimensional spin-echo CMRA, two-dimensional gradient-echo CMRA, and navigator three-dimensional CMRA with or without contrast) to identify CABG occlusion, their use in clinical settings still suffers several limitations, including the inability to differentiate between different degrees of luminal narrowing and the occurrence of local signal loss and artifacts due to nearby implanted metallic objects (sternal wires, hemostatic clips, graft stents, and coexistent prosthetic valves, supporting struts, or rings).

Comparison with Other Noninvasive Techniques

At the moment, CTCA is more widely available and offers better spatial resolution than CMRA. Several studies have shown the excellent negative predictive value of CTCA, making it a valuable tool for ruling out CAD. In contrast, the positive predictive value of CTCA is low [62], due to overestimation of calcified plaques and motion artefacts. Thus, coronary MRA shows a better diagnostic performance than CTCA for the detection of significant stenosis in patients with high calcium scores [63]. Other limitations of CTCA are radiation exposure (considerably higher than standard x-ray angiography) and need for injection of iodinated contrast agents (nephrotoxicity, risk for anaphylactoid reactions). Moreover, patients with heart rates above 60 beats per minute need to receive beta-blockers prior to the examination in order to decrease the frequency and extent of motion artifacts on the images.

Compared to standard x-ray angiography and CTCA, the limitations of CMRA are a lower spatial resolution and the necessity to average data from several cardiac cycles. This probably explains the generally lower reported sensitivity and specificity of CMRA compared with CTA.

Interventional Guidance

Percutaneous and endovascular interventions are becoming increasingly complex and require progressively more sophisticated imaging techniques for guidance and control. The ability of MRI to provide both unprecedented morphology (including vascular wall and surrounding structures) and functional information has created growing interest in MRI-guided interventions in three main settings: endovascular therapy, interventional electrophysiology procedures, and myocardial therapy. For all these purposes, MR images can be combined with other imaging modalities such as x-ray fluoroscopy or—in the particular case of electrophysiology—to electroanatomic mapping systems.

The lack of radiation in CMR may be of special interest for children and younger patients who have to undergo repeated interventional procedures. Although MR guidance needs considerable further development to overcome technical challenges (safety issues, MR-compatible materials), it may offer the benefits of MR for many potential clinical applications, including cardiac catheterization, endovascular therapy, congenital heart disease, and myocardial therapy (transvascular delivery of drugs, genes, angiogenic growth factors, or cells).

Stent deployment under MRI guidance in animals has been achieved in coronary and pulmonary arteries using nitinol or platinum wires and stents, since stainless steel stents create severe artifacts and image distortion. After deployment, localization and function of the stent can be documented together with flow measurements using phase-contrast velocity imaging. Percutaneous placement of closure devices for treatment of atrial septal de-

fects or deployment of pulmonary stents and aortic valve stents have also been successfully guided by MR in animal models.

Finally, different kinds of therapies such as genes or cells can be locally delivered into the myocardium. Due to the potential of producing multiplanar views and excellent soft-tissue contrast, MRI is very well suited for targeting administration sites in the myocardium (eg, infracted areas) as well as for monitoring of the distribution and effects of these therapies. Thus, MR has successfully been used for gene delivery [64] as well as for intramyocardial injection of cells labelled with iron particles [65] in animal models. The site of injection can also be labelled using gadolinium chelates [66].

Clinical Applications

The use of CMR and its clinical applications are broadly supported by the diagnostic accuracy and prognostic value of the different techniques described earlier in this chapter. However, because of its limited clinical availability until now, there are few guidelines for the use of CMR for the evaluation of patients with suspected or declared coronary artery disease (CAD). Not all smaller hospitals are equipped with MR facilities and, unlike echocardiography, MR cannot be used in a private cardiology practice. Today the clinical use of CMR can be supported by the 2006 published appropriateness criteria for CCT and CMR [67]. This report has been initiated by the American College of Cardiology Foundation (ACCF) in collaboration with several societies involved in cardiovascular imaging. Table 14.2 summarizes the appropriateness criteria for CMR. In order to make the table easier to read, the uncertain or inappropriate indications are not listed.

Detection of CAD

Although MRMPI or DSMR are appropriate for the evaluation of patients with intermediate pre-test probability of CAD, their indication is uncertain in patients with high pre-test probability of CAD. In accordance to a 2004 published consensus panel

Table 14.2 Appropriate Indications for CMR

Detection of Coronary Artery Disease in Symptomatic Patients

MRMPI or DSMR in patients with intermediate pre-test probability of CAD and uninterpretable ECG (or patient unable to exercise)

MRA for evaluation of suspected coronary anomalies

Risk Assessment Using MRMPI or DSMR in Patients with Prior Test Results

Coronary angiography (catheterization or CT) with stenosis of unclear significance

Structure and Function—Evaluation of Ventricular and Valvular Function (LV/RV Mass and Volumes, MRA, Assessment of Valves, DCE)

Assessment of complex congenital heart disease including anomalies of coronary circulation, great vessels, and cardiac chambers and valves

Evaluation of LVEF following myocardial infarction or in heart failure patients (1) if echo images are technically limited or (2) if there is discordant information from prior tests

Evaluation of specific cardiomyopathies (infiltrative, HCM, or due to cardiotoxic therapies)

Characterization of native and prosthetic cardiac valves—including planimetry of stenotic disease and quantification of regurgitant disease—in patients with technically limited images from TTE or TEE

Evaluation for arrythmogenic right ventricular cardiomyopathy (ARVC) in patients presenting with syncope or ventricular arrhythmia

Evaluation of myocarditis or myocardial infarction in patients with positive cardiac enzymes without obstructive atherosclerosis on angiography

Structure and Function—Evaluation of Intra- and Extra-Cardiac Structures

Evaluation of cardiac mass (suspected tumor or thrombus), using contrast for perfusion and enhancement

Evaluation of pericardial conditions (pericardial mass, constrictive pericarditis)

Evaluation for aortic dissection

Evaluation of pulmonary veins prior to radiofrequency ablation for atrial fibrillation (left atrial and pulmonary venous anatomy including dimensions of veins for mapping purposes)

Detection of Myocardial Scar and Viability—Evaluation of Myocardial Scar

To determine the location, and extent of myocardial necrosis including "no reflow" regions after acute myocardial infarction

To determine viability prior to revascularization (in order to establish the likelihood of functional recovery with revascularization (PCI or CABG) or medical therapy)

Adapted from [67] Hendel RC, Patel MR, Kramer CM, et al. ACCF/ACR/SCCT/SCMR/ASNC/NASCI/SCAI/SIR 2006 appropriateness criteria for cardiac computed tomography and cardiac magnetic resonance imaging: a report of the American College of Cardiology Foundation Quality Strategic Directions Committee Appropriateness Criteria Working Group, American College of Radiology, Society of Cardiovascular Computed Tomography, Society for Cardiovascular Magnetic Resonance, American Society of Nuclear Cardiology, North American Society for Cardiac Imaging, Society for Cardiovascular Angiography and Interventions, and Society of Interventional Radiology. *J Am Coll Cardiol.* 2006;48:1475–1497.

report [68], the 2006 Guidelines of the European Society of Cardiology (ESC) [69] give a class II recommendation for the use of DSMR or MRMPI in patients with stable angina pectoris. In the setting of acute coronary syndromes in patients with intermediate pre-test probability of CAD without ECG changes and with serial negative cardiac enzymes, the appropriateness of DSMR or MRMPI is still uncertain. However, some organizations like the Dutch Society of Cardiology recommend their use in this setting. Although CT and transesophagial echocardiography are of easier use in emergency settings, CMR is appropriate for the evaluation of aortic dissection.

Before intermediate- or high-risk surgery, the use of CMR as an intermediate perioperative risk predictor is uncertain. However, Rerkpattanapipat and associates [70] showed in patients unable to undergo stress echocardiography that DSMR may be used to identify those at high and low risk for cardiac events during or after noncardiac surgery.

Evaluation of Patients with MI

The evaluation of a patient after MI has several purposes. In the (sub-) acute phase, the determination of infarct size and extent of areas of no-reflow allows for prognostic evaluation of the patient. The technical approaches used are usually bright-blood cine imaging for determination of biventricular global and regional function, STIR imaging (T2-weighted turbo spin-echo sequence along with fat saturation; Fig. 14.1) for visualization of edema, and late enhancement imaging for determination of infarct size and microvascular obstruction (MVO) correlating with areas of no reflow (see also "Scar Detection/Assessment of Viability" earlier in the chapter). Sometimes, rest perfusion imaging is made during administration of contrast, since this technique also allows for identification of areas of MVO. Precise evaluation of possible intraventricular thrombi can be made with these different techniques.

In the evaluation of chronic infarction, CMR allows for follow-up of the infracted area, remodelling assessment, and determination of viability and prognosis. CMR is also used for precise calculation of LVEF, thus helping decision-making processes before cardiac resynchronization (CRT) and/or implantable cardiac defibrillator (ICD) devices, since these therapies are expensive and their therapeutic effect not always conclusive. Moreover, it has been recently reported that scar size, transmurality, and location affect the efficacy of cardiac resynchronization [71]. The 2006 ACC/AHA/ESC guidelines for management of patients with ventricular arrhythmias and the prevention of sudden cardiac death (SCD) recommend (class IIa, level of evidence B) the use of MRI (or CT or SPECT) in patients with ventricular arrhythmias when echocardiography does not provide accurate assessment of LV and RV function and/or evaluation of structural changes [72]. Detection of silent ischemia is recommended in patients with ventricular arrhythmias who have an intermediate probability for CAD by age, symptoms, and gender, and in whom exercise test is not optimally interpretable (class I, level of evidence B).

Conclusion

CMR is a new diagnostic modality in cardiovascular medicine, offering high-quality images and a broad spectrum of anatomic and functional information in acquired and congenital heart disease. In ischemic heart disease, CMR plays a role of growing importance in the assessment of patients before, during, and after interventional procedures. Assessment of cardiac function, myocardial viability after infarction, myocardial ischemia, coronary and noncoronary arteries, and catheter guidance using CMR open perspectives for integrated imaging of the cardiovascular system.

The oncoming developments and challenges in CMR will mainly arise in the fields of coronary artery imaging (including characterization of the atherosclerotic plaque) and MR-guided catheter interventions, using molecular imaging and new contrast agents such as blood pool agents.

Although CMR still suffers limited availability, its integration in clinical practice will further progress. Given the rapid development of new applications for CMR, regular updates of clinical guidelines will be needed.

References

1. Pohost GM, Kim RJ, Kramer CM, Manning WJ. Task Force 12: training in advanced cardiovascular imaging (cardiovascular magnetic resonance [CMR]) endorsed by the Society for Cardiovascular Magnetic Resonance. *J Am Coll Cardiol*. 2008;22;51:404–408.
2. Woodard PK, Bluemke DA, Cascade PN, *et al.* ACR practice guideline for the performance and interpretation of cardiac magnetic resonance imaging (MRI). *J Am Coll Radiol*. 2006;3:665–676.
3. Schellock FG, Spinazzi A. MRI safety update 2008: part 1, MRI contrast agents and nephrogenic systemic fibrosis. *Am J Roentgenol*. 2008;191:1129–1139.
4. Bellenger NG, Burgess MI, Ray SG, *et al.* Comparison of left ventricular ejection fraction and volumes in heart failure by echocardiography, radionuclide ventriculography and cardiovascular magnetic

resonance; are they interchangeable? *Eur Heart J.* 2000;21:1387–1396.

5. Grothues F, Moon JC, Bellenger NG, Smith GS, Klein HU, Pennell DJ. Interstudy reproducibility of right ventricular volumes, function, and mass with cardiovascular magnetic resonance. *Am Heart J.* 2004;147:218–223.

6. Cerqueira MD, Weissman NJ, Dilsizian V, et al. Standardized myocardial segmentation and nomenclature for tomographic imaging of the heart: a statement for healthcare professionals from the Cardiac Imaging Committee of the Council on Clinical Cardiology of the American Heart Association. *Circulation.* 2002;105:539–542.

7. Maceira AM, Prasad SK, Khan M, Pennell DJ. Normalized left ventricular systolic and diastolic function by steady state free precession cardiovascular magnetic resonance. *J Cardiovasc Magn Reson.* 2006;8:417–426.

8. Maceira AM, Prasad SK, Khan M, Pennell DJ. Reference right ventricular systolic and diastolic function normalized to age, gender and body surface area from steady-state free precession cardiovascular magnetic resonance. *Eur Heart J.* 2006;27:2879–2888.

9. Young AA, Axel L. Three-dimensional motion and deformation of the heart wall: estimation with spatial modulation of magnetization—a model-based approach. *Radiology.* 1992;185:241–247.

10. Paelinck BP, Lamb HJ, Bax JJ, Van der Wall EE, de Roos A. Assessment of diastolic function by cardiovascular magnetic resonance. *Am Heart J.* 2002;144:198–205.

11. Rathi VK, Doyle M, Yamrozik J, et al. Routine evaluation of left ventricular diastolic function by cardiovascular magnetic resonance: a practical approach. *J Cardiovasc Magn Reson.* 2008;10:36.

12. Mahrholdt H, Wagner A, Judd RM, Sechtem U, Kim RJ. Delayed enhancement cardiovascular magnetic resonance assessment of non-ischaemic cardiomyopathies. *Eur Heart J.* 2005;26:1461–1474.

13. Ricciardi MJ, Wu E, Davidson CJ, et al. Visualization of discrete microinfarction after percutaneous coronary intervention associated with mild creatine kinase-MB elevation. *Circulation.* 2001;103:2780–2783.

14. Kumar A, Abdel-Aty H, Kriedemann I, et al. Contrast-enhanced cardiovascular magnetic resonance imaging of right ventricular infarction. *J Am Coll Cardiol.* 2006;48:1969–1976.

15. Kim RJ, Fieno DS, Parrish TB, et al. Relationship of MRI delayed contrast enhancement to irreversible injury, infarct age, and contractile function. *Circulation.* 1999;100:1992–2002.

16. Klein C, Nekolla SG, Bengel FM, et al. Assessment of myocardial viability with contrast-enhanced magnetic resonance imaging: comparison with positron emission tomography. *Circulation.* 2002;105:162–167.

17. Kuhl HP, Van der Weerdt A, Beek A, Visser F, Hanrath P, van Rossum A. Relation of end-diastolic wall thickness and the residual rim of viable myocardium by magnetic resonance imaging to myocardial viability assessed by fluorine-18 deoxyglucose positron emission tomography. *Am J Cardiol.* 2006;97:452–457.

18. Setser RM, Kim JK, Chung YC, et al. Cine delayed-enhancement MR imaging of the heart: initial experience. *Radiology.* 2006;239:856–862.

19. Wagner A, Mahrholdt H, Holly TA, et al. Contrast-enhanced MRI and routine single photon emission computed tomography (SPECT) perfusion imaging for detection of subendocardial myocardial infarcts: an imaging study. *Lancet.* 2003;361:374–379.

20. Wu YW, Tadamura E, Kanao S, et al. Myocardial viability by contrast-enhanced cardiovascular magnetic resonance in patients with coronary artery disease: comparison with gated single-photon emission tomography and FDG position emission tomography. *Int J Cardiovasc Imaging.* 2007;23:757–765.

21. Kuhl HP, Lipke CS, Krombach GA, et al. Assessment of reversible myocardial dysfunction in chronic ischaemic heart disease: comparison of contrast-enhanced cardiovascular magnetic resonance and a combined positron emission tomography-single photon emission computed tomography imaging protocol. *Eur Heart J.* 2006;27:846–853.

22. Kitagawa K, Sakuma H, Hirano T, Okamoto S, Makino K, Takeda K. Acute myocardial infarction: myocardial viability assessment in patients early thereafter comparison of contrast-enhanced MR imaging with resting (201)Tl SPECT. Single photon emission computed tomography. *Radiology.* 2003;226:138–144.

23. Gutberlet M, Frohlich M, Mehl S, et al. Myocardial viability assessment in patients with highly impaired left ventricular function: comparison of delayed enhancement, dobutamine stress MRI, end-diastolic wall thickness, and TI201-SPECT with functional recovery after revascularization. *Eur Radiol.* 2005;15:872–880.

24. Srichai MB, Schvartzman PR, Sturm B, Kasper JM, Lieber ML, White RD. Extent of myocardial scarring on nonstress delayed-contrast-enhancement cardiac

magnetic resonance imaging correlates directly with degrees of resting regional dysfunction in chronic ischemic heart disease. *Am Heart J*. 2004;148:342–348.

25. Kim RJ, Wu E, Rafael A, *et al*. The use of contrast-enhanced magnetic resonance imaging to identify reversible myocardial dysfunction. *N Engl J Med*. 2000;343:1445–1453.

26. Schvartzman PR, Srichai MB, Grimm RA, *et al*. Nonstress delayed-enhancement magnetic resonance imaging of the myocardium predicts improvement of function after revascularization for chronic ischemic heart disease with left ventricular dysfunction. *Am Heart J*. 2003;146:535–541.

27. Selvanayagam JB, Kardos A, Francis JM, *et al*. Value of delayed-enhancement cardiovascular magnetic resonance imaging in predicting myocardial viability after surgical revascularization. *Circulation*. 2004;110:1535–1541.

28. Schmidt A, Azevedo CF, Cheng A, *et al*. Infarct tissue heterogeneity by magnetic resonance imaging identifies enhanced cardiac arrhythmia susceptibility in patients with left ventricular dysfunction. *Circulation*. 2007;115:2006–2014.

29. Beek AM, Kuhl HP, Bondarenko O, *et al*. Delayed contrast-enhanced magnetic resonance imaging for the prediction of regional functional improvement after acute myocardial infarction. *J Am Coll Cardiol*. 2003;42:895–901.

30. Rubenstein JC, Ortiz JT, Wu E, *et al*. The use of periinfarct contrast-enhanced cardiac magnetic resonance imaging for the prediction of late postmyocardial infarction ventricular dysfunction. *Am Heart J*. 156:498–505.

31. Lund GK, Stork A, Muellerleile K, *et al*. Prediction of left ventricular remodeling and analysis of infarct resorption in patients with reperfused myocardial infarcts by using contrast-enhanced MR imaging. *Radiology*. 2007;245:95–102.

32. Yan AT, Shayne AJ, Brown KA, *et al*. Characterization of the peri-infarct zone by contrast-enhanced cardiac magnetic resonance imaging is a powerful predictor of post-myocardial infarction mortality. *Circulation*. 114:32–39.

33. Nijveldt R, Beek AM, Hirsch A, *et al*. Functional recovery after acute myocardial infarction: comparison between angiography, electrocardiography, and cardiovascular magnetic resonance measures of microvascular injury. *J Am Coll Cardiol*. 2008;52:181–189.

34. Pijls NH, De Bruyne B, Peels K, *et al*. Measurement of fractional flow reserve to assess the functional severity of coronary-artery stenoses. *N Engl J Med*. 1996;334:1703–1708.

35. Pijls NH, De Bruyne B, Bech GJ, *et al*. Coronary pressure measurement to assess the hemodynamic significance of serial stenoses within one coronary artery: validation in humans. *Circulation*. 2000;102:2371–2377.

36. Pennell DJ, Underwood SR, Manzara CC, *et al*. Magnetic resonance imaging during dobutamine stress in coronary artery disease. *Am J Cardiol*. 1992;70:34–40.

37. Paetsch I, Jahnke C, Wahl A, *et al*. Comparison of dobutamine stress magnetic resonance, adenosine stress magnetic resonance, and adenosine stress magnetic resonance perfusion. *Circulation*. 2004;110:835–842.

38. Schalla S, Klein C, Paetsch I, *et al*. Real-time MR image acquisition during high-dose dobutamine hydrochloride stress for detecting left ventricular wall-motion abnormalities in patients with coronary arterial disease. *Radiology*. 2002;224:845–851.

39. Paetsch I, Foll D, Kaluza A, *et al*. Magnetic resonance stress tagging in ischemic heart disease. *Am J Physiol*. 2005;288:H2708–H2714.

40. Saito I, Watanabe S, Masuda Y. Detection of viable myocardium by dobutamine stress tagging magnetic resonance imaging with three-dimensional analysis by automatic trace method. *Jpn Circ J*. 2000;64:487–494.

41. Wahl A, Paetsch I, Gollesch A, *et al*. Safety and feasibility of high-dose dobutamine-atropine stress cardiovascular magnetic resonance for diagnosis of myocardial ischaemia: experience in 1000 consecutive cases. *Eur Heart J*. 2004;25:1230–1236.

42. Nagel E, Lehmkuhl HB, Bocksch W, *et al*. Noninvasive diagnosis of ischemia-induced wall motion abnormalities with the use of high-dose dobutamine stress MRI: comparison with dobutamine stress echocardiography. *Circulation*. 1999;99:763–770.

43. Hundley WG, Hamilton CA, Thomas MS, *et al*. Utility of fast cine magnetic resonance imaging and display for the detection of myocardial ischemia in patients not well suited for second harmonic stress echocardiography. *Circulation*. 1999;100:1697–1702.

44. Wahl A, Paetsch I, Roethemeyer S, Klein C, Fleck E, Nagel E. High-dose dobutamine-atropine stress cardiovascular MR imaging after coronary revascularization in patients with wall motion abnormalities at rest. *Radiology*. 2004;233:210–216.

45. Nandalur KR, Dwamena BA, Choudhri AF, Nandalur MR, Carlos RC. Diagnostic performance of stress cardiac magnetic resonance imaging in the detection of

coronary artery disease: a meta-analysis. *J Am Coll Cardiol.* 2007;50:1343–1353.

46. Hundley WG, Morgan TM, Neagle CM, Hamilton CA, Rerkpattanapipat P, Link KM. Magnetic resonance imaging determination of cardiac prognosis. *Circulation.* 2002;106:2328–2333.

47. Kuijpers D, van Dijkman PR, Janssen CH, Vliegenthart R, Zijlstra F, Oudkerk M. Dobutamine stress MRI. Part II. Risk stratification with dobutamine cardiovascular magnetic resonance in patients suspected of myocardial ischemia. *Eur Radiol.* 2004;14:2046–2052.

48. Wellnhofer E, Olariu A, Klein C, *et al.* Magnetic resonance low-dose dobutamine test is superior to SCAR quantification for the prediction of functional recovery. *Circulation.* 2004;109:2172–2174.

49. Al-Saadi N, Nagel E, Gross M, *et al.* Noninvasive detection of myocardial ischemia from perfusion reserve based on cardiovascular magnetic resonance. *Circulation.* 2000;101:1379–1383.

50. Futamatsu H, Wilke N, Klassen C, et al. .Evaluation of cardiac magnetic resonance imaging parameters to detect anatomically and hemodynamically significant coronary artery disease. *Am Heart J.* 2007;154:298–305.

51. Gerber BL, Raman SV, Nayak K, *et al.* Myocardial first-pass perfusion cardiovascular magnetic resonance: history, theory, and current state of the art. *J Cardiovasc Magn Reson.* 2008;10:18.

52. Schwitter J, Wacker CM, van Rossum AC, *et al.* MR-IMPACT: comparison of perfusion-cardiac magnetic resonance with single-photon emission computed tomography for the detection of coronary artery disease in a multicentre, multivendor, randomized trial. *Eur Heart J.* 2008;29:480–489.

53. Klem I, Heitner JF, Shah DJ, *et al.* Improved detection of coronary artery disease by stress perfusion cardiovascular magnetic resonance with the use of delayed enhancement infarction imaging. *J Am Coll Cardiol.* 2006;47:1630–1638.

54. Jahnke C, Nagel E, Gebker R, *et al.* Prognostic value of cardiac magnetic resonance stress tests: adenosine stress perfusion and dobutamine stress wall motion imaging. *Circulation.* 2007;115:1769–1776.

55. Ingkanisorn WP, Kwong RY, Bohme NS, *et al.* Prognosis of negative adenosine stress magnetic resonance in patients presenting to an emergency department with chest pain. *J Am Coll Cardiol.* 2006;47:1427–1432.

56. Korosoglou G, Weiss RG, Kedziorek DA, *et al.* Noninvasive detection of macrophage-rich atherosclerotic plaque in hyperlipidemic rabbits using "positive contrast" magnetic resonance imaging. *J Am Coll Cardiol.* 2008;52:483–491.

57. Stuber M, Weiss RG. Coronary magnetic resonance angiography. *J Magn Reson Imaging.* 2007;26: 219–234.

58. Stuber M, Botnar RM, Danias PG, *et al.* Contrast agent-enhanced, free-breathing, three-dimensional coronary magnetic resonance angiography. *J Magn Reson Imaging.* 1999;10:790–799.

59. Post JC, van Rossum AC, Bronzwaer JG, *et al.* Magnetic resonance angiography of anomalous coronary arteries. A new gold standard for delineating the proximal course? *Circulation.* 1995;92:3163–3171.

60. Bunce NH, Lorenz CH, Keegan J, *et al.* Coronary artery anomalies: assessment with free-breathing three-dimensional coronary MR angiography. *Radiology.* 2003;227:201–208.

61. Kim WY, Danias PG, Stuber M, *et al.* Coronary magnetic resonance angiography for the detection of coronary stenoses. *N Engl J Med.* 2001;345:1863–1869.

62. Stein PD, Yaekoub AY, Matta F, Sostman HD. 64-slice CT for diagnosis of coronary artery disease: a systematic review. *Am J Med.* 2008;121:715–725.

63. Liu X, Zhao X, Huang J, *et al.* Comparison of 3D free-breathing coronary MR angiography and 64-MDCT angiography for detection of coronary stenosis in patients with high calcium scores. *Am J Roentgenol.* 2007;189:1326–1332.

64. Yang X, Atalar E, Li D, *et al.* Magnetic resonance imaging permits in vivo monitoring of catheter-based vascular gene delivery. *Circulation.* 2001;104: 1588–1590.

65. Dick AJ, Guttman MA, Raman VK, *et al.* Magnetic resonance fluoroscopy allows targeted delivery of mesenchymal stem cells to infarct borders in swine. *Circulation.* 2003;108:2899–2904.

66. Saeed M, Lee R, Martin A, *et al.* Transendocardial delivery of extracellular myocardial markers by using combination x-ray/MR fluoroscopic guidance: feasibility study in dogs. *Radiology.* 2004;231:689–696.

67. Hendel RC, Patel MR, Kramer CM, et al. ACCF/ACR/SCCT/SCMR/ASNC/NASCI/SCAI/SIR 2006 appropriateness criteria for cardiac computed tomography and cardiac magnetic resonance imaging: a report of the American College of Cardiology Foundation Quality Strategic Directions Committee Appropriateness Criteria Working Group, American College of Radiology, Society of Cardiovascular Computed Tomography, Society for Cardiovascular Magnetic Resonance, American Society of Nuclear

Cardiology, North American Society for Cardiac Imaging, Society for Cardiovascular Angiography and Interventions, and Society of Interventional Radiology. *J Am Coll Cardiol*. 2006;48:1475–1497.

68. Pennell DJ, Sechtem UP, Higgins CB, *et al.* Clinical indications for cardiovascular magnetic resonance (CMR): Consensus Panel report. *Eur Heart J*. 2004;25:1940–1965.

69. Fox K, Garcia MA, Ardissino D, *et al.* Guidelines on the management of stable angina pectoris: executive summary: The Task Force on the Management of Stable Angina Pectoris of the European Society of Cardiology. *Eur Heart J*. 2006;27:1341–1381.

70. Rerkpattanapipat P, Morgan TM, Neagle CM, Link KM, Hamilton CA, Hundley WG. Assessment of preoperative cardiac risk with magnetic resonance imaging. *Am J Cardiol*. 2002;90:416–419.

71. Chalil S, Foley PW, Muyhaldeen SA, *et al.* Late gadolinium enhancement-cardiovascular magnetic resonance as a predictor of response to cardiac resynchronization therapy in patients with ischaemic cardiomyopathy. *Europace*. 2007;9:1031–1037.

72. Zipes DP, Camm AJ, Borggrefe M, et al. ACC/AHA/ESC 2006 guidelines for management of patients with ventricular arrhythmias and the prevention of sudden cardiac death: a report of the American College of Cardiology/American Heart Association Task Force and the European Society of Cardiology Committee for Practice Guidelines (Writing Committee to Develop guidelines for management of patients with ventricular arrhythmias and the prevention of sudden cardiac death) developed in collaboration with the European Heart Rhythm Association and the Heart Rhythm Society. *Europace*. 2006;8:746–837.

CHAPTER 15

Optical Coherence Tomography for Coronary Imaging

Jean-François Surmely
Cardiology, Clinique de la Source, Lausanne, Switzerland

Chapter Overview

- Optical coherence tomography (OCT) is an invasive imaging modality that provides in situ cross-sectional images of tissue with a near histologic resolution.
- The resolution of OCT is about 10 times higher than any other currently available imaging modalities
- OCT allows the in-vivo characterization of coronary atherosclerotic plaque and the detection of vulnerable plaque
- OCT is the only in-vivo imaging method allowing the accurate measurement of the fibrous cap thickness of atherosclerotic plaque
- OCT allows the evaluation of stent deployment characteristics, vessel injury post stent implantation, and intimal healing in the chronic phase

---

Optical coherence tomography (OCT) is an invasive imaging modality that provides high-resolution cross-sectional images of tissue in situ. The basic technical principles are analogous to ultrasound, but as its name indicates, OCT uses an optical signal (near-infrared light) as the signal source. After reflection from the tissue, information gained by the backscattered signal is converted into a tomographic image.

Coronary artery wall imaging by OCT was first reported to be possible in 1991[1]. Since the mid-1990s, ex-vivo studies investigating coronary atherosclerotic plaque characterization have been published. Improvements in technology and devices have led to easier use and more accurate data over the years. In-vivo OCT recording was first shown to be feasible in animal studies and

then performed in humans [2–5]. In order to overcome the signal attenuation caused by red blood cells, a blood free zone is needed. This can be achieved adequately either by proximal balloon occlusion with distal saline flush, or by saline flushing alone. The main advantage of OCT over any other currently available imaging technologies is its high resolution of about 10 to 15 μm. On the other hand, the main limitations of OCT are the need for a blood free zone and a limited penetration depth.

Coronary arteries are medium-sized muscular arteries. The diameters of major epicardial coronary arteries range from about 2 to 5 mm and are therefore in the scan area depth of the OCT system. Normal coronary artery walls have three distinct histologic layers: (1) the intima, with luminal endothelial cells and subendothelial fibroelastic connective tissue; (2) the media, formed of smooth muscle cells and connective tissue; and (3) the adventitia, formed of connective tissue. These three layers

---

Current Best Practice in Interventional Cardiology. Edited by B Meier. © 2010 Blackwell Publishing,

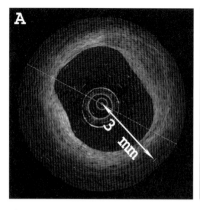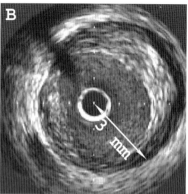

Figure 15.1 Comparison of penetration between OCT (Lightlab Imaging) (A) and grey-scale IVUS (Atlantis pro, Boston, 40 MHz) (B), on corresponding same-scale images of a large proximal LAD artery (lumen 4 × 3 mm, vessel 6 mm). By OCT, adequate penetration over the entire circumference is observed, with a maximum penetration depth of 1.3 mm at the site of maximal plaque burden (2 o'clock). In addition, a large lipid pool with a TCFA can be detected only by OCT. (IVUS, intravascular ultrasound; LAD, left anterior descending; OCT, optical coherence tomography; TCFA, thin cap fibroatheroma.)

are separated by the internal and external elastic membranes. Due to its near-histologic resolution, OCT allows differentiating those three layers and to visualize minute details [6]. The OCT penetration depth of about 1.5 mm raises concern about its ability to completely image the arterial wall. In the context of coronary arteries, however, it is often sufficient, apart from some cases with very large atherosclerotic plaque (Fig. 15.1).

Further signal processing techniques allow gaining additional tissue characterization, such as the intimal collagen content by polarization sensitive OCT, or the tissue tensile properties by OCT–elastography [7,8]. Another important advance is the development of a high-speed OCT system (also named optical frequency domain imaging), which allows reducing the acquisition time and therefore the time of blood clearing by balloon occlusion or saline flushing.

This chapter will summarize the current knowledge about three main OCT applications for coronary imaging, namely the characterization of atherosclerotic plaque and detection of vulnerable plaque, the information gained during PCI, and the follow-up evaluation post stent implantation.

Atherosclerotic Plaque Characterization and Vulnerable Plaque Detection

Vulnerable Plaque Histopathology and Epidemiology

Although atherosclerosis is a pan-coronary syndrome, coronary thrombosis occurs at focal sites of increased vulnerability. Sudden changes in coronary plaque luminal surface morphology consisting of plaque rupture or fissure have been recognized as an important mechanism of thrombosis. The most common cause of coronary thrombosis is plaque rupture, followed by plaque erosion and, infrequently, a calcified nodule [9]. Plaque disruption, like endothelial erosion, is a reflection of enhanced inflammatory activity within the plaque. Necropsy studies of coronary arteries plaques that have undergone disruption have been used to determine the characteristics of currently stable plaques whose structure and composition make them likely to undergo an episode of thrombosis in the future. The risk for a plaque to rupture has been shown to be associated to the plaque composition and include a large lipid core, a reduced number of smooth muscle cells, a thin fibrous cap

($< 65\ \mu m$), and a high macrophage density [10,11]. These features are more frequently found in plaque with positive remodeling [12,13].

About 80% percent of all infarctions result from thrombosis of a lesion that by itself is not hemodynamically significant. This does not mean that mild/moderate stenoses have an increased risk for inducing an acute event compared to severe stenoses, but reflects the fact that mild/moderate lesions outnumber flow-limiting lesions by a factor of about 10. It is therefore the cumulative risk of all the nonsignificant stenoses that prevails [14–18].

Ex-Vivo Histopathologic Validation

Plaque Composition

Plaque components have different echogenicity properties. With OCT, fibrous tissue is characterized by homogeneous high backscattering area, calcification is shown as a well-delineated low backscattering heterogeneous area with sharp border, and lipid pool is a less well-delineated low backscattering homogeneous area with poor border (Fig. 15.2). The first ex-vivo histopathologic validation

study reported a high accuracy for fibrous plaque (OCT reader 1: sensitivity 79 %, specificity 97 %; OCT reader 2: sensitivity 71 %, specificity 98 %), fibrocalcific plaques (OCT reader 1: sensitivity 95 %, specificity 97 %; OCT reader 2: sensitivity 96 %, specificity 97 %), and for lipid-rich plaques (OCT reader 1: sensitivity 90 %, specificity 92 %; OCT reader 2: sensitivity 94 %, specificity 90 %). The interobserver and intraobserver agreements were also high ($\kappa = 0.88$ and $= 0.91$, respectively) [19]. Several studies have since confirmed these initial results (Table 15.1) [20–23]. Characterization of coronary plaque composition has also been shown to be superior with OCT compared to conventional gray-scale IVUS (intravascular ultrasound) or integrated backscatter IVUS, and this particularly for the detection of lipid pools [21,22].

Fibrous Cap Thickness Measurement

TCFA is known to be one of the important features predisposing to plaque rupture and thrombus formation, resulting in an acute coronary event. TCFA is characterized by a lipid pool/necrotic core with a thin overlying fibrous cap measuring

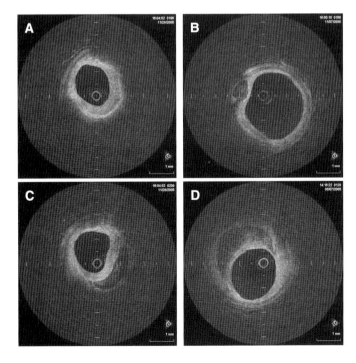

Figure 15.2 Examples of different plaque types. **A.** Plaque with concentric fibrous tissue. **B.** Small calcified nodule. **C.** Calcified plaque (from 3 to 7 o'clock). **D.** Plaque with a large lipid pool with a thin overlying fibrous cap.

Table 15.1 Optical Coherence Tomography Validation Studies

Study	Lipid-rich		Fibrocalcific		Fibrous		Study Design	
	Sensitivity (%)	Specificity (%)	Sensitivity (%)	Specificity (%)	Sensitivity (%)	Specificity (%)	Study Sample Size	Cross-Sections Included in the Accuracy Analysis
Yabushita et al. [19]	90–94	90–92	95–96	97	71–79	97–98	307 sections (L = 68, FC = 162, F = 77)	All
Manfrini et al. [20]	45	83	68	76	83	82	68 sections (L = 38, FC = 19, F = 6)	All
Rieber et al. [21]	77	94	67	97	64	88	117 sections, divided in 468 quadrants (L = 39, FC = 46, F = 97)	Only "assessable" quadrants (323 out of 468 = 69%)
Kawasaki et al. [22]	95	98	100	100	98	94	128 ROI (0.2 × 0.2 mm), within OCT penetration depth (L = 19, FC = 7, F = 88)	Only ROI in which the diagnoses were identical between the two study readers (121 out of 128 = 95 %)
Kume et al. [23]	85	94	96	88	79	99	166 sections (L = 41, FC = 82, F = 43)	All

F, fibrous; FC, fibrocalcific; L, lipid-rich; OCT, optical coherence tomography; ROI, region of interest.

<65 μm. In an ex-vivo study by Kume and associates, 35 lipid-rich plaques from 102 coronary artery segments obtained from 38 human cadavers were examined by OCT (LightLab Imaging system) and histology. Lipid-rich plaques were defined histologicaly as the presence of lipid in ≥ 2 quadrants within a plaque. Fibrous cap thickness between OCT and corresponding histologic images showed an excellent correlation (r = 0.9, $p < 0.001$). Correlation coefficients were also high for repeated measurements by the same observer (r = 0.92) and for measurements by two different observers (r = 0.88) [24]. To date, OCT is the only in-vivo imaging method allowing the accurate measurement of the fibrous cap thickness.

Macrophage Detection

A study by Tearney and colleagues reported the ability of OCT to provide detailed knowledge of the superficial plaque components up to a cellular level, with macrophage detection in the fibrous cap. In this ex-vivo study, a high correlation between OCT and histologic measurements of fibrous cap macrophage density was shown (r = 0.84, $p < 0.0001$) [25].

In-Vivo Coronary Plaque Evaluation

The current understanding of coronary artery disease pathophysiology is based largely on autopsy data. OCT is a validated imaging modality with near-histologic resolution and could therefore increase our understanding in patients.

Plaque Characterization

In a study including 57 patients, coronary plaque characteristics of culprit/target lesions were analyzed and compared according to the clinical presentation. It was found that the frequency of TCFA was significantly higher in acute myocardial infarction and acute coronary syndromes compared to stable angina pectoris (72%, 50%, and 20%, respectively, $p = 0.01$). Lipid-rich plaque was observed in 90%, 75%, and 59%, respectively ($p = 0.09$). The median value of the minimum fibrous cap thickness was 47.0, 53.8, and 102.6 μm, respectively ($p = 0.03$) [26].

Kubo and colleagues performed OCT in 30 patients with acute myocardial infarction and reported that the incidence of plaque rupture at the location of culprit lesions was 73%. In addition, lipid-rich plaque was observed in 93% and the frequency of TCFA was 83% [27]. Chia and coworkers compared culprit plaque characteristics in women and men presenting with acute coronary syndromes and observed no significant sex difference in the plaque characteristics of culprit lesions [28].

Lumen Surface Evaluation

Plaques fulfilling the criteria for vulnerable plaques are relatively frequent, with multiple vulnerable plaque and even multiple ruptured plaques being present in acute coronary syndrome patients. In a coronary angiography study, multiple complex plaques were found in 40% of patients with an acute myocardial infarction [29]. Intravascular studies have since documented the presence of additional plaque rupture at distance from the culprit lesion, as well as in nontarget vessels [30–32].

Endothelial integrity breach (EIB) includes the four following types: rupture (cavity communicating with the lumen), fissure (endothelial disruption involving only the inner surface of the intima and without underlying cavity), intraluminal masses (thrombus or necrotic debris), and surface irregularities (rough intimal surface) (Fig. 15.3).

Due to this near-histologic resolution, OCT allows a minute evaluation of the coronary lumen surface. Compared to IVUS, OCT can provide more detailed and additional structural information such as fissure or surface irregularities. We compared with OCT the prevalence and type of endothelial integrity breaches in acute coronary syndromes versus stable angina pectoris patients [33]. Adequate OCT image quality with ≥ 150 continuous frames in de novo coronary artery lesions were obtained in 29 patients (14 ACS, 15 SAP) before any percutaneous treatments.

The mean number of EIBs was higher in ACS patients compared to SAP patients (48 vs. 25). Multiple EIBs were observed in 13 (93%) ACS patients versus 7 (47%) SAP patients, a single EIB in 1 (7%)

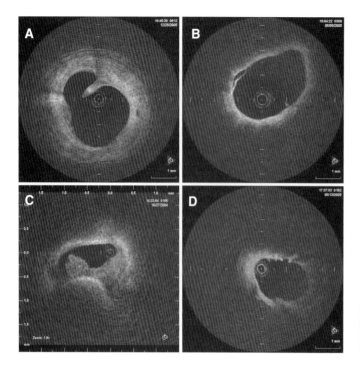

Figure 15.3 Examples of endothelial integrity breaches. **A.** Plaque rupture. **B.** Plaque fissure. **C.** Intraluminal mass. **D.** Surface irregularities.

versus 4 (27%), and none in 0 versus 4 (27%) patients. This higher prevalence was true for all types of EIBs. Ruptures were present in 86% of ACS patients compared to 47% of SAP patients, fissures in 57% versus 20%, and irregularities in 50% versus 27%. EIBs were located outside the lesion segment in 27% for the ACS group, and in 36% for the SAP group. In the nonlesion segment, the number of breachs per centimeter was similar in ACS and SAP patients (0.7 ± 0.82 vs. 0.42 ± 0.65, $p = 0.28$). These results show that endothelial integrity breach is not only frequent but ubiquitous, in both ACS and SAP patients. The severity and number of EIBs was higher in ACS patients compared to SAP patients. The presence of at least one EIB was observed in all ACS patients, and multiple EIBs in 93% of cases. For SAP patients, the presence of at least one EIB was observed in 73%, and multiple EIBs in half of the patients. Another important finding is that EIBs were found not only at the site of the culprit lesion, but also on the adjacent proximal and distal segments.

Guidance of Percutaneous Coronary Intervention

Percutaneous coronary intervention, and in particular stent implantation, has evolved into the commonest treatment for coronary artery disease. Understanding the mechanisms of treatment failure such as in-stent thrombosis or in-stent restenosis is necessary for optimizing the procedure outcome. Most of our knowledge, before OCT utilization, comes from IVUS observations, and can be divided in two main issues: stent deployment characteristics (stent apposition, stent expansion) and vessel injury post stent implantation (tissue prolapse, edge dissection) (Fig. 15.4). Those observations have been shown to correlate with the occurrence of complications/treatment failure and have influenced PCI technique (eg, concept of high-pressure stent deployment) [34].

The introduction of drug-eluting stents and the observation of new entities such as late stent malaposition have shifted the interest towards even

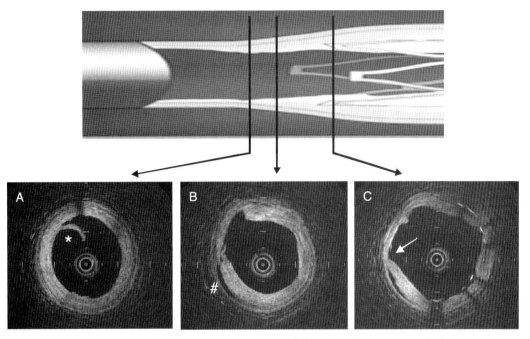

Figure 15.4 Example of stent edge dissection. In **A,** an intimal flap (∗) can be seen. In **B,** the dissection (#) extends deeply through the media and along the media-adventitia border. In **C,** the beginning of the stent can be seen. The origin of the dissection seems to be the impaction of one of the stent struts (*arrow*).

more detailed analysis of the interaction between stent and vessel wall. IVUS is limited by a relatively low resolution, in the range of 150 μm. Due to its high resolution of about 10 μm, OCT can provide more detailed structural information than IVUS. Besides, the high echogenicity of stent struts makes the evaluation of adjacent structures such as small dissections and tissue prolapse difficult by IVUS, but possible by OCT.

Stent Deployment Characteristics and Vessel Injury Post Stent Implantation

Adequate stent deployment is of primordial importance in order to achieve a favorable long-term patency and clinical outcome. Incomplete apposition is defined as a clear separation between at least one stent strut and the vessel wall. This may

cause local flow turbulence and increase the risk for subacute thrombosis. Furthermore, the healing process is delayed, leaving a thrombogenic material uncovered by neointimal tissue formation. Incomplete expansion occurs when a portion of the stent is fully pressed into the vessel wall but inadequately expanded compared with the distal and proximal reference dimensions. Incomplete expansion occurs most frequently in areas of the vessel where dense fibrocalcific or fully calcified plaque is present.

Angiographic guidance does not allow an adequate evaluation. When using intravascular ultrasound, it was shown that despite a successful angiographic result, a large number of stents are not adequately deployed. A number of studies have shown that inadequate stent expansion and apposition as measured by IVUS is a powerful predictor of angiographic or clinical restenosis as well as stent thrombosis following stenting [34–41].

Vessel injury is an unavoidable event occurring during percutaneous coronary intervention. Mechanisms involved in the acute lumen gain post PCI include plaque compression and redistribution, vessel stretching, dissection of the intimal plaque, and partial disruption of the media and adventitia. Thrombus formation at a dissection site is also a common event. The occurrence of tissue prolapse and edge dissection is specifically related to stent implantation [42,43]. Prolapse is defined as a protrusion of tissue between stent struts extending inside a circular or connecting adjacent strut. Those vessel injuries have been shown to be associated with the occurrence of subacute and late stent thrombosis [44,45].

In a study evaluating intracoronary stenting by OCT, stent deployment characteristics and vessel injury post stent implantation were evaluated in 39 patients (42 stents) and a comparison between OCT and IVUS was made. With OCT, only 3 locations within the stents were imaged. Corresponding sites were imaged by IVUS with a margin of 3 mm around the location of OCT imaging. Images were evaluated for the presence of dissection (OCT 8, IVUS 2), tissue prolapse (OCT 29, IVUS 12), incomplete apposition (OCT 7, IVUS 3), and irregular stent strut distribution (18 by OCT and IVUS). The only association found was for tissue prolapse with irregular struts distribution [46]. We obtained similar data in a study comparing OCT with IVUS immediately after high-pressure stent implantation in 18 patients. Incomplete apposition was observed in 5 (28%) stents by OCT and in 1 (6%) by IVUS; tissue prolapse in 14 (78%) cases by OCT and in 8 (44%) with IVUS. The mean magnitude of incomplete apposition was 230 ± 114 μm ($\pm$ SD),

the maximum was 360 μm, and the minimum was 120 μm. [47].

Stent Strut Coverage Post Stent Implantation

In-stent restenosis has been dramatically reduced by the advent of drug-eluting stents, which inhibit the neointimal proliferation. However, the inhibition of stent reendothelialization has been shown in autopsy studies to correlate with the occurrence of in-stent thrombosis. Late or very late thrombosis after placing a drug-eluting stent is related to the percentage of stent strut endothelialization [48,49].

OCT also makes it possible to visualize and quantify the intimal healing post stent implantation. OCT could increase our understanding about the timing for in-vivo complete neointimal coverage, and could influence treatment decision such as the duration of antiplatelet therapy.

We reported data on neointimal coverage 2 and 8 months after implantation of a bare metal stent (BMS) or drug-eluting stent (DES) [50]. With the BMS, neointimal coverage was already completed 2 months post-implantation, with 98% of stent struts covered. On the other hand, only 85% of stent struts were covered at 2 months with the DES, which increased only to 93% at 8 months post-implantation. This discrepancy was even greater for struts located on a side branch. At 8 months, 70% of these bifurcation struts were covered in the DES compared to all of them in the BMS (Fig. 15.5). Similar data have been recently published [51–53]. In the study by Matsumoto and associates [51], the average rate of neointima-covered struts

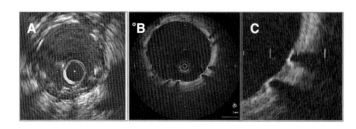

Figure 15.5 Corresponding IVUS **(A)** and OCT **(B)** images 8 months post-implantation of a sirolimus-eluting stent. On the OCT image magnification **(C),** incomplete neointimal coverage is observed.

at 6 months in sirolimus-eluting stents was 89%. Interestingly, only 16% of sirolimus-eluting stents showed a full coverage of all struts by neointima.

Conclusion

The high resolution of OCT, which is about 10 times higher than any other currently available imaging modality, gives a unique opportunity to investigate and clarify our understanding of the mechanisms leading to coronary events. Plaque characterization by OCT has been shown to be highly accurate in ex-vivo histopathologic validation studies, and to be higher than for other imaging modalities.

To date, OCT has been used principally as a research tool. In order to become a modality useful in clinical practice, the clinical relevance and benefit of OCT should be further investigated in prospective studies. Although OCT can identify the morphologic characteristics of vulnerable plaques in vivo, additional information about the fate of such plaques is necessary for potentially initiating specific therapies before a coronary event occurs. In only a few cases does plaque fulfilling the morphologic criteria for vulnerability lead to plaque rupture, and in only a few cases does rupture lead to thrombosis, which may be occlusive or not. Any ulceration or breach of endothelial integrity, mild or severe, may be important in the pathogenesis of acute coronary disease, with or without luminal stenosis. We do not know if these ulcerated plaques resolve and reendothelialize, or if they progress to further stenosis or thrombotic events. Specific preventive therapies for non–flow-limiting vulnerable plaques should have very low risks of complications but far greater efficacy than medical treatment.

In the context of the evaluation of stent deployment characteristics, vessel injury post stent implantation, and intimal healing in the chronic phase, possible practical implications of the detailed OCT findings need also to be determined. In addition, acquisition of adequate image quality over long coronary segments without the need of proximal balloon occlusion should be achieved. Future developments in OCT technology, such as high speed OCT, may be an important step toward this goal.

References

1. Huang D, Swanson EA, Lin CP, *et al.* Optical coherence tomography. *Science.* 1991;254:1178–1181.
2. Fujimoto JG, Boppart SA, Tearney GJ, Bouma BE, Pitris C, Brezinski ME. High resolution in vivo intra-arterial imaging with optical coherence tomography. *Heart.* 1999;82:128–133.
3. Jang IK, Bouma BE, Kang DH, *et al.* Visualization of coronary atherosclerotic plaques in patients using optical coherence tomography: comparison with intravascular ultrasound. *J Am Coll Cardiol.* 2002;39:604-609.
4. Jang IK, Tearney G, Bouma B. Visualization of tissue prolapse between coronary stent struts by optical coherence tomography: comparison with intravascular ultrasound. *Circulation.* 2001;104:2754.
5. Tearney GJ, Jang IK, Kang DH, *et al.* Porcine coronary imaging in vivo by optical coherence tomography. *Acta Cardiol.* 2000;55:233–237.
6. Kume T, Akasak T, Kawamoto T, *et al.* Assessment of coronary intima-media thickness by optical coherence tomography. Comparison with intravascular ultrasound. *Circ J.* 2005;69:903–907.
7. Giattina SD, Courtney BK, Herz PR, *et al.* Assessment of coronary plaque collagen with polarization sensitive optical coherence tomography (PS-OCT). *Int J Cardiol.* 2006;107:400–409.
8. Rogowska J, Patel N, Plummer S, Brezinski ME. Quantitative optical coherence tomographic elastography: method for assessing arterial mechanical properties. *Br J Radiol.* 2006;79:707–711.
9. Virmani R, Burke AP, Farb A, Kolodgie FD. Pathology of the Vulnerable Plaque. *J Am Coll Cardiol.* 2006;47:C13–C18.
10. Davies MJ. Stability and instability: two faces of coronary atherosclerosis. The Paul Dudley White Lecture 1995. *Circulation.* 1996;94:2013–2020.
11. Ross R. Atherosclerosis–an inflammatory disease. *N Engl J Med.* 1999;340:115–126.
12. Varnava AM, Mills PG, Davies MJ. Relationship between coronary artery remodeling and plaque vulnerability. *Circulation.* 2002;105:939–943.
13. Burke AP, Kolodgie FD, Farb A, Weber D, Virmani R. Morphological predictors of arterial remodeling in coronary atherosclerosis. *Circulation.* 2002;105:297–303.

14. Alderman EL, Corley SD, Fisher LD, *et al.* Five-year angiographic follow-up of factors associated with progression of coronary artery disease in the Coronary Artery Surgery Study (CASS). CASS Participating Investigators and Staff. *J Am Coll Cardiol.* 1993;22:1141–1154.

15. Ambrose JA, Tannenbaum MA, Alexopoulos D, *et al.* Angiographic progression of coronary artery disease and the development of myocardial infarction. *J Am Coll Cardiol.* 1988;12:56–62.

16. Giroud D, Li JM, Urban P, Meier B, Rutishauer W. Relation of the site of acute myocardial infarction to the most severe coronary arterial stenosis at prior angiography. *Am J Cardiol.* 1992;69:729–732.

17. Nobuyoshi M, Tanaka M, Nosaka H, *et al.* Progression of coronary atherosclerosis: is coronary spasm related to progression? *J Am Coll Cardiol.* 1991;18:904–910.

18. Falk E, Shah PK, Fuster V. Coronary plaque disruption. *Circulation.* 1995;92:657–671.

19. Yabushita H, Bouma BE, Houser SL, *et al.* Characterization of human atherosclerosis by optical coherence tomography. *Circulation.* 2002;106:1640–1645.

20. Manfrini O, Mont E, Leone O, *et al.* Sources of error and interpretation of plaque morphology by optical coherence tomography. *Am J Cardiol.* 2006;98:156–159.

21. Rieber J, Meissner O, Babaryka G, *et al.* Diagnostic accuracy of optical coherence tomography and intravascular ultrasound for the detection and characterization of atherosclerotic plaque composition in ex-vivo coronary specimens: a comparison with histology. *Coron Artery Dis.* 2006;17:425–430.

22. Kawasaki M, Bouma BE, Bressner J, *et al.* Diagnostic accuracy of optical coherence tomography and integrated backscatter intravascular ultrasound images for tissue characterization of human coronary plaques. *J Am Coll Cardiol.* 2006;48:81–88.

23. Kume T, Akasaka T, Kawamoto T, *et al.* Assessment of coronary arterial plaque by optical coherence tomography. *Am J Cardiol.* 2006;97:1172–1175.

24. Kume T, Akasaka T, Kawamoto T, *et al.* Measurement of the thickness of the fibrous cap by optical coherence tomography. *Am Heart J.* 2006;152:755.el–e4.

25. Tearney GJ, Yabushita H, Houser SL, *et al.* Quantification of macrophage content in atherosclerotic plaques by optical coherence tomography. *Circulation.* 2003;107:113–119.

26. Jang IK, Tearney GJ, MacNeil B, *et al.* In vivo characterization of coronary atherosclerotic plaque by use of optical coherence tomography. *Circulation.* 2005;111:1551–1555.

27. Kubo T, Imanishi T, Takarada S, *et al.* Assessment of culprit lesion morphology in acute myocardial infarction. *J Am Coll Cardiol.* 2007;50:933–939.

28. Chia S, Raffel C, Takano M, *et al.* In-vivo comparison of coronary plaque characteristics using optical coherence tomography in women vs. men with acute coronary syndrome. *Coronary Artery Dis.* 2007;18:423–427.

29. Goldstein JA, Demetriou D, Grines CL, Pica M, Shoukfeh M, O'Neill WW. Multiple complex coronary plaques in patients with acute myocardial infarction. *N Engl J Med.* 2000;343:915–922.

30. Rioufol G, Finet G, Ginon I, *et al.* Multiple atherosclerotic plaque rupture in acute coronary syndrome: a three-vessel intravascular ultrasound study. *Circulation.* 2002;106:804–808.

31. Hong MK, Mintz GS, Lee CW, *et al.* Comparison of coronary plaque rupture between stable angina and acute myocardial infarction: a three-vessel intravascular ultrasound study in 235 patients. *Circulation.* 2004;110:928–933.

32. Schoenhagen P, Stone GW, Nissen SE, *et al.* Coronary Plaque morphology and frequency of ulceration distant from culprit lesions in patients with unstable and stable presentation. *Arterioscler Thromb Vasc Biol.* 2003;23:1895–1900.

33. Surmely JF, Izuka T, Terashima M, *et al.* Multiple coronary endothelial integrity breach: An in-vivo Optical Coherence Tomography study. Abstract ESC 2007.

34. de Jaegere P, Mudra H, Figulla H, *et al.* Intravascular ultrasound-guided optimized stent deployment. Immediate and 6 months clinical and angiographic results from the Multicenter Ultrasound Stenting in Coronaries Study (MUSIC Study). *Eur Heart J.* 1998;19:1214–1223.

35. Colombo A, Hall P, Nakamura S, *et al.* Intracoronary stenting without anticoagulation accomplished with intravascular ultrasound guidance. *Circulation.* 1995;91:1676–1688.

36. Uren NG, Schwarzacher SP, Metz JA, *et al.* Predictors and outcomes of stent thrombosis: an intravascular ultrasound registry. *Eur Heart J.* 2002;23:124–132.

37. Fitzgerald PJ, Oshima A, Hayase M, *et al.* Final results of the Can Routine Ultrasound Influence Stent Expansion (CRUISE) study. *Circulation.* 2000;102:523–530.

38. Kasaoka S, Tobis JM, Akiyama T, *et al.* Angiographic and intravascular ultrasound predictors of in-stent restenosis. *J Am Coll Cardiol.* 1998;32:1630–1635.

39. Mudra H, di Mario C, de Jaegere P, *et al.* Randomized comparison of coronary stent implantation

under ultrasound or angiographic guidance to reduce stent restenosis (OPTICUS Study). *Circulation.* 2001;104:1343–1349.

40. Schiele F, Meneveau N, Vuillemenot A, *et al.* Impact of intravascular ultrasound guidance in stent deployment on 6-month restenosis rate: a multicenter, randomized study comparing two strategies–with and without intravascular ultrasound guidance. RESIST Study Group. REStenosis after Ivus guided STenting. *J Am Coll Cardiol.* 1998;32:320–328.

41. Dirschinger J, Kastrati A, Neumann FJ, *et al.* Influence of balloon pressure during stent placement in native coronary arteries on early and late angiographic and clinical outcome: a randomized evaluation of high-pressure inflation. *Circulation.* 1999;100: 918–923.

42. Hong MK, Park SW, Lee NH, *et al.* Long-term outcomes of minor dissection at the edge of stents detected with intravascular ultrasound. *Am J Cardiol.* 2000;86:791–795, A9.

43. Farb A, Sangiorgi G, Carter AJ, *et al.* Pathology of acute and chronic coronary stenting in humans. *Circulation.* 1999;99:44–52.

44. Farb A, Burke AP, Kolodgie FD, Virmani R. Pathological mechanisms of fatal late coronary stent thrombosis in humans. *Circulation.* 2003;108:1701–1706.

45. Hong MK, Park SW, Lee CW, *et al.* Long-term outcomes of minor plaque prolapsed within stents documented with intravascular ultrasound. *Catheter Cardiovasc Interv.* 2000;51:22–26.

46. Bouma BE, Tearney GJ, Yabushita H, *et al.* Evaluation of intracoronary stenting by intravascular optical coherence tomography. *Heart.* 2003;89:317–320.

47. Takeda Y, Ito T, Tsuchikane E, *et al.* Incomplete apposition and tissue prolapse immediately after stenting evaluated by optical coherence tomography. Abstract AHA 2004.

48. Joner M, Finn AV, Farb A, *et al.* Pathology of drug-eluting stents in humans: delayed healing and late thrombotic risk. *J Am Coll Cardiol.* 2006;48:193–202.

49. Finn AV, Joner M, Nakazawa G, *et al.* Pathological correlates of late drug-eluting stent thrombosis: strut coverage as a marker of endothelialization. *Circulation.* 2007;115:2435–2441.

50. Ito T, Terashima M, Takeda Y, *et al.* Optical coherence tomographic analysis of neointimal stent coverage in sirolimus-eluting stent, compared with bare metal stent. Abstract TCT 2005.

51. Matsumoto D, Shite J, Shinke T, *et al.* Neointimal coverage of sirolimus-eluting stents at 6 month follow-up: evaluated by optical coherence tomography. *Eur Heart J.* 2007;28:961–967.

52. Takano M, Inami S, Jang IK, *et al.* Evaluation by optical coherence tomography of neointimal coverage of sirolimus-eluting stent three months after implantation. *Am J Cardiol.* 2007;99:1033–1038.

53. Chen BX, M FY, Wei L, *et al.* Neointimal coverage of bare metal and sirolimus-eluting stents evaluated with optical coherence tomography. *Heart.* 2008;94:566–570.

CHAPTER 16

Intravascular Ultrasound

Masao Yamasaki[1], Junya Ako[2], Yasuhiro Honda[1], and Peter J. Fitzgerald[1]

[1]Division of Cardiology, Stanford University Medical Center, Stanford, CA, USA
[2]Center for Research in Cardiovascular Interventions, Stanford University Medical Center, Stanford, CA, USA

Chapter Overview

- Intravascular ultrasound (IVUS) is considered useful in PCI (percutaneous coronary intervention) guidance.
- IVUS plays an important role in understanding vessel responses following PCI or pharmacologic interventions.
- IVUS enables detailed analysis on the effect of drug-eluting stents (DES) through volumetric analysis on neointimal hyperplasia.
- Late-acquired incomplete stent apposition, a unique IVUS finding, is brought into focus because of its possible association with stent thrombosis following DES implantation.
- Newer-generation IVUS-based technologies include virtual histology, backscatter analysis, wavelet analysis, elastography, and palpography.

Intravascular ultrasound (IVUS) provides a tomographic perspective from within the vessel wall. Real-time direct image of the vessel wall by IVUS allows detailed comprehensive observation of the vessel structures as a pathologic tool in vivo, offering unmatched guidance in percutaneous coronary interventions (PCI). IVUS is also crucial to understand vessel responses following PCI or pharmacologic interventions.

Drug-Eluting Stents

Drug-eluting stents (DES) have been the mainstay of PCI since their first introduction to clinical use. There are a number of new DES on the horizon, and IVUS has been playing a crucial role in understanding their safety and efficacy profile when first-in-man trials are conducted. In addition, IVUS has been playing an important role in de-

termining the mechanism of untoward long-term clinical events including restenosis and late stent thrombosis.

New-Generation Drug-Eluting Stents

We have been witness to a number of new developments in DES. In the ETHOS trial, 17-beta estradiol-eluting stents did not show significant differences in volume obstruction by IVUS at 6-month follow-up (slow release 31 ± 14%, moderate release 33 ± 11%, bare-metal stent 31 ± 14%) [1]. The Zomaxx stent is a zotarolimus-eluting stent, utilizing biocompatible phosphorylcholine polymer loaded onto a novel, thin, stainless steel stent platform containing a thin inner layer of tantalum. The first-in-man trial of the Zomaxx stent showed a neointimal volume obstruction at 4-month follow-up of 6.2%, with no late-acquired incomplete stent apposition [2]. The ENDEAVOR stent is another zotarolimus-eluting stent, which utilizes a cobalt chromium stent platform. In the ENDEAVOR III trial, this stent showed a percent neointimal volume of 16.1 ± 10.8% at 8 months

Current Best Practice in Interventional Cardiology. Edited by B Meier. © 2010 Blackwell Publishing,

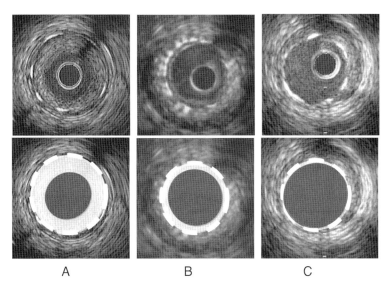

A   B   C

Figure 16.1 Representative cross-sectional IVUS images of intracoronary stents. Lower panels show the stent (*white dotted line*), lumen (dark gray), and neointima (light gray). **A.** bare-metal stent. Lumen area is encroached by abundant neointimal hyperplasia.

B. Endeavor stent (Medtronic, Santa Rosa, CA). The amount of neointima is significantly less than with the bare metal stent. **C.** Xience stent (Abbott Vascular, Santa Clara, CA). Note the minimal amount of neointimal hyperplasia in the Xience stent.

postimplantation, while a sirolimus-eluting stent showed 2.7 ± 3.1% in the same trial ($p < 0.01$). However, the ENDEAVOR stent showed a significantly lower incidence of late-acquired incomplete stent apposition as compared with sirolimus-eluting stents [3]. The SPIRIT III trial has shown

excellent results for an everolimus-eluting stent (Xience, Abbott Vascular, Santa Clara, CA), with neointimal volume obstruction of 6.9 ± 6.4% at 8-month IVUS follow-up (Figs. 16.1 and 16.2) [4].

One IVUS observation showed interesting results from a self-expanding nitinol DES. The AXXESS

Figure 16.2 Comparison of percentage of neointimal obstruction (neointimal volume divided by stent volume) among different type of stents. The following stents were used in the trials. ASPECT used a paclitaxel-eluting stent (Cook Cardiology); TAXUS used the Taxus paclitaxel-eluting stent (Boston Scientific); Zomaxx used the zotarolimus-eluting Trimaxx stent (Abbott Vascular); ENDEAVOR used the zotarolimus-eluting Endeavor stent; RESOLUTE used the zotarolimus-eluting Resolute stent (Medtronic); SPIRIT III used the everolimus-eluting Xience stent; FUTURE used an everolimus-eluting stent (Biosensors); and SIRIUS and RAVEL used the sirolimus-eluting Cypher stent (Cordis). (BMS, bare metal stents.)

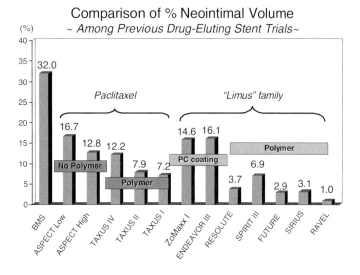

stent is a novel dedicated bifurcation stent comprised of a self-expanding flare-shaped stent platform and a bioabsorbable polymer coating that releases Biolimus A9. In the AXXESS Plus trial, this stent showed a percent neointimal volume of 2.3 ± 2.2% at 6-months follow-up, proving its safety and efficacy for the treatment of bifurcation lesions [5].

Failure Mode of Drug-Eluting Stents

Although DES has a great impact on the prevention of restenosis after PCI, the restenosis issue after DES implantation is not completely addressed. It is well known that stent underexpansion is the most common mechanism of restenosis in the Cypher stent. According to Hong and associates [6], independent predictors of angiographic restenosis after Cypher implantation were postprocedural final minimum stent area by IVUS and IVUS-measured stent length. The angiographic restenosis rate was highest in lesions with stent area <5.5 mm^2 and stent length >40 mm. On the other hand, in an analysis of 48 Cypher restenoses, a minimum lumen area was located at the minimum stent site in less than 50% cases [7]. Furthermore the neointimal hyperplasia (NIH) at the minimal lumen site was greater in the group with a stent area >5.0 mm^2 than the group with a stent area <5.0 mm^2. Circumferential stent strut distribution may affect the dose of sirolimus delivered to the arterial wall and therefore the amount of NIH. In addition to nonuniform stent strut distribution, the gap between stents and stent fractures, both of which are also detectable by IVUS, should be taken into account when arguing restenosis in DES.

Stent Thrombosis: Possible Connection with Late-Acquired Incomplete Stent Apposition?

It has been increasingly known that stent thrombosis (ST) may occur unusually late in patients treated with DES, a phenomenon often referred to as very late ST [8,9]. Several observational studies linked an IVUS finding of late incomplete stent apposition (ISA) and late ST in DES patients (Fig. 16.3). Siqueira and coworkers reported that late-acquired ISA was observed in 5.1% of patients after DES implantation, and that there was a signif-

icantly high incidence (20%) of late ST in patients with this IVUS finding [10]. Cook and colleagues also found that ISA is highly prevalent in patients with very late ST after DES implantation [11]. They also found that there was a significantly larger external elastic membrane area, which suggested that the ISA was mainly late-acquired ISA, which may be consistent with the report by Siqueira and associates. Possible association between ST and ISA should be further investigated with careful long-term follow-up on DES patients.

Late-acquired ISA (LISA) is not an uncommon finding [12]. In a real-world experience, Hong and coworkers [13] reported LISA occurred in 13.2% of 538 Cypher stents versus 8.4% of 167 Taxus stents ($p = 0.12$) at a 6-month follow-up after DES implantation. The frequency of LISA was 32% in acute myocardial infarction (AMI), 28% in chronic total occlusions (CTOs), and 25% of stenting after directional coronary atherectomy. Independent predictors of LISA were total stent length, primary stenting in AMI, and CTO. Considering its implication of future risk of ST, this IVUS finding may deserve more clinical attention.

Drug-Eluting Balloons

In-stent restenosis remains one of the most difficult challenges in the treatment of coronary artery disease even in the drug-eluting stent era. The drug-eluting balloon is an emerging treatment option for these complex lesion subsets. A study has shown a significant reduction in the incidence of restenosis using a paclitaxel-eluting balloon [14]. Another study has shown a promising result with this technology in the treatment of peripheral artery disease [15]. Future clinical trials using IVUS will elucidate the detailed vascular responses to this novel therapeutic choice.

Beyond Gray-Scale IVUS

While gray-scale IVUS imaging allows morphologic assessment of lesions, it is not sufficient in detecting clinically relevant vulnerable plaque. Attempts to identify the vulnerability of atherosclerotic plaques

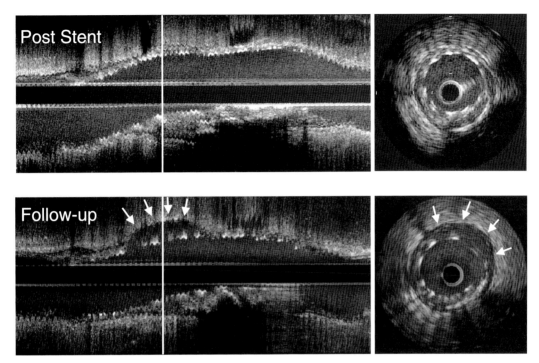

Figure 16.3 A case of late-acquired incomplete stent apposition (ISA) following drug-eluting stent implatation. *Upper panels* show images at postintervention; *lower panels* show 8-month follow-up. Detachment of the vessel wall (*arrows*) from stent strut was observed in cross-sectional image (*right*) and longitudinal image (*left*).

have been made by several novel imaging modalities using an IVUS system such as virtual histology (VH), IVUS with integrated backscatter (IB-IVUS), wavelet analysis of radiofrequency (RF) IVUS signals, elastography, and palpography.

VH and IB-IVUS apply spectral analysis of the IVUS backscatter RF signal to characterize plaque components via computerized color-coded image on the basis of tissue characteristics. RF signals are digitized at 1 or 2 GHz in IB-IVUS using a conventional 40-MHz IVUS catheter. Nasu and associates [16] showed that in vivo tissue characterization by VH favorably correlated with the results of in vitro histopathologic examination of tissue samples obtained by DCA. This is the first VH clinical study to assess the accuracy of in vivo histology for the diagnosis of plaque composition. Kawasaki and colleagues [17] compared the diagnostic accuracy for characterizing tissue types among optical coherence tomography (OCT), IB-IVUS, and con-

ventional IVUS (C-IVUS) using histologic images as a gold standard. They reported OCT had a best potential for tissue characterization of coronary plaques within the penetration depth of OCT, and IB-IVUS had a better potential for characterizing fibrous lesions and lipid pools than C-IVUS. By using IB-IVUS, Sano and associates [18] showed the differences in percentage lipid area ($72 \pm 10\%$ vs. $50 \pm 16\%$; $p < 0.0001$) and percentage fibrous area ($23 \pm 6\%$ vs. $47 \pm 14\%$; $p < 0.0001$) between vulnerable plaques and stable plaques in moderate coronary lesions.

Wavelet analysis is a new mathematical model for assessing local changes in the geometrical profile of time-series signals. This method discriminates a local unique wave pattern within a complex signal. Murashige and coworkers [19] demonstrated the detection of not only lipid-laden plaque with a sensitivity of 83% and a specificity of 82% in vitro, but also fatty plaque with a sensitivity of

81% and a specificity of 85% in vivo with this method.

Elastography is a technique that assesses the local elasticity (strain and modulus) of tissue. It is based on the principle that the deformation of tissue by an intracoronary pressure is directly related to the mechanical properties of the tissue. The radial strain in the tissue is obtained by cross-correlation techniques on the radiofrequency signals. The strain is color-coded and plotted as a complimentary image to the IVUS echogram. Palpography applies the same principle, but this technique provides a surface-based assessment of the mechanical properties in contrast to elastography, which assesses the entire plaque. Palpography derives mechanical information of the surface of the plaque, where the rupture may happen. According to Schaar and colleagues [20], palpography showed a highly significant difference in strain ($p = 0.0012$) between fibrous and fatty tissue in vitro. In vivo animal study also revealed higher strain values in fatty than in fibrous plaques ($p < 0.001$). The presence of a high-strain region at the lumen–plaque interface had a high predictive value to identify macrophages. Van Mieghem and associates [21] reported that palpography detected a significant reduction in abnormal strain pattern after 6-months interval in patients with ST-segment elevation myocardial infarction.

These novel imaging modalities might provide insights into plaque biology and might allow identification of vulnerable plaque in the near future. However, the clinical utility of these techniques is not yet established, and more investigation is needed.

References

1. Abizaid A, Chaves AJ, Leon MB, et al. Randomized, double-blind, multicenter study of the polymer-based 17-beta estradiol-eluting stent for treatment of native coronary artery lesions: six-month results of the ETHOS I trial. *Catheter Cardiovasc Interv.* 2007;70:654–660.

2. Abizaid A, Lansky AJ, Fitzgerald PJ, et al. Percutaneous coronary revascularization using a trilayer metal phosphorylcholine-coated zotarolimus-eluting stent. *Am J Cardiol.* 2007;99:1403–1408.

3. Miyazawa A, Ako J, Hongo Y, et al. Comparison of vascular response to zotarolimus-eluting stent versus sirolimus-eluting stent: intravascular ultrasound results from ENDEAVOR III. *Am Heart J.* 2008;155:108–113.

4. Stone GW, Midei M, Newman W, et al. Comparison of an everolimus-eluting stent and a paclitaxel-eluting stent in patients with coronary artery disease: a randomized trial. *JAMA.* 2008;299:1903–1913.

5. Miyazawa A, Ako J, Hassan A, et al. Analysis of bifurcation lesions treated with novel drug-eluting dedicated bifurcation stent system: intravascular ultrasound results of the AXXESS PLUS trial. *Catheter Cardiovasc Interv.* 2007;70:952–957.

6. Hong MK, Mintz GS, Lee CW, et al. Intravascular ultrasound predictors of angiographic restenosis after sirolimus-eluting stent implantation. *Eur Heart J.* 2006;27:1305–1310.

7. Sano K, Mintz GS, Carlier SG, et al. Volumetric intravascular ultrasound assessment of neointimal hyperplasia and nonuniform stent strut distribution in sirolimus-eluting stent restenosis. *Am J Cardiol.* 2006;98:1559–1562.

8. McFadden EP, Stabile E, Regar E, et al. Late thrombosis in drug-eluting coronary stents after discontinuation of antiplatelet therapy. *Lancet.* 2004;364:1519–1521.

9. Ong AT, McFadden EP, Regar E, de Jaegere PP, van Domburg RT, Serruys PW. Late angiographic stent thrombosis (LAST) events with drug-eluting stents. *J Am Coll Cardiol.* 2005;45:2088–2092.

10. Siqueira DA, Abizaid AA, Costa Jde R, et al. Late incomplete apposition after drug-eluting stent implantation: incidence and potential for adverse clinical outcomes. *Eur Heart J.* 2007;28:1304–1309.

11. Cook S, Wenaweser P, Togni M, et al. Incomplete stent apposition and very late stent thrombosis after drug-eluting stent implantation. *Circulation.* 2007;115:2426–2434.

12. Ako J, Morino Y, Honda Y, et al. Late incomplete stent apposition after sirolimus-eluting stent implantation: a serial intravascular ultrasound analysis. *J Am Coll Cardiol.* 2005;46:1002–1005.

13. Hong MK, Mintz GS, Lee CW, et al. Late stent malapposition after drug-eluting stent implantation: an intravascular ultrasound analysis with long-term follow-up. *Circulation.* 2006;113:414–419.

14. Scheller B, Hehrlein C, Bocksch W, et al. Treatment of coronary in-stent restenosis with a paclitaxel-coated

balloon catheter. *N Engl J Med.* 2006;355: 2113–2124.

15. Tepe G, Zeller T, Albrecht T, *et al.* Local delivery of paclitaxel to inhibit restenosis during angioplasty of the leg. *N Engl J Med.* 2008;358:689–699.

16. Nasu K, Tsuchikane E, Katoh O, *et al.* Accuracy of in vivo coronary plaque morphology assessment: a validation study of in vivo virtual histology compared with in vitro histopathology. *J Am Coll Cardiol.* 2006;47:2405–2412.

17. Kawasaki M, Bouma BE, Bressner J, *et al.* Diagnostic accuracy of optical coherence tomography and integrated backscatter intravascular ultrasound images for tissue characterization of human coronary plaques. *J Am Coll Cardiol.* 2006;48:81–88.

18. Sano K, Kawasaki M, Ishihara Y, *et al.* Assessment of vulnerable plaques causing acute coronary syndrome using integrated backscatter intravascular ultrasound. *J Am Coll Cardiol.* 2006;47:734–741.

19. Murashige A, Hiro T, Fujii T, *et al.* Detection of lipid-laden atherosclerotic plaque by wavelet analysis of radiofrequency intravascular ultrasound signals: in vitro validation and preliminary in vivo application. *J Am Coll Cardiol.* 2005;45:1954–1960.

20. Schaar JA, Van Der Steen AF, Mastik F, Baldewsing RA, Serruys PW. Intravascular palpography for vulnerable plaque assessment. *J Am Coll Cardiol.* 2006;47(suppl):C86–C91.

21. Van Mieghem CA, McFadden EP, de Feyter PJ, *et al.* Noninvasive detection of subclinical coronary atherosclerosis coupled with assessment of changes in plaque characteristics using novel invasive imaging modalities: the Integrated Biomarker and Imaging Study (IBIS). *J Am Coll Cardiol.* 2006;47: 1134–1142.

Index

Note: Italicized page numbers refer to figures and tables